S0-BMG-628

VITAMINS AND HORMONES

VOLUME 30

VITAMINS AND HORMONES

ADVANCES IN RESEARCH AND APPLICATIONS

Edited by

ROBERT S. HARRIS
Massachusetts Institute of Technology
Cambridge, Massachusetts

PAUL L. MUNSON
University of North Carolina
Chapel Hill, North Carolina

EGON DICZFALUSY
Karolinska Sjukhuset
Stockholm, Sweden

JOHN GLOVER
University of Liverpool
Liverpool, England

Consulting Editors

KENNETH V. THIMANN
University of California, Santa Cruz
Santa Cruz, California

IRA G. WOOL
University of Chicago
Chicago, Illinois

JOHN A. LORAINE
Medical Research Council
Edinburgh, Scotland

Volume 30
1972

ACADEMIC PRESS, New York and London

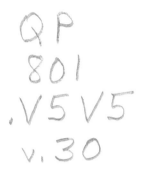

Copyright © 1972, by Academic Press, Inc.
ALL RIGHTS RESERVED.
NO PART OF THIS PUBLICATION MAY BE REPRODUCED OR
TRANSMITTED IN ANY FORM OR BY ANY MEANS, ELECTRONIC
OR MECHANICAL, INCLUDING PHOTOCOPY, RECORDING, OR ANY
INFORMATION STORAGE AND RETRIEVAL SYSTEM, WITHOUT
PERMISSION IN WRITING FROM THE PUBLISHER.

ACADEMIC PRESS, INC.
111 Fifth Avenue, New York, New York 10003

United Kingdom Edition published by
ACADEMIC PRESS, INC. (LONDON) LTD.
24/28 Oval Road, London NW1

LIBRARY OF CONGRESS CATALOG CARD NUMBER: 43-10535

PRINTED IN THE UNITED STATES OF AMERICA

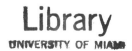
Library
UNIVERSITY OF MIAMI

Contents

Biological Hydroxylations and Ascorbic Acid with Special Regard to Collagen Metabolism

M. J. BARNES AND E. KODICEK

Effect of Vitamin E Deficiency on Cellular Membranes

I. MOLENAAR, J. VOS, AND F. A. HOMMES

FSH-Releasing Hormone and LH-Releasing Hormone

A. V. SCHALLY, A. J. KASTIN, AND A. ARIMURA

Hypothalamic Control of Prolactin Secretion

Joseph Meites and James A. Clemens

Comparative Endocrinology of Gestation

I. John Davies and Kenneth J. Ryan

Hormonal Changes in Pathological Pregnancy

Hubertus A. Van Leusden

Contributors to Volume 30

Numbers in parentheses indicate the pages on which the authors' contributions begin.

A. Arimura, *Department of Medicine, Tulane University School of Medicine, New Orleans, Louisiana* (83)

M. J. Barnes, *Dunn Nutritional Laboratory, University of Cambridge and Medical Research Council, Cambridge, United Kingdom* (1)

James A. Clemens, *Department of Physiological Research, Eli Lilly and Company, Indianapolis, Indiana* (165)

I. John Davies, *Department of Obstetrics and Gynecology, University of California, San Diego, School of Medicine, La Jolla, California* (223)

F. A. Hommes, *Department of Pediatrics, University of Groningen, School of Medicine, Groningen, The Netherlands* (45)

A. J. Kastin, *Department of Medicine, Tulane University School of Medicine, New Orleans, Louisiana* (83)

E. Kodicek, *Dunn Nutritional Laboratory, University of Cambridge and Medical Research Council, Cambridge, United Kingdom* (1)

Joseph Meites, *Department of Physiology, Michigan State University, East Lansing, Michigan* (165)

I. Molenaar, *Centre for Medical Electron Microscopy, University of Groningen, School of Medicine, Groningen, The Netherlands* (45)

Kenneth J. Ryan, *Department of Obstetrics and Gynecology, University of California, San Diego, School of Medicine, La Jolla, California* (223)

A. V. Schally, *Endocrine and Polypeptide Laboratories and Endocrinology Section of the Medical Service, Veterans Administration Hospital, New Orleans, Louisiana* (83)

HUBERTUS A. VAN LEUSDEN, *University Department of Obstetrics and Gynecology, St. Radboud Ziekenhuis, Nijmegen, The Netherlands* (281)

J. VOS, *Centre for Medical Electron Microscopy, University of Groningen, School of Medicine, Groningen, The Netherlands* (45)

Preface

Thirty years have passed since the first volume of *Vitamins and Hormones* was published in 1942. To mark that occasion the Editors invited Professor E. V. McCollum, renowned discoverer of vitamin A and a pioneer in the exciting new field of vitamins, to write the Foreword for this new series. He wrote in part:

> The time is ripe for the founding of such a venture, since it is no longer possible for anyone to read sufficient of the current papers and the library files dealing with these two classes of substances to assimilate all the knowledge which has accumulated. We must increasingly depend upon our colleagues who maintain mastery of specialized experimentation, to appraise for us the numerous contributions which they alone can interpret, sifting error from truth and assembling scattered data to make a connected account which places a body of related facts in proper perspective. This is the function of the new publication. . . .
>
> This first volume of *Vitamins and Hormones* appears at a time when clinicians are cautiously attempting to apply both vitamins and hormones for the benefit of their patients. The future of preventive and curative medicine is filled with promise in these departments of learning.
>
> The editing of a publication and the preparation of carefully prepared digests of researches by men actively engaged in productive research are labors of love. Workers in many fields of science will be grateful to the editors and contributors for furthering the cause of education by giving of their time and labor to the making of this new publication. They will have many appreciative readers and well-wishers.

Vitamins and Hormones was one of the first in pioneering the publication of serial volumes which were scholarly and critical reviews of advances in scientific research. Today there are several hundred publications of this type covering many areas of biological science. The previous twenty-nine volumes of *Vitamins and Hormones* have proved to be valuable especially to professors, scientific investigators, graduate students, and young biomedical research scientists.

The present volume contains six critical reviews of recent progress in vitamin and hormone research: Biological Hydroxylations and Ascorbic Acid with Special Regard to Collagen Metabolism (Barnes and Kodicek); Effect of Vitamin E Deficiency on Cellular Membranes (Molenaar, Vos, and Hommes); FSH-Releasing Hormone and LH-Releasing Hormone (Schally, Kastin, and Arimura); Hypothalamic Control of Prolactin Secretion (Meites and Clemens); Comparative Endocrinology of Gestation (Davies and Ryan); and Hormonal Changes in Pathological Pregnancy (Van Leusden). This broad spectrum of subjects is consonant with the original objectives when this serial was started and reflects some of the contemporary themes which are of great interest to current investigators laboring in this research area.

The Editors greatly appreciate the fine efforts of the thirteen authors who wrote this volume.

ROBERT S. HARRIS
PAUL MUNSON
EGON DICZFALUSY
JOHN GLOVER

Biological Hydroxylations and Ascorbic Acid with Special Regard to Collagen Metabolism

M. J. BARNES AND E. KODICEK

Dunn Nutritional Laboratory, University of Cambridge and Medical Research Council, Cambridge, United Kingdom

I. INTRODUCTION

A direct involvement of ascorbic acid in collagen metabolism has been recognized for many years, and it is not the purpose of this article to relate the process whereby this relationship was established. The reader is referred to the review by Gould (1960) when this subject was last considered in *Vitamins and Hormones* and to the more recent reviews elsewhere of Gould (1968b), Chvapil and Hurych (1968), and Barnes (1969). It is the authors' intention rather to discuss the evidence that has accumulated since Gould's (1960) article concerning the actual site of action of ascorbic acid in collagen metabolism. This relates essentially to the possible role of ascorbic acid in collagen proline and lysine hydroxylation, and we shall attempt to consider these particular hydroxylations in the context of a more general consideration of the role of ascorbic acid in biological hydroxylation reactions.

1

II. Collagen Synthesis

In order to discuss the role of ascorbic acid in collagen metabolism, it is necessary first to describe briefly certain important features of collagen and its synthesis. This subject has been recently reviewed by Udenfriend (1966, 1970), Prockop and Kivirikko (1967, 1968a), Gould (1968a,b), Chvapil and Hurych (1968), Juva (1968), Rosenbloom and Prockop (1969), and Prockop (1970).

Collagen contains two unusual amino acids, hydroxyproline and hydroxylysine, that apart from a small quantity of hydroxyproline in elastin, occur only rarely if at all elsewhere in other animal proteins. Collagen hydroxyproline and hydroxylysine are not, as might have been anticipated, derived from their respective free amino acids, which fail to be incorporated into collagen. They have been shown to arise from free proline and lysine, respectively (Stetten and Schoenheimer, 1944; Stetten, 1949; Sinex and Van Slyke, 1955; Piez and Likins, 1957; Van Slyke and Sinex, 1958; Sinex et al., 1959). These findings implied not only that collagen hydroxyproline and hydroxylysine are derived by hydroxylation of proline and lysine, but further that this hydroxylation occurred at a level other than that of the free amino acid. It was shown that the oxygen of the hydroxyl group in both instances is derived from atmospheric oxygen (rather than water) (Fujimoto and Tamiya, 1962; Prockop et al., 1963, 1966; Popenoe et al., 1966), and this indicated that the hydroxylations could be regarded as mixed-function oxidase reactions. It was at one time considered that hydroxylation may occur at the level of prolyl (or lysyl) adenylate or prolyl (or lysyl)-sRNA. Although several laboratories reported the presence of hydroxyprolyl-sRNA in systems synthesizing collagen (Manner and Gould, 1963; Coronado et al., 1963; Jackson et al., 1964; Urivetsky et al., 1965), it was subsequently demonstrated that this compound is not a precursor of collagen hydroxyproline (Urivetsky et al., 1966).

It is now agreed (for reasons that will be described in some detail later) that hydroxylation occurs after incorporation of proline and lysine into peptide linkage. It is still a subject of some debate whether this hydroxylation occurs primarily after release from polyribosomes of unhydroxylated but otherwise fully synthesized collagen α-chains or whether it occurs during the actual course of synthesis of the α-chains while still attached to the polyribosome structure (see Lazarides et al., 1971; Lane et al., 1971a). It has been established, however, that the hydroxylation can be inhibited, for example, by inclusion of the chelating agent, α,α'-dipyridyl, or by the exclusion of oxygen, in isolated collagen-forming systems, and under these circumstances an unhydroxylated polypeptide is formed and released from the ribosome (Lazarides and Lukens, 1971a).

This polypeptide can, at least in certain situations, be regarded as of a size equivalent to an unhydroxylated collagen α-chain or its higher-molecular weight precursor (Lukens, 1966, 1970; Kivirikko and Prockop, 1967a; Müller et al., 1971). Collagen synthesized under conditions in which hydroxylation is prevented has been termed protocollagen (Juva and Prockop, 1965).

It is in the hydroxylation of collagen proline and lysine that ascorbic acid is thought to be involved.

III. Evidence for the Participation of Ascorbic Acid in Collagen Proline Hydroxylation

A. Whole-Cell Preparations from Scorbutic Guinea Pigs

Although Robertson and Schwartz (1953) mooted that the function of ascorbic acid in collagen metabolism may be in the conversion by hydroxylation of a proline-rich, hydroxyproline-free collagen precursor to collagen, perhaps the first definitive evidence for such a role of the vitamin arose from the studies of Stone and Meister (1962). These authors induced granulomas in normal and scorbutic guinea pigs by injection of carrageenin as described by Robertson and Schwartz (1953). They demonstrated that when minces of granulomas from vitamin-deficient animals were incubated in the presence of radioactively labeled proline, incorporation of radioactivity into collagen hydroxyproline was greatly diminished in comparison to controls whereas incorporation into collagen proline was little affected (Table I). In the light of subsequent

TABLE I

Incorporation of [14C]Proline into the Collagen Proline and Hydroxyproline of Granulomas from Normal and Scorbutic Guinea Pigs[a]

| Expt. No. | Specific activity (dpm/μmole) | | | |
| | Normal | | Deficient | |
	Proline	Hydroxyproline	Proline	Hydroxyproline
1	790	697	787	<10
2	745	680	530	10

[a] Granuloma mince (2 gm) was incubated with 5 ml of medium containing 1 μCi of DL-[1-14C]proline. Incubation was carried out for 30 minutes at 37°C under 95% O_2/5% CO_2. Granulomas were obtained after 6 days of growth: deficient animals were deprived of ascorbic acid for 2 weeks. Proline and hydroxyproline were assayed colorimetrically after separation from collagen hydrolyzates by paper chromatography. Radioactivity was determined by liquid scintillation counting [Stone and Meister, 1962, by permission of Nature (London)].

studies by Peterkofsky and Udenfriend (1963), who, as described below, were able to demonstrate that collagen hydroxyproline arose from the hydroxylation of proline previously incorporated into peptide linkage, the findings of Stone and Meister could be regarded as indicative of the formation of an unhydroxylated collagen by the tissue from the scorbutic animals. Upon addition of ascorbic acid to the incubation medium containing the granuloma preparation from the ascorbic acid-deficient animals, incorporation of radioactivity into collagen hydroxyproline was appreciably stimulated.

Robertson and Hewitt (1961) similarly reported that the formation *in vitro* of collagen hydroxyproline, as measured by incorporation of isotopically labeled, proline into collagen hydroxyproline, using isolated whole-cell preparations of carrageenin granuloma from ascorbic acid deficient guinea pigs, was augmented upon addition of ascorbic acid to the incubation mixture. These authors, however, did not report collagen proline-specific activities, and so evidence for the formation of unhydroxylated material in the preparation from deficient animals incubated directly without addition of the vitamin could not be deduced from their studies.

Subsequently Udenfriend and his colleagues demonstrated, in a number of collagen-forming systems, the formation *in vitro* of a proline-rich, hydroxyproline-deficient polypeptide that was, like collagen, soluble in hot trichloroacetic acid and degraded by collagenase and was presumed to be a collagen precursor. Thus this polypeptide was formed when tissues were incubated under anaerobic conditions and, particularly pertinent to the present considerations, during incubation of tissues with a

TABLE II

SYNTHESIS OF HYDROXYPROLINE-DEFICIENT, COLLAGENASE-DEGRADABLE
PROTEIN BY NORMAL AND SCORBUTIC GUINEA PIG GRANULOMAS[a]

	Proline (cpm/flask)	Hydroxyproline (cpm/flask)	Proline:hydroxyproline ratio
Normal	644	564	1.1
	8994	3888	2.3
	4860	1870	2.6
Scorbutic	684	6	114
	212	0	α

[a] Granuloma minces were incubated, in the presence of L-[U-^{14}C]proline for 90 minutes at 37°C. Minces were then extracted with hot trichloroacetic acid. Extracts were digested with collagenase and then precipitated with tannic acid. Proline and hydroxyproline radioactivity were estimated in the supernatant which contained collagen-derived peptides released by the action of collagenase (Gottlieb *et al.*, 1966, by permission of The American Society of Biological Chemists, Inc., Bethesda, Maryland).

low ascorbic acid concentration, such as granuloma tissue from scorbutic guinea pigs (Table II) (Gottlieb *et al.*, 1966).

Manning and Meister (1966) extended the studies of Stone and Meister (1962) and confirmed the synthesis in isolated scorbutic granuloma tissue of a protein resembling collagen, inasmuch as it was soluble in hot trichloroacetic acid and precipitable with tannic acid, but into the hydroxyproline of which radioactive proline was incorporated only very slightly. Thus incorporation of labeled proline into bound proline was approximately 65% of that in control granuloma, but incorporation into hydroxyproline was only 14%.

B. CELL AND TISSUE CULTURE STUDIES

Convincing evidence for the participation of ascorbic acid in the hydroxylation of peptide-bound proline to collagen hydroxyproline during collagen biosynthesis has arisen from studies using isolated connective tissue cells grown in culture.

Several investigators have reported a stimulation of collagen formation in these cell culture systems when ascorbic acid was added to the growth medium (Green and Goldberg, 1964; Schimizu *et al.*, 1965; Birge and Peck, 1966; Priest and Bublitz, 1967; Schafer *et al.*, 1967; Levene and Bates, 1970). Priest and Bublitz (1967), studying collagen formation by cultured 3T6 mouse fibroblasts, demonstrated that the stimulation of collagen formation by ascorbic acid was not affected when RNA synthesis was inhibited by actinomycin D and further that stimulation was observed also when ascorbic acid was replaced by the unconjugated pteridine, 2-amino-4-hydroxy-6,7-dimethyl-5,6,7,8-tetrahydropteridine.

Bates *et al.* (1972a) have investigated by use of radioactive proline the level of proline hydroxylation in macromolecular collagenase-susceptible material synthesized by cultured 3T6 mouse fibroblasts at various stages of growth and at various levels of ascorbic acid. Cells in the stationary phase of growth produced a fully hydroxylated collagen when ascorbic acid was included in the growth medium at 50 μg/ml. When ascorbic acid was not added to the growth medium, the total incorporation of radioactivity into collagenase-susceptible polypeptide was not reduced, but the proline:hydroxyproline radioactivity ratio in such material rose to values greater than 2:1, in contrast to the ratio of unity in supplemented cells. At intermediate levels of ascorbic acid, intermediate values for the radioactivity ratio were obtained (Fig. 1). It was concluded that at very low levels of ascorbic acid microsomal synthesis of protocollagen polypeptide was unimpaired, except for the hydroxylation of prolyl residues which was reduced by 50–75%. An underhydroxylated collagen containing only one-quarter to one-half of the normal level of hydroxyproline was thereby

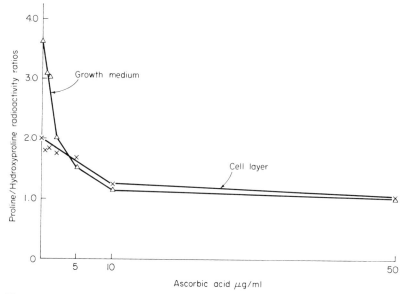

Fig. 1. Effect of ascorbic acid status on the degree of hydroxylation of proline in collagen synthesized by 3T6 mouse fibroblast cultures (Bates et al., 1972a, by permission of Elsevier, Amsterdam).

produced. This material could be detected in both cell layer and growth medium.

Tissue culture studies by Jeffrey and Martin (1966a,b) and Reynolds (1967) have demonstrated the requirement for ascorbic acid in the synthesis of bound hydroxyproline (i.e., collagen) by isolated embryonic chick bone rudiments grown in a chemically defined medium. Jeffrey and Martin (1966a,b) demonstrated that in the presence of puromycin, to inhibit protein synthesis, incorporation of [14C]proline into bound hydroxyproline was inhibited to a greater extent than incorporation into bound proline and concluded that incorporation of proline into peptide linkage preceded hydroxylation. Upon addition of ascorbic acid to the medium, the formation of peptide-bound [14C]hydroxyproline in vitamin C-depleted bones prelabeled with [14C]proline, was stimulated. Since this effect occurred even in the presence of puromycin it was concluded that ascorbic acid stimulated hydroxylation of peptidylproline (formed prior to the introduction of puromycin during the prelabeling with [14C]proline).

C. Direct Enzymatic Studies

The ability of ascorbic acid to participate in the enzymatic hydroxylation of peptide-bound proline during formation of collagen hydroxyproline has been demonstrated unequivocally in studies which first demonstrated the existence of a hydroxylase in various collagen-forming tissues which could hydroxylate peptidylproline and eventually led to the isolation of the purified enzyme and establishment of the cofactors necessary for the expression of enzymatic activity.

The studies of Peterkofsky and Udenfriend (1963) using a cell-free system from chick embryo were the first to indicate clearly that collagen synthesis consisted of two separate processes: first, a process common to all protein synthesis, namely, ribosomal amino acid incorporation into a polypeptide structure of amino acid sequence specific to the protein being synthesized, and then second the formation of collagen hydroxyproline by the hydroxylation of specific prolyl residues already incorporated into peptide linkage. Thus Peterkofsky and Udenfriend observed that when a system composed of microsomal and soluble fractions from chick embryo homogenates, supplemented with an adenosine triphosphate-generating system and magnesium ions, was incubated with labeled proline, incorporation of radioactivity into protein-bound proline occurred immediately, whereas incorporation into protein-bound hydroxyproline was delayed by approximately 30 minutes (the delay was attributed to the time required for the regeneration of cofactors essential for the hydroxylation, and which were lost by dialysis during preparation of the cell-free system). If anaerobic conditions were imposed throughout the incubation or introduced after the lag period, incorporation into hydroxyproline was inhibited, but if the anaerobiosis was limited only to the lag period, then incorporation was unaffected. Inhibition of protein synthesis by means of either puromycin or ribonuclease, caused an inhibition of incorporation of radioactivity into hydroxyproline when these compounds were included at the beginning of the incubation, but caused little or no effect when they were introduced at the end of the lag phase. The authors concluded as inferred above that the substrate for hydroxylation was peptide-bound proline.

Juva and Prockop (1964) studying collagen synthesis in cartilaginous tibiae from chick embryos by means of labeled proline demonstrated that puromycin caused a greater inhibition of collagen hydroxyproline formation than the inhibition of general amino acid incorporation and presented evidence for the release into the soluble fraction of the cells, of proline-enriched peptides. They also concluded that collagen hydroxyproline occurred as a product of the hydroxylation of peptide bound-proline in a hydroxyproline-free collagen precursor.

There followed a series of publications from various laboratories, all indicating that when conditions for hydroxylation were impaired an unhydroxylated polypeptide was synthesized (Hurych and Chvapil, 1965;

Gottlieb *et al.*, 1965, 1966; Lukens, 1965, 1966; Peterkofsky and Udenfriend, 1965; Prockop and Juva, 1965a,b; Hutton and Udenfriend, 1966; Jeffrey and Martin, 1966a,b; Juva and Prockop, 1966; Manning and Meister, 1966). Hydroxylation could be prevented by incubation under nitrogen or by means of the chelating agent, α,α'-dipyridyl. By these means it was possible to obtain incorporation of labeled proline into peptide-bound proline with negligible incorporation into hydroxyproline (Table III). The labeled material, which behaved in many ways like collagen, could be extracted into solution (with preformed collagen) or isolated in subcellular fractions prepared from homogenates by differential centrifugation and then subsequently utilized as a substrate for enzymatic hydroxylation in studies directed at establishing the nature of the enzyme involved and identification of the cofactors required. Udenfriend and his colleagues and Prockop and co-workers have been particularly active in this area.

Prockop and Juva (1965a,b) thus observed the formation of labeled hydroxyproline upon aerobic incubation of cartilage fractions, prelabeled with radioactive proline under anaerobic conditions. The hydroxylation was enzymatic as evidenced by the reduced activity in hydroxyproline when the fractions were boiled. The system also required unidentified heat-stable dialyzable cofactors contained in chick embryonic extracts. The authors were able to establish a requirement for ferrous ion.

TABLE III

EFFECT OF α,α'-DIPYRIDYL ON THE INCORPORATION OF (A) [¹⁴C]PROLINE INTO
COLLAGEN PROLINE AND HYDROXYPROLINE AND (B) [¹⁴C]LYSINE INTO
COLLAGEN LYSINE AND HYDROXYLYSINE[a]

(A)	Proline (cpm/μmole)	Hydroxyproline (cpm/μmole)
Control	16,400	14,000
1 mM α,α'-Dipyridyl	37,700	143

(B)	Lysine (dpm/μmole)	Hydroxylysine (dpm/μmole)
Control	37,800	32,800
1 mM α,α'-Dipyridyl	50,000	0

[a] Chick embryo skin slices were incubated for 2 hours at 37°C in a medium containing labeled proline or lysine and, in the case of test samples, 1 mM α,α'-dipyridyl. After incubation, samples were homogenized, and extracted with 0.2 M NaCl; collagen was then extracted from the residue with hot trichloroacetic acid. Collagen proline, hydroxyproline, lysine, and hydroxylysine specific activities were determined after acid hydrolysis (Hurych and Chvapil, 1965; Hurych and Nordwig, 1967, by permission of Elsevier, Amsterdam).

Particularly pertinent in relation to the role of ascorbic acid, Peterkofsky and Udenfriend (1965) prelabeled the microsomal fraction from chick embryos with [^{14}C]proline by incubation under nitrogen. They were able to demonstrate the formation of labeled hydroxyproline upon incubation of these microsomal preparations with a heat-stable soluble protein fraction and a boiled supernatant fraction prepared from the 105,000 g supernatant obtained from chick embryo homogenates. Significantly the latter fraction could be replaced in the incubation mixture by ascorbic acid, optimally at 1 μmole/ml. At this state of purity of the hydroxylating system, the ascorbic acid could be replaced by 2-amino-4-hydroxy-6,7-dimethyltetrahydropteridine (DMPH$_4$). The maximal activity, occurring at a concentration of 0.2 μmole/ml, was just less than the maximal activity of ascorbic acid.

Hutton et al. (1967) made the important observation, using purified dialyzed preparations of hydroxylase from chick embryo, that the heat-stable, dialyzable cofactors in addition to ferrous ion and a reducing agent such as ascorbic acid included α-ketoglutarate (Table IV). Activity lost on dialysis could be regained by a combination of these cofactors.

The enzyme protocollagen proline hydroxylase has now been isolated in highly purified form and extensively characterized (Halme et al., 1970; Olsen et al., 1970; Pankalainen et al., 1970; Rhoads and Udenfriend, 1970). With purified preparations of the enzyme it has been observed that activity is stimulated by catalase, by bovine serum albumin, and by dithiothreitol. The requirement for both ferrous ion and α-ketoglutarate

TABLE IV

DEPENDENCE OF PROTOCOLLAGEN PROLINE HYDROXYLASE ACTIVITY ON
α-KETOGLUTARATE, FERROUS ION AND ASCORBATE[a]

	Tritiated water formed (cpm)		
Omission from complete hydroxylating system	Chick embryo enzyme	Rat skin enzyme	Granuloma enzyme
None	982	850	600
α-Ketoglutarate	40	68	71
Ascorbate	0	47	0
Ferrous ion	153	323	0

[a] Complete hydroxylating system (volume 2 ml) contained (in μmoles): Tris · HCl, pH 7.5, 200; α-ketoglutarate, 0.2; ascorbate, 1.0; ferrous ion, as Fe(NH4)$_2$(SO$_4$)$_2$, 0.2; plus [3,4-^{3}H]proline-labeled peptidylproline substrate (as 0.5 mg protein), containing 800,000 dpm. Enzyme (as dialyzed 105,000 g supernatant of tissue homogenates) added as follows (as mg protein): chick embryo 2.0; fetal rat skin, 0.4; guinea pig granuloma 1.4. Hydroxylase activity was estimated as tritium released from the labeled substrate, counted at 8% efficiency (Hutton et al., 1967, by permission of Academic Press, New York).

TABLE V
Specificity of Ascorbate Requirement by
Protocollagen Proline Hydroxylase[a]

Substance replacing ascorbate	μMoles added	Tritiated water formed (cpm)	Relative activity (%)
None	—	0	0
Ascorbate	1	880	100
Isoascorbate	1	920	104
Mercaptoethanol	20	53	6
Tetrahydropteridine (DMPH₄)	1	490	56
Tetrahydrofolate	1	375	43
NADH	1	0	0
NADPH	1	0	0
Dihydroxymaleate	1	165	19
Piperidinohexose reductone	1	171	19

[a] Hydroxylating system contained 4 mg (as protein) of chick embryo enzyme partially purified by ammonium sulfate precipitation. Apart from the omission of ascorbate, the system was otherwise as described in Table IV (Hutton *et al.*, 1967, by permission of Academic Press, New York).

is specific. However, the requirement for ascorbic acid can be replaced by tetrahydrofolate or more easily by DMPH₄ (Table V). In either case, however, these compounds, even at much higher concentrations, are not so effective as ascorbic acid. The requirement for a reducing agent can also be met by dithiothreitol, and Udenfriend (1970) claims that with a suitable mixture of dithiothreitol and a protein such as bovine serum albumin in addition to α-ketoglutarate and ferrous ion, almost full hydroxylase activity can be obtained without ascorbic acid.

IV. Collagen Lysine Hydroxylation

The formation of collagen hydroxylysine has been shown to be analogous to that of collagen hydroxyproline. Collagen hydroxylysine arises by the hydroxylation of specific lysyl residues bound in peptide linkage. Molecular oxygen is required (Popenoe *et al.*, 1966; Prockop *et al.*, 1966). Hydroxylation can be prevented by anaerobiosis or use of the chelator α,α'-dipyridyl (Hurych and Nordwig, 1967). Under these conditions it is possible to obtain incorporation of radioactive lysine into peptide-bound lysine with little if any incorporation into peptidylhydroxylysine (see Table III). The subsequent enzymatic conversion of such peptide-bound labeled lysine to labeled hydroxylysine has been shown to require ferrous ion, α-ketoglutarate, and ascorbic acid (Table VI) (Hausmann, 1967; Kivirikko and Prockop, 1967b,c).

TABLE VI
COFACTOR REQUIREMENTS FOR THE HYDROXYLATION OF
[^{14}C]LYSINE IN PROTOCOLLAGEN[a]

Incubation conditions	[^{14}C]Hydroxylysine (dpm)
Substrate alone	500
Complete system	10,600
Complete system minus Fe^{2+}	800
Complete system minus α-ketoglutarate	900
Complete system minus ascorbate	500

[a] Complete system contained 200,000 dpm [^{14}C]lysine-labeled protocollagen as substrate; 50 mg ammonium sulfate precipitated chick embryo extract as enzyme; 0.01 mM FeSO$_4$; 0.5 mM α-ketoglutarate; 1 mM ascorbic acid; 0.05 M Tris buffer, pH 7.6; and 0.1 M KCl in a volume of 8 ml. After incubation at 37°C, the incubation mixture was hydrolyzed and the extent of hydroxylation was determined by measuring the [^{14}C]hydroxylysine content of the hydrolyzates. Supplementation of the complete system with an ethanolic extract of chick embryo homogenate as a source of possible additional cofactors did not increase the amount of hydroxylation (Kivirikko and Prockop, 1967c, by permission of The National Academy of Sciences, Washington, D.C.).

Highly purified preparations of protocollagen proline hydroxylase were found to contain no lysine hydroxylating activity (Halme et al., 1970), indicating that two separate enzymes were involved, a conclusion reached by Weinstein et al. (1969) from inhibition studies. R. L. Miller (1971), Kivirikko and Prockop (1972) and Popenoe and Aronson (1972) have since reported on the purification of protocollagen lysine hydroxylase free from protocollagen proline hydroxylase activity.

V. MIXED-FUNCTION OXIDATION: ROLE OF ASCORBIC ACID

With the requirement for molecular oxygen and a reducing agent, protocollagen proline hydroxylase could be regarded as a mixed function oxidase (Mason, 1965) in which, according to the following equation, one atom of molecular oxygen is incorporated into the hydroxyl group of the substrate R undergoing hydroxylation and the other atom is reduced to water by the cosubstrate XH$_2$.

$$R + XH_2 + O_2 \rightarrow ROH + X + H_2O \tag{1}$$

An example of such a hydroxylase which requires ascorbic acid as the cosubstrate is dopamine-β-hydroxylase.

A. DOPAMINE-β-HYDROXYLASE

Dopamine-β-hydroxylase is a copper-containing, mixed-function oxidase (Levin et al., 1960; Goldstein, 1966) that catalyzes the conversion of dopamine (3,4-dihydroxyphenylethylamine) to norepinephrine according to the following equation:

Dopamine + ascorbic acid + O_2 $\xrightarrow{\text{fumarate}}$

norepinephrine + dehydroascorbic acid + H_2O (2)

The mechanism of action has been studied in some detail by Kaufman and his colleagues. Ascorbic acid can be replaced by D-ascorbic acid, iso-ascorbic acid, or glucoascorbic acid (Levin et al., 1960). Otherwise, other ene-diols, SH-compounds, reduced pteridines (tetrahydrofolate or $DMPH_4$), NAD, and NADP have little if any activity. Ascorbic acid can be substituted by certain catechols, but the latter have much less activity than ascorbic acid (Levin and Kaufman, 1961). Catalase stimulates the hydroxylation, and this has been attributed to a protection of the enzyme from loss of activity due to the formation of hydrogen peroxide during incubation in the presence of substrate and ascorbic acid (Levin and Kaufman, 1961). In addition, the reaction is stimulated by fumarate and to a lesser extent by certain other dicarboxylic acids, including α-ketoglutarate [which appears to possess about two-thirds the activity of fumarate (Levin et al., 1960)]. It is believed that the fumarate acts by favoring the oxidation of enzyme-bound copper to the cupric state (Friedman and Kaufman, 1966).

Friedman and Kaufman (1966) have shown that the enzyme-bound copper undergoes a cyclic oxidation and reduction while hydroxylation of substrate is proceeding. They have demonstrated that copper on the enzyme undergoes a stoichiometric reduction by ascorbic acid. Most of the copper on the enzyme can be reduced by ascorbic acid, and this reduction can occur anaerobically. The reduced enzyme complex can then participate in hydroxylation in the presence of substrate and molecular oxygen. Once the enzyme has been reduced, ascorbic acid is no longer required for hydroxylation to proceed. Thus after reduction of enzyme, excess ascorbic acid could be removed with ascorbic acid oxidase, and the reduced enzyme was able to hydroxylate an equivalent amount of substrate when oxygen was present (Friedman and Kaufman, 1965a,b).

Goldstein (1966) confirmed that, once reduced, the enzyme could catalyze hydroxylation in the absence of ascorbate. Cysteine could reduce cupric copper on the enzyme, and upon removal of excess cysteine with p-chloromercuribenzoate, the reduced enzyme could catalyze hydroxylation without addition of ascorbate. Goldstein and Joh (1967) reported that $DMPH_4$ exhibited some slight activity in respect to reduction of the enzyme and that a mixture of $DMPH_4$ and $NADH_2$ was about half as active as ascorbic acid.

The reaction mechanism outlined in Fig. 2 has been proposed by Friedman and Kaufman (1966).

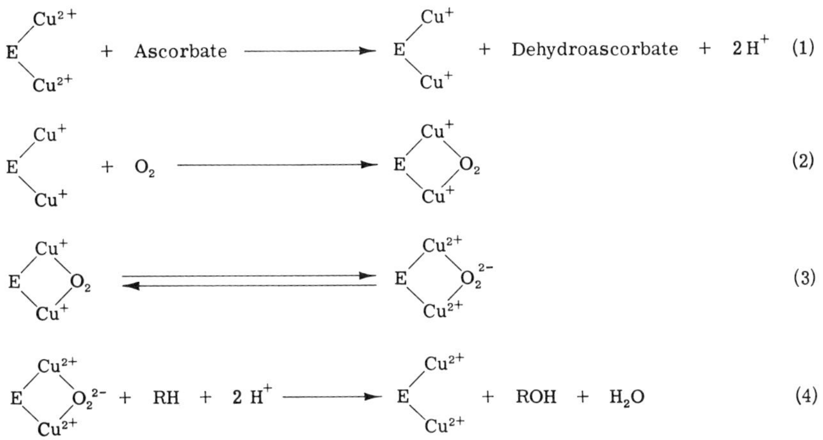

$$E\underset{Cu^{2+}}{\overset{Cu^{2+}}{\diagdown}} + \text{Ascorbate} \longrightarrow E\underset{Cu^{+}}{\overset{Cu^{+}}{\diagdown}} + \text{Dehydroascorbate} + 2\,H^{+} \quad (1)$$

$$E\underset{Cu^{+}}{\overset{Cu^{+}}{\diagdown}} + O_2 \longrightarrow E\underset{Cu^{+}}{\overset{Cu^{+}}{\diamondsuit}}O_2 \quad (2)$$

$$E\underset{Cu^{+}}{\overset{Cu^{+}}{\diamondsuit}}O_2 \rightleftharpoons E\underset{Cu^{2+}}{\overset{Cu^{2+}}{\diamondsuit}}O_2^{2-} \quad (3)$$

$$E\underset{Cu^{2+}}{\overset{Cu^{2+}}{\diamondsuit}}O_2^{2-} + RH + 2\,H^{+} \longrightarrow E\underset{Cu^{2+}}{\overset{Cu^{2+}}{\diagdown}} + ROH + H_2O \quad (4)$$

Fig. 2. Proposed reaction mechanism for the hydroxylation of dopamine (RH) to norepinephrine (ROH) by dopamine β-hydroxylase. E = Enzyme (Friedman and Kaufman, 1966, by permission of The American Society of Biological Chemists, Inc., Bethesda, Maryland).

B. PROTOCOLLAGEN PROLINE AND LYSINE HYDROXYLASES

At first sight, it was a reasonable assumption that these enzymes might have a mechanism of action similar to that just outlined for dopamine-β-hydroxylase. The requirement for molecular oxygen and a reducing agent, the most effective of which seemed to be ascorbic acid, suggested a mixed-function oxidation in which oxidation of ascorbic acid was coupled to hydroxylation of proline or lysine. This was proposed by Hutton et al. (1967). α-Ketoglutarate was considered to act as an allosteric activator. However, Prockop and Kivirikko (1968b) reported that, after reduction of enzyme by ascorbic acid and removal of excess ascorbic acid with ascorbic acid oxidase, attempts to demonstrate subsequently hydroxylation in the absence of ascorbic acid were unsuccessful [in contrast to the case with dopamine-β-hydroxylase (Friedman and Kaufman, 1965a,b)].

It subsequently emerged that, in fact, the second substrate or electron donor in the mixed-function oxidation was a α-ketoglutarate itself. It was shown that during the course of hydroxylation of peptidylproline by protocollagen proline hydroxylase, there occurred a stoichiometric decarboxylation of α-ketoglutarate to succinate (Rhoads and Udenfriend, 1968). Cardinale et al. (1971) demonstrated that one atom of molecular oxygen is incorporated into collagen hydroxyproline while the other is incorporated into succinate. It is proposed by these authors that a hydro-

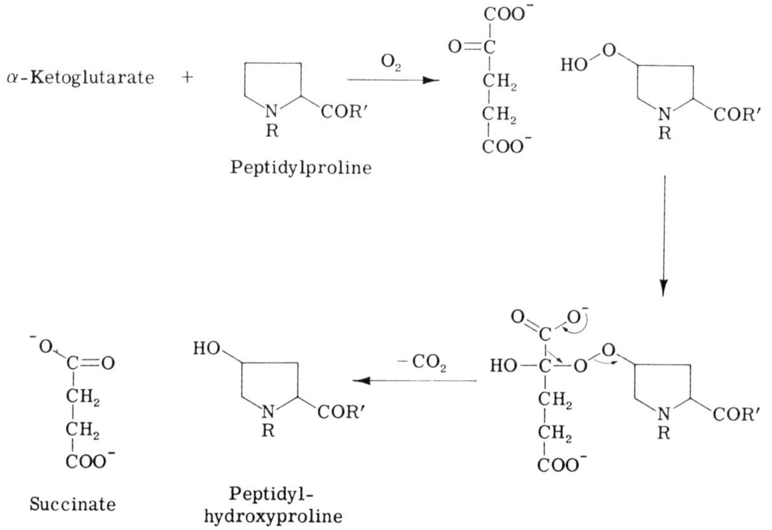

FIG. 3. Proposed reaction mechanism for the hydroxylation of peptidylproline by protocollagen proline hydroxylase (Cardinale *et al.*, 1971, by permission of Academic Press, New York).

peroxide at C-4 of proline may be an intermediate in the hydroxylation reaction, as indicated above (Fig. 3).*

Kivirikko *et al.* (1972) have also shown that the enzymatic hydroxylation of lysine in synthetic peptides by protocollagen lysine hydroxylase is coupled to the decarboxylation of α-ketoglutarate.

With the role of cosubstrate firmly ascribed to α-ketoglutarate, the role of ascorbic acid as a reductant remains obscure. The requirement for a reducing agent by protocollagen proline hydroxylase is an absolute one, but not highly specific. The various stereoisomers of ascorbic acid are all equally active in a cell-free system (Kutnink *et al.*, 1969). Tetra-hydropteridine (DMPH₄) is about half as active as ascorbic acid (Hutton *et al.*, 1967). It would be of considerable interest to know the activity of tetrahydrobiopterin, the natural cofactor for phenylalanine hydroxylase (Kaufman, 1971). Dithiothreitol can be used to replace ascorbic acid, but at best it appears to be only approximately one-third as active as ascorbic acid (Rhoads and Udenfriend, 1970). Dithiothreitol has a stimulatory effect at low concentrations in the presence of saturating levels of ascorbic acid and this has been ascribed to a protective effect toward essential SH groups in the enzyme. This effect of dithiothreitol appears

* More recently, Dr. S. Udenfriend (1972) has indicated that the primary attachment of oxygen may be to α-ketoglutarate, and that a peroxyketoglutarate (or succinate) may be an intermediate rather than a peroxyproline.

to be very dependent upon the ferrous ion concentration (Popenoe et al., 1969).

Rhoads and Udenfriend (1970) considered that the effectiveness of ascorbic acid as a reductant might lie in the ability of the reducing agent to act as a cyclic electron carrier between α-ketoglutarate and enzyme. However, they ruled this possibility out by showing that dehydroascorbic acid was ineffective as a replacement for ascorbic acid.

The stimulation by proteins such as bovine serum albumin is still not properly understood (Rhoads et al., 1967; Popenoe et al., 1969; Rhoads and Udenfriend, 1970).

The stimulatory effect of catalase (Kivirikko and Prockop, 1967d) may be attributable in part to a general protein effect similar to that exerted by bovine serum albumin and in part to its enzymatic activity toward hydrogen peroxide thereby affording protection against loss of activity due to peroxides formed during the course of the reaction (Rhoads and Udenfriend, 1970). A similar effect of catalase is seen in the case of dopamine-β-hydroxylase (Levin and Kaufman, 1961) and phenylalanine hydroxylase (Kaufman, 1959, 1971; Bublitz, 1969; Jacubovic et al., 1971).

C. Other 2-Ketoacid-Dependent Hydroxylations

Protocollagen proline and lysine hydroxylases appear to be members of a newly recognized class of mixed function oxidases, all of which require molecular oxygen, ferrous ion, a 2-ketoacid, a reductant, the most effective of which is ascorbic acid, and all of which are stimulated by catalase.

Thus the hydroxylation of γ-butyrobetaine (4-trimethylaminobutyrate) to carnitine (3-hydroxy-4-trimethylaminobutyrate) by the enzyme γ-butyrobetaine hydroxylase of either bacterial or animal origin requires all the factors outlined above (Lindstedt, 1967a; Lindstedt et al., 1967a,b). Using a partially purified enzyme preparation from rat liver, Lindstedt and Lindstedt (1970) demonstrated that the requirement for α-ketoglutarate was highly specific. There occurred a stoichiometric degradation of α-ketoglutarate relative to the amount of γ-butyrobetaine hydroxylated. α-Ketoglutarate underwent an oxidative decarboxylation to succinate (see Lindstedt et al., 1968). Succinic semialdehyde was ruled out as a possible free intermediate in the formation of succinate from α-ketoglutarate (Holme et al., 1968).

The requirement for ascorbic acid as a reductant could be easily well met by isoascorbic acid and to a lesser extent by $DMPH_4$, tetrahydrofolate or the nonphysiological reducing agent, 2,6-dichlorophenolindophenol. Oxidation products of ascorbic acid including dehydroascorbic acid and the reduced pyridine nucleotides were inactive (Lindstedt and Lindstedt, 1970).

Lindblad *et al.* (1969) demonstrated, using a preparation of γ-butyrobetaine hydroxylase from *Pseudomonas* AKl and conducting the hydroxylation in an $^{18}O_2$-enriched atmosphere that while one atom of molecular oxygen is incorporated into the new hydroxyl group of carnitine (Lindstedt, 1967b; Lindstedt and Lindstedt, 1962) the other is incorporated into succinate. A reaction mechanism is proposed (Holme *et al.*, 1968; Lindstedt and Lindstedt, 1970) as outlined below (Fig. 4), in which the anion of the substrate to be hydroxylated (I) reacts with a ferrous ion–oxygen complex. There follows a nucleophilic attack by the resultant hydroperoxide anion (II) upon the C-2 atom of α-ketoglutarate. The resulting peroxide (III) then rearranges with the formation of carnitine anion, succinate, and carbon dioxide. Peroxide intermediates have also been postulated in the enzymatic hydroxylation of phenylalanine by phenylalanine hydroxylase (Kaufman, 1971; Woolf *et al.*, 1971).

It will be noted that in this scheme the iron does not undergo cyclic oxidation and reduction as occurs with the enzyme-bound copper during the hydroxylation of dopamine by dopamine-β-hydroxylase. Further, there is no requirement for an exogenous reducing cofactor in the scheme and the precise role of ascorbic acid in this type of hydroxylation reaction

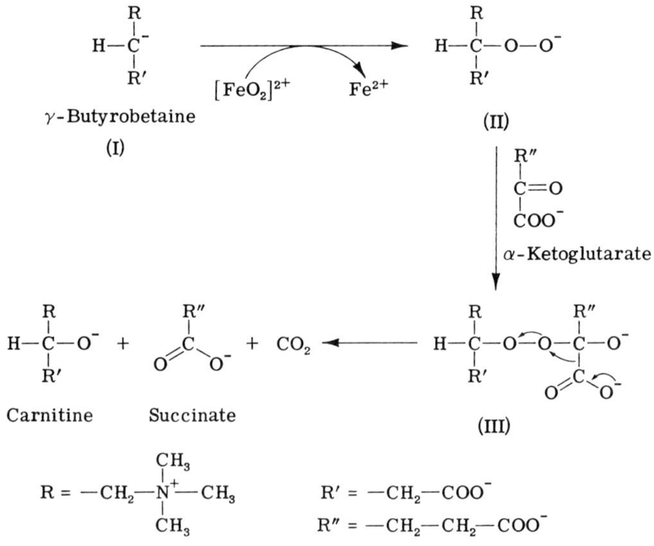

FIG. 4. Proposed reaction mechanism for the enzymatic hydroxylation of γ-butyrobetaine to carnitine (Holme *et al.*, 1968, by permission of North-Holland Publ., Amsterdam; Lindstedt and Lindstedt, 1970, by permission of The American Society of Biological Chemists, Inc., Bethesda, Maryland).

remains ill-defined. Holme *et al.* (1968) and Lindstedt and Lindstedt (1970) proposed that ascorbic acid may function by keeping iron in the ferrous state or alternatively by protecting essential SH groups from oxidation. It is also suggested that catalase stimulates the hydroxylation by protecting the enzyme from inactivation, probably by peroxides, during incubation. Preincubation of the enzyme with ascorbate and ferrous ion without catalase caused loss of activity. If catalase was included, the enzyme activity was retained (Lindstedt and Lindstedt, 1970).

The sequential oxygenation of thymine to 5-hydroxymethyluracil, 5-formyluracil, and finally 5-carboxyuracil by extracts of *Neurospora crassa*, reactions which are intermediate in the conversion of thymine to the pyrimidines of RNA in this organism, have also been shown to require atmospheric oxygen, ferrous ion, α-ketoglutarate, and ascorbate and to be stimulated by catalase (Abbott *et al.*, 1967, 1968; Watanabe *et al.*, 1970; Holme *et al.*, 1970, 1971). Holme *et al.* (1971) showed that α-ketoglutarate underwent decarboxylation and that one atom of molecular oxygen was incorporated into the resultant succinate during each oxygenation. These authors proposed a reaction mechanism similar to that outlined above for γ-butyrobetaine hydroxylase. Bankel *et al.* (1972) have reported that the three oxygenations are catalyzed by a single enzyme. The same enzyme catalyzes the conversion of 1-methyluracil to uracil.

The conversion of thymidine to thymine riboside and deoxyuridine to uridine are two further oxygenase reactions occurring in *N. crassa* and also requiring ferrous ion, α-ketoglutarate, and ascorbate but which are catalysed by an enzyme different from thymine-7-hydroxylase (Shaffer *et al.*, 1968, 1972; Bankel *et al.*, 1972).

The conversion of *p*-hydroxyphenylpyruvate to homogentisic acid is also believed to represent another example of a mixed-function oxidation in which a 2-ketoacid acts as specific cosubstrate. In this case both the 2-ketoacid and the C atom to be hydroxylated are contained within the same substrate molecule, i.e., hydroxylation of the aromatic ring is coupled to oxidative decarboxylation of the α-keto side chain. Ascorbic acid was at one time thought to be a specific cofactor in this hydroxylation. It was then concluded that ascorbic acid protected the enzyme, *p*-hydroxyphenylpyruvic acid oxidase, from inhibition by its substrate, *p*-hydroxyphenylpyruvic acid, when the latter is present in relatively high concentration (La Du and Zannoni, 1961; Knox and Goswami, 1961). It seems reasonable to suppose that the function of ascorbic acid in this hydroxylation reaction will prove to be similar to the as yet ill-defined function of the vitamin in the other 2-ketoacid-dependent hydroxylations already cited. The nature of the inhibition of *p*-hydroxyphenylpyruvic acid oxidase by excess substrate is not understood, but it is thought to be an inactivation of enzyme by small amounts of an inhibitory product that does not form when lower substrate concentrations are used (Zannoni and La Du, 1959). 2,6-Dichlorophenolindophenol can both protect the enzyme from substrate inhibition and also reactivate enzyme preparations previously inhibited by substrate provided this inhibition was not complete.

Interestingly, Mussini et al. (1967) have reported that extracts from guinea pig granuloma normally containing high levels of protocollagen proline hydroxylase, contain very little such activity when granuloma from scorbutic guinea pigs are used. It would appear here that in the absence

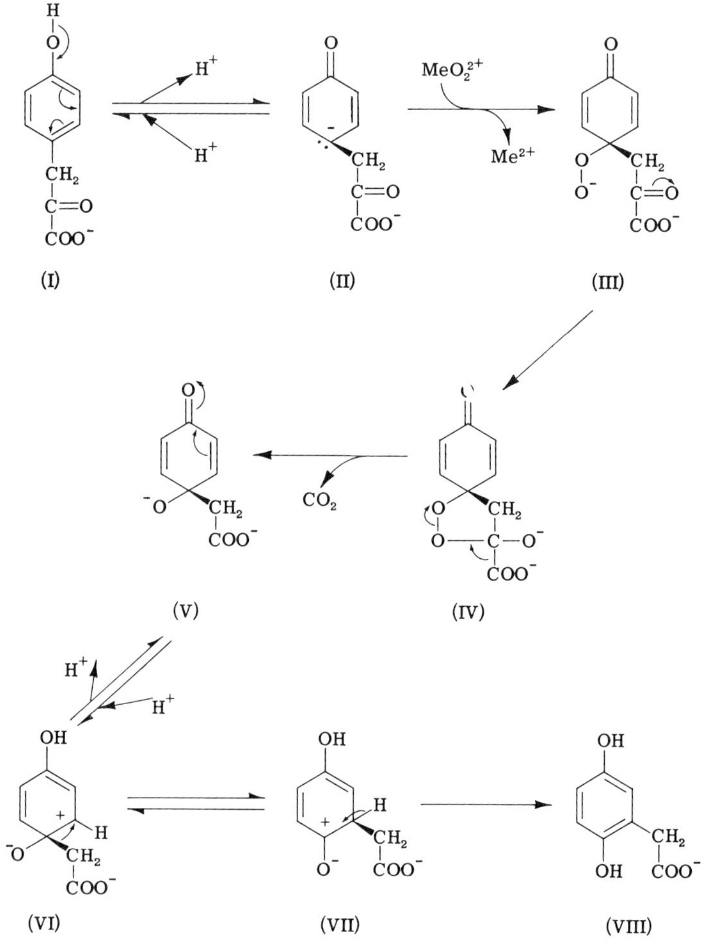

FIG. 5. Proposed reaction mechanism for the enzymatic formation of homogentisate from p-hydroxyphenylpyruvate (Lindblad et al., 1970, reprinted from J. Amer. Chem. Soc. 92, 7446; copyright 1970 by the American Chemical Society. Reprinted by permission of the copyright owner).

of ascorbic acid, the enzyme becomes irreversibly inactivated. The stimulation of hydroxylation observed upon addition of ascorbic acid to ascorbic acid-deficient cells in the studies of Stone and Meister (1962), Robertson and Hewitt (1961), and Jeffrey and Martin (1966a,b) must presumably involve new synthesis of protocollagen proline hydroxylase. Bhatnagar et al. (1968) have also reported that protocollagen proline hydroxylase is irreversibly inactivated when α,α'-dipyridyl is used to prevent hydroxylation.

Lindblad et al. (1970) have suggested the mechanism shown in Fig. 5 for p-hydroxyphenylpyruvic acid oxidase. In support of this mechanism, they have shown that oxygen from molecular oxygen is incorporated into the new hydroxyl group and into the carboxyl group of homogentisic acid.

Catalase stimulates the hydroxylation by p-hydroxyphenylpyruvic acid oxidase (La Du and Zannoni, 1956), and recently Lindblad et al. (1971), using a highly purified preparation of human liver p-hydroxyphenylpyruvate hydroxylase, have concluded that there is a requirement for ferrous ion.

It is interesting to note that the α-oxidation or 1 C degradation of long-chain α-hydroxy fatty acids that occurs in mammalian brain and involves oxidation to an α-keto acid followed by decarboxylation, has been shown to require molecular oxygen, ferrous ion, and ascorbic acid (see Mead and Hare, 1971).

VI. Function of Ascorbic Acid in Collagen Metabolism in Vivo

Studies have been undertaken in this laboratory, the purpose of which was to attempt to establish whether the role of ascorbic acid in collagen metabolism in vivo could be regarded as one solely in the hydroxylation of protocollagen proline and lysine or whether there was evidence for the involvement of ascorbic acid at some other site of action in collagen formation. As will be discussed below, investigations in vivo have sometimes given rise to doubts as to whether the primary lesion in collagen metabolism in scurvy is one of impaired hydroxylation.

Thus, it might seem reasonable in view of the foregoing evidence for the ability of ascorbic acid to participate in the hydroxylation of protocollagen proline and lysine, to anticipate the formation and accumulation of protocollagen in the tissues of scorbutic animals. However, past attempts to identify a proline-enriched, hydroxyproline-deficient collagen in such animals have been unrewarding.

Robertson and Schwartz (1953) induced granulomas in guinea pigs by the subcutaneous injection of a 1% suspension of carrageenin. Granulomas in scorbutic guinea pigs contained protein that, like collagen, was extractable by autoclaving, soluble in hot trichloroacetic acid and precipitable with tannic acid. The concentration of hydroxyproline, however, was low. It was suggested that this protein, present in amounts similar to the amount of collagen in normal granulomas, was a hydroxyproline-deficient collagen precursor. However, Robertson *et al.* (1959) subjected the protein to amino acid analysis and concluded that it could not be a collagen precursor. It did not exhibit particularly high concentrations of proline or glycine and revealed an amino acid composition very different from that anticipated for such a collagen precursor.

Similarly, Gould and Woessner (1957), studying changes in the amino acid composition in skin wound granulation tissue in response to the administration of ascorbic acid to scorbutic animals (wounded 10–12 days previously and fed a scorbutogenic diet for 1 week before wounding), were led to conclude that the rapid appearance of collagen following such administration of the vitamin may be due to the conversion to collagen of a hydroxyproline-deficient collagen precursor previously accumulated in the tissue in the absence of the vitamin. However, Gould *et al.* (1960) were unsuccessful in their attempts to isolate such a proline-rich collagen precursor from either granulation tissue or subcutaneous polyvinyl sponge implants from scorbutic guinea pigs.

Gross (1959) demonstrated that in severely scorbutic guinea pigs the skin contained no detectable neutral-salt extractable collagen. However, fractionation of neutral-salt extracts of skin from scorbutic animals failed to reveal any evidence for the replacement of neutral-salt soluble collagen by an equivalent amount of an unhydroxylated form of soluble collagen.

Relevant to this discussion, Robertson *et al.* (1959) and Gould *et al.* (1960) concluded from radioisotopic studies that the rapid synthesis of collagen observed in carrageenin granulomas or polyvinyl sponge implants in scorbutic guinea pigs after administration of ascorbic acid must arise, primarily, by complete protein synthesis and not by hydroxylation of a preexisting precursor accumulated during the period of ascorbic acid deprivation.

A. ISOTOPE INCORPORATION STUDIES IN
   SCORBUTIC GUINEA PIGS

One explanation for the failure to detect, by chemical analysis, the accumulation of unhydroxylated material in scorbutic tissues, might be that protocollagen is formed in scorbutic guinea pigs only for a limited period following the decline in ascorbic acid concentration and that a continuing deprivation of ascorbic acid then leads to an inhibition of its formation. Alternatively, protocollagen may be formed but rapidly degraded.

As an approach to exploring this problem further, it was considered that low levels of protocollagen would be more readily detectable by radioisotope techniques. The authors decided to examine the situation in scorbutic guinea pigs by these techniques at varying periods of ascorbic acid deficiency.

Normally hydroxylation occurs either as the collagen polypeptide is formed on the ribosome or almost immediately after its release from the ribosome (see Lazarides et al., 1971; Lane et al., 1971a). This means that, if collagen is isolated after administration of radioactive proline, the collagen proline:hydroxyproline specific activity ratio is 1:1 (indicative of the same level of hydroxylation in the newly synthesized labeled collagen as in the preformed unlabeled collagen) even when collagen is isolated shortly after administration of the isotope (Hausmann and Neuman, 1961). If, however, hydroxylation is impaired and protocollagen is formed, then upon isolation, after administration of radioactive proline, of the labeled protocollagen with the preformed unlabeled collagen the proline:hydroxyproline specific activity ratio will be greater than 1:1, approaching infinity, if impairment of hydroxylation is complete.

Robertson et al. (1959) had previously studied the incorporation of radioactive proline into the collagen of granuloma induced in scorbutic guinea pigs. Labeled proline was administered at 12-hour intervals during days 11–14 of granuloma development (and ascorbic acid deprivation), and the animals were sacrificed 12 hours after the last injection of isotope. The authors found that the collagen hydroxyproline specific activity was only about 50% of that in collagen from control granuloma whereas there was little difference in the proline specific activity. The proline:hydroxyproline specific activity ratio was thus approximately 2:1.

Mitoma and Smith (1960), in a similar study, isolated collagen from scorbutic granuloma 24 hours after the administration of radioactive proline in three 12-hour doses on days 9 and 10 of granuloma development (and ascorbic acid deprivation). They found that the collagen proline and hydroxyproline specific activities were both appreciably reduced, and to a similar degree in comparison to controls. Nevertheless, inspection of their data shows that the collagen proline:hydroxyproline specific activity ratio was rather greater than unity (1.14 and 1.36 in two separate experiments), control values being somewhat less than unity.

In both these cases it is tempting to suggest that the elevated ratios are indicative of impaired hydroxylation. However in both instances, it is not certain to what extent the increased ratio can be attributed to the presence of [^{14}C]proline-labeled noncollagenous protein. The same holds

true for the studies of Richmond and Stokstad (1969). Robertson *et al.*
(1959) concluded that in their case collagen from scorbutic granuloma
was probably contaminated with noncollagen protein.

In our studies (Barnes *et al.*, 1969a, 1970) we attempted to overcome
this problem by the use of collagenase. Collagen proline and hydroxyproline specific activities were determined in the diffusible products
obtained by collagenase digestion of collagen extracted from skin of
guinea pigs with hot trichloroacetic acid.

For comparison, the incorporation of labeled proline into elastin isolated from aorta was also examined, since elastin also contains some
hydroxyproline (see Barnes *et al.*, 1969a; Bentley and Hanson, 1969;
Sandberg *et al.*, 1969) although at a concentration of approximately
1.5% (about 12 residues/1000 residues) much less than in collagen.
Elastin hydroxyproline is derived from free proline rather than hydroxyproline (Barnes *et al.*, 1969a; Bentley and Hanson, 1969), and it seems
probable that it is formed by the hydroxylation of a limited number of
prolyl residues in elastin that occur within a sequence that fulfills the
substrate specificity requirements of collagen proline hydroxylase. Rhoads
and Udenfriend (1969) have reported that the level of hydroxyproline in
elastin can be slightly increased (by approximately 5 residues/1000) by

TABLE VII

INCORPORATION OF TRITIATED PROLINE *in Vivo* INTO ELASTIN IN
CONTROL AND SCORBUTIC GUINEA PIGS[a]

| | Day of experiment | No. of animals | Specific radioactivity (cpm/μmole) | | Proline/ hydroxyproline specific radioactivity ratio |
			Proline	Hydroxyproline	
Ascorbic acid-	6	6	222	149	1.5
deficient group	8	6	132	62	2.1
	10	5	142	15	9.5
	12	6	61	3	20.3
Control group	6	6	129	125	1.0
	8	6	111	131	0.9
	10	5	80	57	1.4
	12	5	35	31	1.1

[a] Each animal received, on the appropriate day of the experiment, 0.1 mCi of L-
[G-^{3}H]proline in a single dose. Animals were killed 24 hours later and the aortas were
removed and combined within each set of animals before the isolation of elastin. Elastin
proline and hydroxyproline were separated, after hydrolysis, by ion-exchange chromatography, estimated with ninhydrin and the radioactivity measured by liquid scintillation
counting. Controls were individually pair-fed with animals in the ascorbic acid-deficient
group after day 8. The number of animals refers to the number available at the time of
killing from an original total of six (Barnes *et al.*, 1970, by permission of *Biochem. J.*).

incubation with collagen proline hydroxylase and the appropriate cofactors, ascorbic acid, ferrous ion, and α-ketoglutarate. Incorporation of labeled proline into collagen and elastin proline and hydroxyproline was studied over the period of from 6 to 14 days of ascorbic acid deprivation. As shown in Table VII, the effect of ascorbic acid deprivation on elastin biosynthesis could be readily interpreted in terms of an increasing elimination of hydroxylation of elastin proline and the formation of a hydroxyproline-free polymer (Barnes et al., 1970). As judged by incorporation of radioactivity into elastin proline, there was no reduction in elastin synthesis. However, incorporation into elastin hydroxyproline rapidly declined and was negligible after 12 days of ascorbic acid deprivation. The elastin proline:hydroxyproline specific activity ratio, 1:1 in controls, was 1.5:1 after 6 days of vitamin deprivation, and 20:1 after 12 days. Formation of the elastin cross-links, desmosine and isodesmosine, was not impaired in ascorbic acid deficiency (Barnes et al., 1969a). This is in accord with the formation and retention of elastin in normal amounts despite the lack of hydroxylation.

Results for skin collagen (Barnes et al., 1970) are shown in Table VIII and are in sharp contrast to those for elastin. At no period of ascorbic acid deficiency was a high incorporation into collagen proline with low incorporation into hydroxyproline observed. The incorporation into both

TABLE VIII

INCORPORATION OF TRITIATED PROLINE in Vivo INTO DORSAL SKIN
COLLAGEN IN CONTROL AND SCORBUTIC GUINEA PIGS[a]

	Day of experiment	Specific activity (cpm/μmole) Proline	Hydroxyproline	Proline/hydroxyproline specific activity ratio
Ascorbic acid-	6	739	667	1.11 ⎫
deficient group	8	357	289	1.24 ⎪ Mean
	10	74	69	1.07 ⎬ 1.15
	12	21	17	1.24 ⎪
	14	13	12	1.08 ⎭
Control group	6	614	583	1.05 ⎫
	8	785	828	0.95 ⎪
	10	553	563	0.98 ⎬ 1.0
	12	224	217	1.03 ⎪
	14	415	417	1.0 ⎭

[a] The results are for the same animals as are listed in Table VII. Approximately equal samples of dorsal skin were combined within each set of animals. Collagen was extracted with hot trichloroacetic acid. Extracts, after dialysis, were digested with collagenase and the specific activities of proline and hydroxyproline determined in the resulting diffusible material.

proline and hydroxyproline rapidly declined around day 8 to day 10 of ascorbic acid deprivation. Nevertheless the proline:hydroxyproline specific activity ratio was consistently slightly above unity in contrast to the ratio of 1:1 in controls. Thus the mean of all control values, measured at both 4.5 and 24 hours after administration of isotope, was 1.00 (SEM ± 0.013) and for the ascorbic acid-deficient group, 1.16 (SEM ± 0.021), $P < 0.001$. This effect was noted as early as day 6 of vitamin deficiency. We interpreted these results as reflecting the appearance in place of collagen, but in rapidly diminishing amounts of a slightly under-hydroxylated collagen in which the level of hydroxylation of proline is of the order of 5–10% less than that normally occurring in collagen.

The aggregation and cross-linking of this collagen did not appear to be very different from that of normal collagen. Thus proline and hydroxy-proline specific activity values measured at varying periods of time after the administration of radioactive proline, did not indicate any significant increase in turnover. The slightly increased specific activity ratio was observed at all time periods (Barnes et al., 1970). The relative distribution of incorporated radioactivity between neutral salt-soluble, acid-soluble, and insoluble skin collagen fractions, measured 48 hours after the administration of the isotope, was similar to that occurring in controls. The increased specific activity ratio was present in all three fractions (Barnes et al., 1972). It would seem that the degree of hydroxylation (of proline and/or lysine, see below) is not sufficiently reduced to affect appreciably the rate of aggregation or cross-linking. Bentley and Jackson (1965) reached a similar conclusion from a study of the distribution in scorbutic guinea pigs of incorporated radioactive glycine between 0.14 M and 1.0 M sodium chloride-extractable collagen.

The constancy of the collagen proline:hydroxyproline specific activity ratio in these scorbutic animals, irrespective of either the duration of ascorbic acid deficiency or the time interval between administration of isotope and isolation of collagen or whether soluble or insoluble collagen fractions are examined, we consider implies most probably that a slightly underhydroxylated collagen is formed. Nevertheless, we cannot exclude the alternative that the slightly increased ratio represents a mixture of newly synthesized, fully hydroxylated collagen together with a trace of protocollagen and that both are accumulated in the skin in rapidly diminishing amounts. However, the extent of hydroxylation, at least of certain proline and lysine residues, is known to vary normally, either according to age or to the nature of the tissue from which the collagen is derived (Bornstein, 1967; E. J. Miller et al., 1969; Lane and Miller, 1969; Barnes et al., 1971a,b) and thus there is no need to regard hydroxylation as an all-or-nothing phenomenon.

During incorporation studies with labeled lysine, comparable to those with labeled proline, it was found, as anticipated, that incorporation of radioactivity into both collagen lysine and hydroxylysine fell rapidly in ascorbic acid deficiency. However, preliminary observations indicate that the collagen lysine:hydroxylysine radioactivity ratio may not differ from that in controls (Barnes *et al.*, 1972), implying that the labeled collagen, although known to be slightly underhydroxylated with respect to proline, may be hydroxylated to the normal extent with respect to lysine. This would suggest that lysine hydroxylation is perhaps less sensitive to ascorbic acid deficiency than proline hydroxylation.

We regard the slightly elevated collagen proline:hydroxyproline specific activity ratio in scurvy as indicative of the participation of ascorbic acid in collagen proline hydroxylation *in vivo*. The question that arises is why, unlike elastin, collagen does not accumulate in a form increasingly deficient in hydroxyproline (and hydroxylysine). This of course may be no more than a reflection of the essential nature of the hydroxylation in collagen metabolism *in vivo*.

One possible explanation could be that once hydroxylation is impaired beyond a certain point, the partially hydroxylated or unhydroxylated polypeptide then synthesized *in vivo* is completely degraded. Such degradation, however, would have to be very rapid since neither the proline:hydroxyproline specific radioactivity ratio nor changes in the actual specific activity values with time provided evidence for the occurrence of such a material undergoing degradation even when the skin was examined as soon as 2 hours after administration of isotope (Barnes *et al.*, 1970).

Hydroxylysine is known to be involved in the formation of intermolecular cross-links in collagen (Bailey and Peach, 1968; Bailey *et al.*, 1969, 1970; Kang *et al.*, 1970; Mechanic and Tanzer, 1970; Tanzer *et al.*, 1970; Davis and Bailey, 1971; Mechanic *et al.*, 1971), and it might be presumed therefore that in ascorbic acid deficiency, formation of cross-links would be impaired and the uncross-linked material removed by degradation. Levene *et al.* (1972a,b) have found a reduction in the formation of hydroxylysine-derived cross-links in ascorbic acid-deficient cultures of 3T6 mouse fibroblasts. However, it would seem unlikely that, solely as a result of a failure in cross-linking, degradation would be so rapid as to exclude the detection, except possibly in trace amounts, of this material in an undegraded form in the tissues. In other conditions where cross-linking is known to be impaired, as in lathyrism, copper deficiency, and after the administration of penicillamine (Levene and Gross, 1959; Weissman *et al.*, 1963; Chou *et al.*, 1969; Rucker *et al.*, 1969; Deshmukh and Nimni, 1969), there is an accumulation of the uncross-linked material as neutral salt-soluble collagen. We consider that the rapid degradation, if it occurs, must reflect some other consequence of reduced hydroxylation.

Alternatively, partially hydroxylated or unhydroxylated peptides may even be released from the ribosome before attaining any significant (nondiffusible) size. A further alternative is that in addition to impairment of hydroxylation, there may occur an inhibition of collagen protein synthesis, i.e., ribosomal amino acid incorporation. This may not necessarily be the direct consequence of impaired hydroxylation.

These possibilities will be discussed in more detail below.

B. HYDROXYPROLINE EXCRETION IN SCURVY

Changes in the excretion of hydroxyproline are regarded as a reflection of changes in the anabolism and catabolism of collagen (see Prockop and Kivirikko, 1968a; Kivirikko, 1970). An appreciable proportion of excreted hydroxyproline is derived from the turnover of newly synthesized collagen. When this synthesis is curtailed, it would be anticipated that hydroxyproline excretion would be reduced. In accord with this reasoning, Martin et al. (1961) reported a reduction in hydroxyproline excretion in scorbutic guinea pigs, compatible with reduced collagen synthesis or, more accurately, reduced formation of collagen hydroxyproline in this condition. However, this reduction did not occur until after 20 days of ascorbic acid deprivation. This is some considerable time after collagen synthesis is first affected by the avitaminosis which can occur as early as days 4–6 of vitamin deprivation [at least in tissues where rapid synthesis normally occurs (Gould, 1968a,b; Chvapil and Hurych, 1968)].

As shown in Table IX, we have not found any change in hydroxyproline

TABLE IX

EXCRETION OF HYDROXYPROLINE (BOUND PLUS FREE) BY SCORBUTIC GUINEA PIGS[a]

Day of experiment	Ascorbic acid-deficient group	Pair-fed control group
6	2.3	2.3
8	2.5	2.5
10	2.4	1.7
12	2.3	1.7
14	2.3	2.1

[a] Hydroxyproline (expressed as milligrams per 24 hours per animal) was determined colorimetrically in urine hydrolyzates as described by Barnes et al. (1969b). Pair-feeding was introduced after day 8. Each result represents the mean for six animals.

excretion in scorbutic guinea pigs during the period when incorporation of radioactive proline into skin collagen showed such a rapid decline. Similarly, the concentration in the skin of diffusible hydroxyproline and hydroxylysine [the occurrence of which is considered attributable to the degradation of collagen and might be expected to reflect, like urinary hydroxyproline, changes in collagen metabolism (Prockop and Kivirikko, 1968a)] was not significantly changed during this period. The incorporation of labeled proline or labeled lysine into, respectively, diffusible hydroxyproline or hydroxylysine in the skin was also relatively constant over this period and similar to that occurring in controls (see Barnes *et al.*, 1970).

A fall in hydroxyproline excretion in scorbutic guinea pigs in our studies (Barnes *et al.*, 1969b) commenced around day 15 of ascorbic acid deprivation and continued thereafter until at death (around day 21 of vitamin deprivation) it had fallen by approximately 50%. A comparable fall, however, occurred in the total excretion of all amino acids. Furthermore a similar situation was observed in pair-fed control animals and therefore it is possible that the eventual reduction in hydroxyproline excretion in scorbutic guinea pigs is due to the inanition accompanying this condition rather than the ascorbic acid deficiency per se.

Mitoma and Smith (1960) measured the specific activity of proline and hydroxyproline in urine collected for 48 hours from guinea pigs on days 10 and 11 of ascorbic acid deprivation, following administration of radioactive proline in three 12-hourly doses, commencing on day 9. They concluded that there was no significant difference from control values and considered that their results did not support the contention that impaired hydroxylation was the main defect in ascorbic acid deficiency.

Burkley (1968) studied hydroxyproline excretion in human scurvy. Four healthy men were fed a diet deficient in ascorbic acid for 29 weeks. The subjects were considered, on the basis of clinical signs and body pool size of ascorbic acid, to be scorbutic by week 14. Repletion commenced at this time by daily dosage with ascorbic acid. Urinary hydroxyproline was found to increase as subjects became scorbutic and to gradually return to normal levels upon repletion. This elevation in urinary hydroxyproline excretion appeared as early as 1 week after the introduction of the ascorbic acid-free diet.

Efron *et al.* (1968) studied a human patient exhibiting hydroxyprolinemia. This condition is characterized by a high concentration in the plasma and a large urinary excretion of free hydroxyproline and is due to a deficiency of the enzyme hydroxyproline oxidase. They noted that when the patient was fed a scorbutic diet, there was a 2- to 3-fold increase in both free and peptide-bound hydroxyproline excretion. A further increase in excretion occurred upon administration of ascorbic acid after the period of depletion, before a return to more normal levels of excretion. Windsor and Williams (1970) have reported that administration of ascorbic acid to elderly patients showing a low leukocyte ascorbic acid level (less than 15 $\mu g/10^8$ white blood cells) caused an increased excretion of hydroxyproline. No increase was observed in patients with higher leukocyte ascorbic acid levels. Hydroxyproline excretion before treatment was lower in the patients with low leukocyte ascorbic acid levels. In this respect, their results differ from those of Burkley and Efron et al. The difference may be related to the fact that the subjects of Windsor and Williams were probably of a long-standing partial deficiency, whereas in the other studies the subjects were exposed to an acute deficiency.

In general, the studies on hydroxyproline excretion in scurvy indicate that despite the marked impairment in collagen formation in scurvy as reflected, for example, in the large decrease in incorporation of radioactivity into skin collagen of scorbutic guinea pigs (Table VIII) (Barnes et al., 1970), this impairment is not, as might have been anticipated, accompanied by a comparable fall in hydroxyproline excretion, which in most cases remains normal or even increases. These observations are not readily compatible with impaired collagen proline hydroxylation in scurvy. There is no evidence that preformed collagen is degraded more rapidly in scurvy (see Gould, 1968b), and the explanation may lie, as suggested by Efron et al. (1968), in the excretion of partially hydroxylated peptides derived from underhydroxylated collagen synthesized as a consequence of the ascorbic acid deficiency.

C. Urinary Fractionation Studies

In order to seek evidence for the occurrence of a greater degree of impairment of hydroxylation than the slight impairment only that could be inferred, with certainty, from a study of the incorporation of labeled proline into skin collagen, we elected to examine the urine of scorbutic guinea pigs; we wished to establish whether changes occurred in the excretion pattern that could be regarded as indicative of the synthesis and degradation of a collagen becoming increasingly deficient in hydroxyproline as the deficiency of ascorbic acid became more severe.

Urine was collected for 24 hours after administration of radioactive proline to guinea pigs deprived of ascorbic acid for a varying period of 6–14 days. These studies are still under investigation, but findings so far are summarized below (Barnes et al., 1972).

Approximately one-third of the total hydroxyproline excretion in guinea pigs is nondiffusible (using Visking 18/32 dialysis tubing). High molecular weight, nondiffusible polypeptides containing hydroxyproline have also been shown to occur in human urine (see Krane et al., 1970). The nondiffusible hydroxyproline excretion did not significantly change in scorbutic guinea pigs over the period examined and was similar to that in controls. Incorporation of radioactivity into the nondiffusible hydroxyproline was also not significantly altered. Collagenase digestion of the nondiffusible fraction of urine rendered only one-quarter to one-third of the hydroxyproline diffusible. Proline and hydroxyproline radioactivity levels in the products rendered diffusible by collagenase suggested a slight reduction in the level of hydroxylation in this fraction of urine from scorbutic guinea pigs as was the case, of course, for the nondiffusible collagen fraction from the skin of scorbutic animals.

Diffusible hydroxyproline in the urine of scorbutic guinea pigs also remained relatively constant at a level comparable to that of controls and incorporation of radioactivity into this hydroxyproline also showed little change. Incorporation of radioactivity into the dipeptide prolyl-hydroxyproline appeared to be somewhat elevated. Interestingly, incorporation of radioactivity into diffusible proline showed an increase (of the order of 100%) for a short period around days 6–8, i.e., at a time when incorporation of radioactivity into skin collagen of scorbutic guinea pigs first began to decline. In confirmation of this finding, a 2- to 3-fold increase in free-proline radioactivity was observed over this same period followed by a return to near normal levels. Barnes et al. (1970) found that the incorporation of radioactive proline into diffusible proline of skin showed a temporary increase in scorbutic guinea pigs. Furthermore, Hornig et al. (1971) reported a very large increase in the concentration of free proline in guinea pig plasma after 8 days of ascorbic acid deprivation. At day 12, when the next determination was made, the level was nearly normal. These observations would seem to imply that, at least for a period, there may be appreciable formation and degradation of hydroxyproline-free or hydroxyproline-deficient collagen. As already pointed out, since the presence of such material in an undegraded form cannot be detected in any amount in the skin, degradation must be very rapid.

The increase in free-proline radioactivity must be interpreted with caution since it may not necessarily be derived from collagenous protein. Examination of the excretion of the dipeptide prolylproline relative to that of prolylhydroxyproline may provide useful information. Nevertheless, in view of the temporary nature of the increase in labeled diffusible proline excretion, the data at present do not support the contention that the almost complete cessation in the deposition of collagen in the tissues, as reflected in the negligible incorporation of radioactivity into skin collagen by days 12–14 of ascorbic acid deficiency, can be accounted for simply and solely in terms of the continual excretion of underhydroxylated material. It is necessary to consider that an inhibition of microsomal collagen protein synthesis occurs.

The constancy in the excretion of labeled hydroxyproline in both diffusible and nondiffusible forms is difficult to explain in the face of only a temporary increase in diffusible labeled proline excretion. If there is only a temporary elevated excretion of underhydroxylated peptides, around days 6–8, as implied from the labeled diffusible proline excretion, it might be anticipated that as the excretion of these peptides declined, the excretion of labeled hydroxyproline would also decline at the same time. It may be that the labeled hydroxyproline is derived primarily from the slightly underhydroxylated collagen, a constant amount of which may be degraded despite the rapidly falling levels in the tissue.

D. INHIBITION OF COLLAGEN PROTEIN SYNTHESIS
   IN SCURVY

As already inferred, the probability is that although the initial effect in scurvy may be a reduction of hydroxylation and the degradation and excretion of underhydroxylated material, the continuous lack of accumulation of either collagen or protocollagen in the tissues must be attributed to impaired collagen protein synthesis, i.e., interference in the actual process of amino acid incorporation.

The incorporation studies of Stone and Meister (1962), Manning and Meister (1966), and Gottlieb et al. (1966) already referred to, using isolated whole cell preparations from scorbutic granuloma, all revealed, not only evidence of impaired hydroxylation by virtue of a high incorporation of radioactivity into collagen proline relative to that into hydroxyproline, but also, as in vivo, a reduction in the overall level of incorporation. This could be indicative of reduced collagen protein synthesis, although it should be borne in mind that this reduction may also be at least partly attributable to increased degradation, resulting in an increased level of radioactivity in low molecular weight degradation products in the incubation medium. Further the studies of Bates et al. (1972a) with mouse fibroblasts suggest that reduced hydroxylation of collagen proline, as a result of ascorbic acid deficiency, can occur without reduced collagen protein synthesis.

A disturbance in ribosomal function in vivo in scurvy is inferred in the electron microscope studies of Ross and Benditt (1964), who observed, in fibroblasts from wounds of scorbutic guinea pigs, a change in the configuration of the ribosomes attached to the membranes of the rough endoplasmic reticulum, and also a marked increase in the number of free ribosomes in the cytoplasm. In contrast, changes were not seen in the macrophages present in the wound tissue.

The question arises whether this effect upon collagen protein synthesis in ascorbic acid deficiency is to be regarded as a consequence of impaired hydroxylation or whether in fact ascorbic acid has some additional role in collagen metabolism.

It is not unreasonable, for example, to question whether if tetrahydrofolate, or perhaps more likely tetrahydrobiopterin, may be able *in vivo* to participate in the hydroxylation of protocollagen proline and lysine. Then the collagen lesion in scurvy may be regarded as not primarily related to impaired hydroxylation. The relationship between ascorbic acid and folic acid is still obscure. Gould (1970) has recently reported a reduction in collagen formation, as measured by collagen hydroxyproline synthesis, in folate deficiency induced in rats by the use of methotrexate, and in guinea pigs by use of a folate-deficient diet. It would seem unlikely, however, that this could be due to impaired hydroxylation when ascorbic acid is present.

In our own recent studies with folate-deficient rats in which the deficiency was obtained by feeding a folate-free diet containing 1% sulfasuxidine, we concluded (Hautvast and Barnes, 1972) that there appeared to be only a relatively small and unspecific effect on collagen synthesis that could be attributed directly to the folate deficiency. The main effect on collagen synthesis in these animals appeared to be related to the relatively poor growth rate since a marked effect was noted in pair-fed controls with the same growth rate when compared to animals fed ad libitum and exhibiting a normal growth rate. However, whether folate has an effect or not in the presence of ascorbate, it remains a possibility that in the absence of ascorbate the presence of folate could still ensure adequate hydroxylation. There is evidence, however, that a folate deficiency may accompany an ascorbic acid deficiency, as witnessed by the occurrence sometimes of a megoloblastic anemia in scurvy (see Cox, 1968). It has been postulated (Vilter *et al.*, 1963; Vilter, 1964) that dihydrofolate reductase, an enzyme whose activity is essential to maintain an adequate level of reduced folates and related unconjugated pteridines (sec Kaufman, 1967, 1971) is protected by ascorbic acid. Thus it might be argued that these compounds would be at a low level in ascorbic acid deficiency (see Nichol and Welch, 1950; Broquist *et al.*, 1951; Gabuzda *et al.*, 1951; Welch *et al.*, 1951; May *et al.*, 1952). In this situation a maintenance of a normal level of hydroxylation of protocollagen proline and lysine in scurvy by reduced folates or relates compounds would seem unlikely. However, it is not clear that if such a reduction in folate level occurs, that its occurrence is coincident with the impairment in collagen synthesis commencing around days 4–6 of ascorbic acid deficiency. It is possible that a folate deficiency, if it occurs, would be manifested at a later stage in ascorbic acid deficiency. In any event there seems to be little doubt from the results with elastin that hydroxylation of peptidylproline is impaired in scurvy, and this would rule out, in this case, any consideration that hydroxylation is maintained by reduced folates in scurvy. By analogy, it would seem unlikely that the apparently slight impairment only in collagen hydroxylation is due to the support of hydroxylation by folates. The question remains open whether *in vivo* the reduced folates can and do participate in the hydroxylation of collagen and whether the impaired hydroxylation in scurvy is contributed to by a folate deficiency.

Other reasons for believing that ascorbic acid is involved in collagen metabolism at a level other than that of hydroxylation have also been advanced. Fernández-Madrid and Pita (1970) incubated guinea pig granuloma slices in the presence of labeled proline and then studied the distribution of incorporated radioactivity in ribosomal aggregates separated from granuloma homogenates by sucrose density gradient centrifugation. They observed, in preparations from scorbutic granuloma, a shift in the size of aggregates from large to small. Total incorporation of radioactivity incorporated was mostly into collagenase-resistant material. Upon addition of ascorbic acid, there was a shift in the pattern toward larger aggregates, which were shown to incorporate radioactivity into collagenase-susceptible material. This shift was prevented if collagenase was present, and it was therefore deduced that the formation of the large polyribosomes was dependent upon collagen synthesis. The effect of ascorbic acid could be explained on the basis of stimulation of collagen synthesis secondary to a stimulation of hydroxylation. However, the authors stated that blocking hydroxylation with α,α'-dipyridyl did not cause any change in the pattern of ribosomal aggregates, and they concluded that the stimulation of collagen synthesis by ascorbic acid is probably due to a direct influence of ascorbic acid upon polyribosomal formation or stability. However it is not clear how rapidly disaggregation of polyribosomes occurs once hydroxylation is inhibited. It may not necessarily be an instantaneous effect and the disaggregation occurring in scorbutic granuloma *in vivo* may be a consequence of a relatively prolonged period of inhibition of hydroxylation in comparison to the much shorter period of inhibition occurring in short-term incubations, employing α,α'-dipyridyl as inhibitor.

Caygill and Clucas (1971), studying the influence of ascorbic acid on collagen fibril formation *in vitro*, have made the suggestion that the role of ascorbic acid may be to prevent collagen fibril formation within the cell. It is maintained that outside the cell the ascorbic acid concentration will be reduced and that fibril formation can then occur.

In studies in the authors' laboratory, it was considered that if ascorbic acid was involved independently in both hydroxylation and ribosomal synthesis of collagen then it might be possible, on the assumption that the maintenance of hydroxylation required the higher level of the vitamin, to impair this function without impairment of the other by reducing the ascorbic acid to an appropriate level. Under these conditions formation of protocollagen might then be detectable. Guinea pigs were maintained on a low level of ascorbic acid (0.5 mg per day) just sufficient to achieve a constant body weight. Skin collagen was isolated following administration of labeled proline. It was found (Barnes et al., 1972) that collagen proline and hydroxyproline specific activities were both reduced by approximately 50%. The proline:hydroxyproline specific activity ratio was, as in acute scurvy, slightly elevated at about 1.2. The results suggested the formation, at a rate approximately half that of normal collagen synthesis, of a slightly underhydroxylated collagen. This rate of synthesis appeared to be maintained throughout the entire period of chronic partial deficiency. No change in hydroxyproline excretion was observed. We were thus unable to obtain evidence from this experiment that one could achieve in vivo a separation of the process of hydroxylation from that of amino acid incorporation. The failure to do so, as in acute scurvy, could be regarded as indicative of the fact that impaired collagen protein synthesis was a direct consequence of impaired hydroxylation.

It is interesting to speculate why, although there occurs, as in vivo, a reduction in the overall level of incorporation into collagen when isolated connective tissues from scorbutic animals are incubated in the presence of labeled proline in vitro (Stone and Meister, 1962; Manning and Meister, 1966; Gottlieb et al., 1966), the proline:hydroxyproline specific activity ratio is much greater than the slightly elevated ratio observed in vivo. In our experience, the incorporation of radioactivity into collagen proline is reduced to a comparable extent (in comparison to controls) in both in vivo and in vitro situations, but incorporation into collagen hydroxyproline shows a greater reduction in vitro. We consider that the residual hydroxylation occurring in vivo is more or less eliminated under in vitro conditions, possibly because of a greater sensitivity under these conditions to the deficiency of the vitamin. It might be expected that the additional reduction in hydroxylation in vitro would lead to a further reduction in collagen protein synthesis. However, as already suggested in relation to polyribosomal disaggregation, this may not occur as an immediate consequence of impaired hydroxylation and may therefore not be observed in short-term in vitro incubations.

A comparison of the effects of ascorbic acid deficiency on collagen metabolism to those produced by inhibiting hydroxylation with α,α'-dipyridyl suggests a similarity between the two and further indicates that impaired hydroxylation may lead, most noticeably *in vivo*, to decreased collagen protein synthesis.

Thus Chvapil and his associates were able to demonstrate formation *in vitro* of protocollagen by incubating chick embryo skin slices in the presence of α,α'-dipyridyl. At the same time, there was little loss in overall rate of collagen protein synthesis (Hurych and Chvapil, 1965; Chvapil *et al.*, 1967; Hurych and Nordwig, 1967). However, when this reagent was used under *in vivo* conditions, by local application to a skin wound through a chamber fixed to the margin of the wound, they could only detect impaired collagen protein synthesis or deposition, not impaired hydroxylation; i.e., incorporation of radioactivity into collagen proline and hydroxyproline was equally reduced [by approximately 30% (Chvapil *et al.*, 1968)].

Ramaley and Rosenbloom (1971) studied the synthesis of collagen in 3T6 mouse fibroblasts grown in culture. They demonstrated the presence in the medium of a high molecular weight collagenous component (somewhat greater in size than a β-chain when examined by gel filtration in $1\,M$ calcium chloride buffer) and collagenase-susceptible peptides of molecular weight in the region of 10,000–50,000. In the presence of an increasing concentration of α,α'-dipyridyl, incorporation of radioactive proline into the high molecular weight fraction decreased until, at a concentration of $10^{-4}\,M$, incorporation into this fraction was negligible. However, the degree of hydroxylation in this material was always high.

The reduction in overall incorporation of radioactivity into the lower molecular weight peptides, with increasing α,α'-dipyridyl concentration, was much less. However, in these peptides the degree of hydroxylation was low.

These results appear to show a strong resemblance to the situation *in vivo* in scorbutic guinea pigs, since in both instances it appears that a slightly underhydroxylated collagen is produced in rapidly diminishing amounts as the severity of the inhibition of hydroxylation is increased. Evidence was presented to show that unhydroxylated molecules accumulated within the cell. The authors concluded that inhibition of hydroxylation prevented normal extrusion and that some of the retained molecules were partially degraded and the products of degradation were extruded. Margolis and Lukens (1971), studying 3T6 mouse fibroblasts in cell culture, also concluded that inhibition of hydroxylation of collagen by means of α,α'-dipyridyl caused an impairment in extrusion.

The studies of Prockop and his group with the proline analog azetidine-2-carboxylic acid, also indicate that interference with hydroxylation may lead *in vivo* primarily to arrest of collagen accumulation. Thus embryonic chick cartilage incubated with azetidine-2-carboxylic acid resulted in its incorporation into collagen with a concomitant reduction in the amount of both hydroxyproline and hydroxylysine formed. This apparently led to reduced transport of the collagen from the cell (Takeuchi and Prockop, 1969; Takeuchi et al., 1969). In vivo, the most marked effect of the analog was upon the synthesis or accumulation of collagen. The concentration of collagen in chick embryos, after administration of azetidine-2-carboxylic acid, was greatly reduced, but a change in the level of hydroxylated residues could not be detected by amino acid analysis, although it was noted that the collagen contained a low level of this analog (about 4 residues/1000 residues of amino acid). It was concluded that intracellular accumulation of the altered collagen led to a marked inhibition of further synthesis (Lane et al., 1971b,c).

It would appear that interference with hydroxylation may lead to impaired transport and hence accumulation of underhydroxylated material within the cells. This material may undergo intracellular degradation as appears to occur in other instances where transport of an extracellular protein is apparently affected by synthesis of an abnormal structure. Schubert and Cohn (1968), for example, have shown that certain mouse myeloma mutants produce a defective immunoglobulin heavy-chain component that is unable to associate with light-chain subunits to produce the normal immunoglobulin structure. Free light chains are secreted, but the heavy chains undergo intracellular degradation.

Accumulation of the underhydroxylated material could also lead to impaired synthesis, and this would become particularly noticeable in vivo. Prockop and colleagues have presented evidence that hydroxylation of both proline and lysine is essential for normal extrusion of collagen (Rosenbloom and Prockop, 1971; Rosenbloom and Christner, 1971). It is known that some of the hydroxylysine of collagen is glycosylated (Butler and Cunningham, 1966; Cunningham and Ford, 1968; Spiro, 1969; Morgan et al., 1970), and it has been suggested that this glycosylation, which occurs on the plasma membrane, is necessary for extrusion (Hagopian et al., 1968). This would offer an explanation for the need for hydroxylation of lysine for collagen transport.

Complete hydroxylation at least of collagen proline, may not be an absolute requirement for collagen transport since work in this laboratory has shown (Bates et al., 1972b) that collagenase-susceptible material appears in the medium of cultures of mouse fibroblasts grown in the absence of ascorbic acid. This material after dissociation has a molecular weight greater than collagen α-chains (and presumably therefore represents undegraded material) and is also substantially underhydroxylated (as determined by examination of the products rendered diffusible by collagenase) with respect to proline. Gribble et al. (1969) and Margolis and Lukens (1971) have also reported the presence of underhydroxylated material in the medium of fibroblast cell cultures, but in their studies it is not certain whether the material represents the products of intracellular degradation.

Several laboratories have now reported on the existence of a precursor of collagen of higher molecular weight than collagen (Layman *et al.*, 1970, 1971; Bellamy and Bornstein, 1971; Church *et al.*, 1971; Jimenez *et al.*, 1971; Lapiere *et al.*, 1971; Lazarides and Lukens, 1971b; Lenaers *et al.*, 1971; Müller *et al.*, 1971; Ramaley and Rosenbloom, 1971; Bates *et al.*, 1972b; Clark and Veis, 1972; Dehm *et al.*, 1972). It is believed that this precursor may be involved in the transport of collagen from the cell or in the control of chain association and fibril formation (see Speakman, 1971). It may be that hydroxylation of specific proline and lysine residues is essential for the fulfillment of the role of this precursor.

VII. SUMMARY

Collagen hydroxyproline and hydroxylysine are formed by the enzymatic hydroxylation of specific proline and lysine residues previously incorporated into peptide linkage. When, in isolated collagen-forming systems, hydroxylation is prevented by the exclusion of oxygen or by means of the chelating agent α,α'-dipyridyl, an unhydroxylated polypeptide termed protocollagen is produced.

Studies with whole-cell preparations from scorbutic tissues, with fibroblast cell cultures, with organ cultures, and more especially with cell-free systems employing a purified enzyme preparation and appropriate cofactors, all indicate that ascorbic acid can and does participate in the hydroxylation of protocollagen proline and lysine.

Separate enzymes are involved in the formation of collagen hydroxyproline and hydroxylysine and are known, respectively, as protocollagen proline and lysine hydroxylase. They may be regarded as belonging to a class of hydroxylases, members of which all require for activity, molecular oxygen, ferrous ion, a 2-ketoacid (generally α-ketoglutarate), and a reductant, the most effective being ascorbic acid. The α-ketoacid is the cosubstrate in the mixed function oxidation, and undergoes a stoichiometric decarboxylation during the course of the hydroxylation. The role of ascorbic acid in the hydroxylation reaction remains undefined.

Despite the evidence for the ability of ascorbic acid to participate in the hydroxylation of protocollagen proline and lysine, protocollagen does not accumulate *in vivo* in connective tissues of scorbutic animals.

In scorbutic guinea pigs, incorporation studies have been interpreted as indicating the appearance, in the place of collagen, but in rapidly diminishing amounts as ascorbic acid deprivation continues, of a slightly underhydroxylated collagen in which the level of hydroxylation of proline is of the order of 5–10% less than that normally occurring in collagen. The reduction in hydroxylation is regarded as direct evidence for the participation of ascorbic acid in the hydroxylation of protocollagen proline *in vivo*. The synthesis, in scorbutic guinea pigs, of an elastin becoming increasingly deficient in hydroxyproline as the vitamin deficiency becomes increasingly severe, is further evidence for the involvement *in vivo* of ascorbic acid in the hydroxylation of peptidylproline.

The failure of protocollagen to accumulate within the tissues of scorbutic animals may be attributable in part to its degradation. It has been observed in particular that an increased proportion of [^{3}H]proline administered to guinea pigs 6 to 8 days after ascorbic acid deprivation, is excreted in urine 24 hours later either as the free amino acid or in the form of low molecular weight diffusible peptides.

The occurrence in ascorbic acid deficiency of a normal or even increased hydroxyproline excretion is not immediately reconcilable with inhibited hydroxylation. It may reflect the formation and degradation in scurvy of partially hydroxylated species rather than (or as well as) formation and degradation of protocollagen. It is suggested that, at least in the guinea pig, normal hydroxyproline excretion in ascorbic acid deficiency may occur through degradation, at a constant rate, of the slightly underhydroxylated collagen detected by isotope incorporation studies, despite its rapidly diminishing rate of formation (or deposition) within the tissues.

The continuous lack of accumulation of protocollagen within the tissues of scorbutic animals is considered to be attributable mostly to an inhibition of ribosomal collagen protein synthesis. For reasons which are given, this inhibition is regarded as a consequence of inhibited hydroxylation. [See Addendum on p. 43.]

REFERENCES

Abbott, M. T., Schandl, E. K., Lee, R. F., Parker, T. S., and Midgett, R. J. (1967). *Biochim. Biophys. Acta* 132, 525.
Abbott, M. T., Dragila, T. A., and McCroskey, R. P. (1968). *Biochim. Biophys. Acta* 169, 1.
Bailey, A. J., and Peach, C. M. (1968). *Biochem. Biophys. Res. Commun.* 33, 812.
Bailey, A. J., Fowler, L. J., and Peach, C. M. (1969). *Biochem. Biophys. Res. Commun.* 35, 663.
Bailey, A. J., Peach, C. M., and Fowler, L. J. (1970). *Biochem. J.* 117, 821.
Bankel, L., Holme, E., Lindstedt, G., and Lindstedt, S. (1972). *FEBS Lett.* 21, 135.
Barnes, M. J. (1969). *Bibl. "Nutr. Dieta"* 13, 86.
Barnes, M. J., Constable, B. J., and Kodicek, E. (1969a). *Biochem. J.* 113, 387.
Barnes, M. J., Constable, B. J., and Kodicek, E. (1969b). *Biochim. Biophys. Acta* 184, 358.

Barnes, M. J., Constable, B. J., Morton, L. F., and Kodicek, E. (1970). *Biochem. J.* **119**, 575.

Barnes, M. J., Constable, B. J., Morton, L. F., and Kodicek, E. (1971a). *Biochem. J.* **125**, 433.

Barnes, M. J., Constable, B. J., Morton, L. F., and Kodicek, E. (1971b). *Biochem. J.* **125**, 925.

Barnes, M. J., Constable, B. J., Morton, L. F., and Kodicek, E. (1972). To be published.

Bates, C. J., Prynne, C., and Levene, C. I. (1972a). *Biochim. Biophys. Acta* **263**, 397.

Bates, C. J., Bailey, A. J., Prynne, C., and Levene, C. I. (1972b). *Biochim. Biophys. Acta* **278**.

Bellamy, G., and Bornstein, P. (1971). *Proc. Nat. Acad. Sci. U. S.* **68**, 1138.

Bentley, J. P., and Hanson, A. N. (1969). *Biochim. Biophys. Acta* **175**, 339.

Bentley, J. P., and Jackson, D. S. (1965). *Biochim. Biophys. Acta* **107**, 519.

Bhatnagar, R. S., Kivirikko, K. I., and Prockop, D. J. (1968). *Biochim. Biophys. Acta* **154**, 196.

Birge, S. J., and Peck, W. A. (1966). *Biochem. Biophys. Res. Commun.* **22**, 532.

Bornstein, P. (1967). *Biochemistry* **6**, 3082.

Broquist, H. P., Stokstad, E. L. R., and Jukes, T. H. (1951). *J. Lab. Clin. Med.* **38**, 95.

Bublitz, C. (1969). *Biochim. Biophys. Acta* **191**, 249.

Burkley, K. (1968). M.Sc. Thesis, University of Iowa, Iowa City.

Butler, W. T., and Cunningham, L. W. (1966). *J. Biol. Chem.* **241**, 3882.

Cardinale, G. J., Rhoads, R. E., and Udenfriend, S. (1971). *Biochem. Biophys. Res. Commun.* **43**, 537.

Caygill, J. C., and Clucas, I. J. (1971). *Z. Klin. Chem. Klin. Biochem.* **1**, 63.

Chou, W. S., Savage, J. E., and O'Dell, B. L. (1969). *J. Biol. Chem.* **244**, 5785.

Church R. L., Pfeiffer, S. E., and Tanzer, M. L. (1971). *Proc. Nat. Acad. Sci. U. S.* **68**, 2638.

Chvapil, M., and Hurych, J. (1968). *Int. Rev. Connect. Tissue Res.* **4**, 67.

Chvapil, M., Hurych, J., Ehrlichova, E., and Cmuchalova, B. (1967). *Biochim. Biophys. Acta* **140**, 339.

Chvapil, M., Hurych, J., and Ehrlichova, E. (1968). *Hoppe-Seyler's Z. Physiol. Chem.* **349**, 218.

Clark, C. C., and Veis, A. (1972). *Biochemistry* **11**, 494.

Coronado, A., Mardones, E., and Allende, J. E. (1963). *Biochem. Biophys. Res. Commun.* **13**, 75.

Cox, E. V. (1968). *Vitam. Horm.* **26**, 635.

Cunningham, L. W., and Ford, J. D. (1968). *J. Biol. Chem.* **243**, 2390.

Davis, N. R., and Bailey, A. J. (1971). *Biochim. Biophys. Res. Commun.* **45**, 1416.

Dehm, P., Jimenez, S. A., Olsen, B. R., and Prockop, D. J. (1972). *Proc. Nat. Acad. Sci. U. S.* **69**, 60.

Deshmukh, K., and Nimni, M. E. (1969). *J. Biol. Chem.* **244**, 1787.

Efron, M. L., Bixby, E. M., Hockaday, T. D. R., Smith, L. H., and Meshorer, E. (1968). *Biochem. Biophys. Acta* **165**, 238.

Fernández-Madrid, F., and Pita, J. Jr. (1970). *In* "Chemistry and Molecular Biology of the Intercellular Matrix" (E. A. Balazs, ed.), Vol. 1, p. 439. Academic Press, New York.

Friedman, S., and Kaufman, S. (1965a). *J. Biol. Chem.* **240**, PC352.

Friedman, S., and Kaufman, S. (1965b). *J. Biol. Chem.* **240,** 4763.

Friedman, S., and Kaufman, S. (1966). *J. Biol. Chem.* **241,** 2256.

Fujimoto, D., and Tamiya, N. (1962). *Biochem. J.* **84,** 333.

Gabuzda, C. J., Philips, G. B., Schilling, R. F., and Davidson, C. J. (1951). *J. Clin. Invest.* **31,** 756.

Goldstein, M. (1966). *In* "Biochemistry of Copper" (J. Peisach, P. Aisen, and W. E. Blumberg, eds.), p. 443. Academic Press, New York.

Goldstein, M., and Joh, T. H. (1967). *Mol. Pharmacol.* **3,** 396.

Gottlieb, A. A., Peterkofsky, B., and Udenfriend, S. (1965). *J. Biol. Chem.* **240,** 3099.

Gottlieb, A. A., Kaplan, A., and Udenfriend, S. (1966). *J. Biol. Chem.* **241,** 1551.

Gould, B. S. (1960). *Vitam. Horm. (New York)* **18,** 89.

Gould, B. S. (1968a). *In* "Treatise on Collagen" (B. S. Gould, ed.), Vol. 2, Part A, p. 139. Academic Press, New York.

Gould, B. S. (1968b). *In* "Treatise on Collagen" (B. S. Gould, ed.), Vol. 2, Part A, p. 323. Academic Press, New York.

Gould, B. S. (1970). *In* "Chemistry and Molecular Biology of the Intercellular Matrix" (E. A. Balazs, ed.), Vol. 1, p. 431. Academic Press, New York.

Gould, B. S., and Woessner, J. F. (1957). *J. Biol. Chem.* **226,** 289.

Gould, B. S., Manner, G., Goldman, H. M., and Stolman, J. (1960). *Ann. N. Y. Acad. Sci.* **85,** 385.

Green, H., and Goldberg, B. (1964). *Proc. Soc. Exp. Biol. Med.* **117,** 258.

Gribble, T. J., Comstock, J. P., and Udenfriend, S. (1969). *Arch. Biochem. Biophys.* **129,** 308.

Gross, J. (1959). *J. Exp. Med.* **109,** 557.

Hagopian, A., Bosmann, H. B., and Eylar, E. H. (1968). *Arch. Biochem. Biophys.* **128,** 387.

Halme, J., Kivirikko, K. I., and Simons, K. (1970). *Biochim. Biophys. Acta* **198,** 460.

Hausmann, E. (1967). *Biochim. Biophys. Acta* **133,** 591.

Hausmann, E., and Neuman, W. F. (1961). *J. Biol. Chem.* **236,** 149.

Hautvast, J., and Barnes, M. J. (1972). *Proc. IXth Int. Congr. Nutr., Mexico City, Mexico* (in press).

Holme, E., Lindstedt, G., Lindstedt, S., and Tofft, M. (1968). *FEBS Lett.* **2,** 29.

Holme, E., Lindstedt, G., Lindstedt, S., and Tofft, M. (1970). *Biochim. Biophys. Acta* **212,** 50.

Holme, E., Lindstedt, G., Lindstedt, S., and Tofft, M. (1971). *J. Biol. Chem.* **246,** 3314.

Hornig, D., Weber, F., and Wiss, O. (1971). *Int. J. Vitamin Nutr. Res.* **41,** 86.

Hurych, J., and Chvapil, M. (1965). *Biochim. Biophys. Acta* **97,** 361.

Hurych, J., and Nordwig, A. (1967). *Biochim. Biophys. Acta* **140,** 168.

Hutton, J. J., and Udenfriend, S. (1966). *Proc. Nat. Acad. Sci. U. S.* **56,** 198.

Hutton, J. J., Tappel, A. L., and Udenfriend, S. (1967). *Arch. Biochem. Biophys.* **118,** 231.

Jackson, D. S., Watkins, D., and Winkler, A. (1964). *Biochim. Biophys. Acta* **87,** 152.

Jacubovic, A., Woolf, L. I., and Chan-Henry, E. (1971). *Biochem. J.* **125,** 563.

Jeffrey, J. J., and Martin, G. R. (1966a). *Biochim. Biophys. Acta* **121,** 269.

Jeffrey, J. J., and Martin, G. R. (1966b). *Biochim. Biophys. Acta* **121,** 281.

Jimenez, S. A., Dehm, P., and Prockop, D. J. (1971). *FEBS Lett.* **17,** 245.

Juva, K. (1968). *Acta Physiol. Scand., Suppl.* **308,** 1.

Juva, K., and Prockop, D. J. (1964). *Biochim. Biophys. Acta* **91,** 174.

Juva, K., and Prockop, D. J. (1965). *In* "Biochemie et Physiologie du Tissu

Conjonctif" (P. Compte, ed.), p. 417. Société Ormeco et Imprimerie du Sud-Est à Lyon, Lyon.

Juva, K., and Prockop, D. J. (1966). *J. Biol. Chem.* **241**, 4419.

Kang, A. H., Faris, B., and Franzblau, C. (1970). *Biochem. Biophys. Res. Commun.* **39**, 175.

Kaufman, S. (1959). *J. Biol. Chem.* **234**, 2677.

Kaufman, S. (1967). *J. Biol. Chem.* **242**, 3934.

Kaufman, S. (1971). *Advan. Enzymol.* **35**, 245.

Kivirikko, K. I. (1970). *Int. Rev. Connect. Tissue Res.* **5**, 93.

Kivirikko, K. I., and Prockop, D. J. (1967a). *Biochem. J.* **102**, 432.

Kivirikko, K. I., and Prockop, D. J. (1967b). *Arch. Biochem. Biophys.* **118**, 611.

Kivirikko, K. I., and Prockop, D. J. (1967c). *Proc. Nat. Acad. Sci. U. S.* **57**, 782.

Kivirikko, K. I., and Prockop, D. J. (1967d). *J. Biol. Chem.* **242**, 4007.

Kivirikko, K. I., and Prockop, D. J. (1972). *Biochim. Biophys. Acta* **258**, 366.

Kivirikko, K. I., Bright, H. J., and Prockop, D. J. (1968). *Biochim. Biophys. Acta* **151**, 558.

Kivirikko, K. I., Shudo, K., Sakakibara, S., and Prockop, D. J. (1972). *Biochemistry* **11**, 122.

Knox, W. E., and Goswami, M. N. D. (1961). *Ann. N. Y. Acad. Sci.* **92**, 192.

Krane, S. M., Muñoz, A. J., and Harris, E. D. (1970). *J. Clin. Invest.* **49**, 716.

Kutnink, M. A., Tolbert, B. M., Richmond, V. L., and Baker, E. M. (1969). *Proc. Soc. Exp. Biol. Med.* **132**, 440.

La Du, B. N., and Zannoni, V. G. (1956). *Nature (London)* **177**, 574.

La Du, B. N., and Zannoni, V. G. (1961). *Ann. N. Y. Acad. Sci.* **192**, 175.

Lane, J. M., and Miller, E. J. (1969). *Biochemistry* **8**, 2134.

Lane, J. M., Rosenbloom, J., and Prockop, D. J. (1971a). *Nature (London)* **232**, 191.

Lane, J. M., Dehm, P., and Prockop, D. J. (1971b). *Biochim. Biophys. Acta* **236**, 517.

Lane, J. M., Parkes, L. J., and Prockop, D. J. (1971c). *Biochim. Biophys. Acta* **236**, 528.

Lapiere, C. M., Lenaers, A., and Kohn, L. D. (1971). *Proc. Nat. Acad. Sci. U. S.* **68**, 3054.

Layman, D. L., McGoodwin, E., and Martin, G. R. (1970). *Fed. Proc., Fed. Amer. Soc. Exp. Biol.* **29**, 668 (Abstr.).

Layman, D. L., McGoodwin, E., and Martin, G. R. (1971). *Proc. Nat. Acad. Sci. U. S.* **68**, 454.

Lazarides, E., and Lukens, L. N. (1971a). *Science* **173**, 723.

Lazarides, E., and Lukens, L. N. (1971b). *Nature (London)* **232**, 37.

Lazarides, E., Lukens, L. N., and Infante, A. A. (1971). *J. Mol. Biol.* **58**, 831.

Lenaers, A., Ansay, M., Nusgens, B. V., and Lapiere, C. M. (1971). *Eur. J. Biochem.* **23**, 533.

Levene, C. I., and Bates, C. J. (1970). *J. Cell Sci.* **7**, 671.

Levene, C. I., and Gross, J. (1959). *J. Exp. Med.* **110**, 771.

Levene, C. I., Shoshan, S., and Bates, C. J. (1972a). *Biochim. Biophys. Acta* **257**, 384.

Levene, C. I., Bates, C. J., and Bailey, A. J. (1972b). *Biochim. Biophys. Acta* **263**, 574.

Levin, E. Y., and Kaufman, S. (1961). *J. Biol. Chem.* **236**, 2043.

Levin, E. Y., Levenberg, B., and Kaufman, S. (1960). *J. Biol. Chem.* **235**, 2080.

Lindblad, B., Lindstedt, S., and Omfelt, M. (1971). Unpublished data quoted by Holme *et al.* (1971).

Lindblad, B., Lindstedt, G., Tofft, M., and Lindstedt, S. (1969). *J. Amer. Chem. Soc.* **91**, 4604.

Lindblad, B., Lindstedt, G., and Lindstedt, S. (1970). *J. Amer. Chem. Soc.* **92**, 7446.

Lindstedt, G. (1967a). Ph.D. Dissertation, Karolinska Institute, Stockholm.

Lindstedt, G. (1967b). *Biochemistry* **6**, 1271.

Lindstedt, G., and Lindstedt, S. (1962). *Biochem. Biophys. Res. Commun.* **7**, 394.

Lindstedt, G., and Lindstedt, S. (1970). *J. Biol. Chem.* **245**, 4178.

Lindstedt, G., Lindstedt, S., Tofft, M., and Midtvedt, T. (1967a). *Biochem. J.* **103**, 19P.

Lindstedt, G., Lindstedt, S., Midtvedt, T., and Tofft, M. (1967b). *Biochemistry* **6**, 1262.

Lindstedt, G., Lindstedt, S., Olander, B., and Tofft, M. (1968). *Biochim. Biophys. Acta* **158**, 503.

Lukens, L. N. (1965). *J. Biol. Chem.* **240**, 1661.

Lukens, L. N. (1966). *Proc. Nat. Acad. Sci. U. S.* **55**, 1235.

Lukens, L. N. (1970). *J. Biol. Chem.* **245**, 453.

Manner, G., and Gould, B. S. (1963). *Biochim. Biophys. Acta* **72**, 243.

Manning, J. M., and Meister, A. (1966). *Biochemistry* **5**, 1154.

Margolis, R. L., and Lukens, L. N. (1971). *Arch. Biochem. Biophys.* **147**, 612.

Martin, G. R., Mergenhagen, S. E., and Prockop, D. J. (1961). *Nature (London)* **191**, 1007.

Mason, H. S. (1965). *Annu. Rev. Biochem.* **34**, 595.

May, C. D., Hamilton, A., and Stewart, C. T. (1952). *Blood* **7**, 978.

Mead, J. F., and Hare, R. S. (1971). *Biochem. Biophys. Res. Commun.* **45**, 1451.

Mechanic, G., and Tanzer, M. L. (1970). *Biochem. Biophys. Res. Commun.* **41**, 1597.

Mechanic, G., Gallop, P. M., and Tanzer, M. L. (1971). *Biochem. Biophys. Res. Commun.* **45**, 644.

Miller, E. J., Lane, J. M., and Piez, K. A. (1969). *Biochemistry* **8**, 30.

Miller, R. L. (1971). *Arch. Biochem. Biophys.* **147**, 339.

Mitoma, C., and Smith, T. E. (1960). *J. Biol. Chem.* **235**, 426.

Morgan, P. H., Jacobs, H. G., Segrest, J. P., and Cunningham, L. W. (1970). *J. Biol. Chem.* **245**, 5042.

Müller, P. K., McGoodwin, E., and Martin, G. R. (1971). *Biochem. Biophys. Res. Commun.* **44**, 110.

Mussini, E., Hutton, J. J., and Udenfriend, S. (1967). *Science* **157**, 927.

Nichol, C. A., and Welch, A. D. (1950). *Proc. Soc. Exp. Biol. Med.* **74**, 52.

Olsen, B. R., Jimenez, S. A., Kivirikko, K. I., and Prockop, D. J. (1970). *J. Biol. Chem.* **245**, 2649.

Pankalainen, M., Aro, H., Simms, K., and Kivirikko, K. I. (1970). *Biochim. Biophys. Acta* **221**, 559.

Peterkofsky, B., and Udenfriend, S. (1963). *J. Biol. Chem.* **238**, 3966.

Peterkofsky, B., and Udenfriend, S. (1965). *Proc. Nat. Acad. Sci. U. S.* **53**, 335.

Piez, K. A., and Likins, R. C. (1957). *J. Biol. Chem.* **229**, 101.

Popenoe, E. A., and Aronson, R. B. (1972). *Biochim. Biophys. Acta* **258**, 380.

Popenoe, E. A., Aronson, R. B., and Van Slyke, D. D. (1966). *Proc. Nat. Acad. Sci. U. S.* **55**, 393.

Popenoe, E. A., Aronson, R. B., and Van Slyke, D. D. (1969). *Arch. Biochem. Biophys.* **133**, 286.

Priest, R. E., and Bublitz, C. (1967). *Lab. Invest.* **17**, 371.

Prockop, D. J. (1970). *In* "Chemistry and Molecular Biology of the Intercellular Matrix" (E. A. Balazs, ed.), Vol. 1, p. 335. Academic Press, New York.

Prockop, D. J., and Juva, K. (1965a). *Biochem. Biophys. Res. Commun.* **18**, 54.

Prockop, D. J., and Juva, K. (1965b). *Proc. Nat. Acad. Sci. U. S.* **53**, 661.

Prockop, D. J., and Kivirikko, K. I. (1967). *Ann. Intern. Med.* **66**, 1243.

Prockop, D. J., and Kivirikko, K. I. (1968a). In "Treatise on Collagen" (B. S. Gould, ed.), Vol. 2, Part A, p. 215. Academic Press, New York.

Prockop, D. J., and Kivirikko, K. I. (1968b). Unpublished data quoted by Kivirikko *et al.* (1968).

Prockop, D. J., Kaplan, A., and Udenfriend, S. (1963). *Arch. Biochem. Biophys.* **101**, 499.

Prockop, D. J., Weinstein, E., and Mulveny, T. (1966). *Biochem. Biophys. Res. Commun.* **22**, 124.

Ramaley, P. B., and Rosenbloom, J. (1971). *FEBS Lett.* **15**, 59.

Reynolds, J. J. (1967). *Exp. Cell Res.* **47**, 42.

Rhoads, R. E., and Udenfriend, S. (1968). *Proc. Nat. Acad. Sci. U. S.* **60**, 1473.

Rhoads, R. E., and Udenfriend, S. (1969). *Arch. Biochem. Biophys.* **133**, 108.

Rhoads, R. E., and Udenfriend, S. (1970). *Arch. Biochem. Biophys.* **139**, 329.

Rhoads, R. E., Hutton, J. J., and Udenfriend, S. (1967). *Arch. Biochem. Biophys.* **122**, 805.

Richmond, V., and Stokstad, E. L. R. (1969). *J. Dent. Res.* **48**, 83.

Robertson, W. van B., and Hewitt, J. (1961). *Biochim. Biophys. Acta* **49**, 404.

Robertson, W. van B., Hewitt, J., and Herman, C. (1959). *J. Biol. Chem.* **234**, 105.

Robertson, W. van B., and Schwartz, B. (1953). *J. Biol. Chem.* **281**, 689.

Rosenbloom, J., and Christner, P. (1971). *Fed. Proc., Fed. Amer. Soc. Exp. Biol.* **30**, 1195 (Abstr.).

Rosenbloom, J., and Prockop, D. J. (1969). In "Repair and Regeneration. The Scientific Basis of Surgical Practice" (J. E. Dunphy and W. Van Winkle, Jr., eds.), p. 117. McGraw-Hill, New York.

Rosenbloom, J., and Prockop, D. J. (1971). *J. Biol. Chem.* **246**, 1549.

Ross, R., and Benditt, E. P. (1964). *J. Cell Biol.* **22**, 365.

Rucker, R. B., Parker, H. E., and Rogler, J. C. (1969). *J. Nutr.* **98**, 57.

Sandberg, L. B., Weissman, N., and Smith, D. W. (1969). *Biochemistry* **8**, 2940.

Schafer, I. A., Silverman, L., Sullivan, J. C., and Robertson, W. van B. (1967). *J. Cell Biol.* **34**, 83.

Schimizu, Y., McCann, D. S., and Keech, M. K. (1965). *J. Lab. Clin. Med.* **65**, 286.

Schubert, D., and Cohn, M. (1968). *J. Mol. Biol.* **38**, 273.

Shaffer, P. M., McCroskey, R. P., Palmatier, R. D., Midgett, R. J., and Abbott, M. T. (1968). *Biochem. Biophys. Res. Commun.* **33**, 806.

Shaffer, P. M., McCroskey, R. P., and Abbott, M. T. (1972). *Biochim. Biophys. Acta* **258**, 387.

Sinex, F. M., and Van Slyke, D. D. (1955). *J. Biol. Chem.* **216**, 245.

Sinex, F. M., Van Slyke, D. D., and Christman, D. R. (1959). *J. Biol. Chem.* **234**, 918.

Speakman, P. T. (1971). *Nature (London)* **229**, 291.

Spiro, R. G. (1969). *J. Biol. Chem.* **244**, 602.

Stetten, M. R. (1949). *J. Biol. Chem.* **181**, 31.

Stetten, M. R., and Schoenheimer, R. (1944). *J. Biol. Chem.* **153**, 113.

Stone, N., and Meister, A. (1962). *Nature (London)* **194**, 555.

Takeuchi, T., and Prockop, D. J. (1969). *Biochim. Biophys. Acta* **175**, 142.

Takeuchi, T., Rosenbloom, J., and Prockop, D. J. (1969). *Biochim. Biophys. Acta* **175**, 156.

Tanzer, M. L., Mechanic, G., and Gallop, P. M. (1970). *Biochim. Biophys. Acta* **207**, 548.
Udenfriend, S. (1966). *Science* **152**, 1335.
Udenfriend, S. (1970). *In* "Chemistry and Molecular Biology of the Intercellular Matrix" (E. A. Balazs, ed.), Vol. 1, p. 371. Academic Press, New York.
Udenfriend, S. (1972). Personal communication.
Urivetzky, M., Frei, J. M., and Meilman, E. (1965). *Arch. Biochem. Biophys.* **109**, 480.
Urivetzky, M., Frei, J. M., and Meilman, E. (1966). *Arch. Biochem. Biophys.* **117**, 224.
Van Slyke, D. D., and Sinex, F. M. (1958). *J. Biol. Chem.* **232**, 797.
Vilter, R. W. (1964). *Medicine (Baltimore)* **43**, 727.
Vilter, R. W., Will, J. J., Wright, T., and Rullman, D. (1963). *Amer. J. Clin. Nutr.* **12**, 130.
Watanabe, M. S., McCroskey, R. P., and Abbott, M. T. (1970). *J. Biol. Chem.* **245**, 2023.
Weinstein, E., Blumenkranz, N., and Prockop, D. J. (1969). *Biochim. Biophys. Acta* **191**, 747.
Weissman, N., Shields, G. S., and Carnes, W. H. (1963). *J. Biol. Chem.* **238**, 3115.
Welch, A. D., Nichol, C. A., Anker, R. M., and Boehne, J. W. (1951). *J. Pharmacol. Exp. Ther.* **103**, 403.
Windsor, A. C. W., and Williams, C. B. (1970). *Brit. Med. J.* **1**, 732.
Woolf, L. I., Jacubovic, A., and Chan-Henry, E. (1971). *Biochem. J.* **125**, 569.
Zannoni, V. G., and La Du, B. N. (1959). *J. Biol. Chem.* **234**, 2925.

ADDENDUM

Dr. Josef Hurych and his colleagues (1972) have recently presented spectrophotometric data in support of their contention that ferrous iron bound to protocollagen hydroxylase is oxidized to ferric iron after interaction with molecular oxygen [*Sigrid Jusélius Found. Symp. Biol. Fibroblast, Turku, 1972* Academic Press, New York (in press)]. It is postulated that an OOH moiety is formed and first interacts with α-ketoglutarate (see footnote on p. 14). Hydroxylation of peptidylproline then follows. In this scheme, ascorbic acid would be required to regenerate ferrous iron from ferric and should be utilized in a stoichiometric manner.

Effect of Vitamin E Deficiency on Cellular Membranes

I. MOLENAAR, J. VOS, AND F. A. HOMMES

Centre for Medical Electron Microscopy and Department of Pediatrics, University of Groningen, School of Medicine, Groningen, The Netherlands

I. Introduction

Despite a continuous stream of publications on vitamin E leading to about 8000 papers in the last 20 years (Herting, 1971), no clear insight into the biological function of this vitamin has been obtained. Symposium proceedings as published in Volume 20 of this series in 1962, and reviews by Horwitt *et al.* (1968), Fitch (1968), and Boguth (1969), may give the reader an idea of the vast sources of literature on this subject.

Although obviously no consensus could be attained, it is remarkable that the number of papers dealing with a relation between vitamin E and cellular membranes* gradually increases. In view of the basic importance of membranes in cell biology, it seems justifiable to screen the recent experimental data on vitamin E as far as they are relevant for membranes, which form the ultrastructural basis for many specific metabolic activities (cf. Lucy, 1964).

---

* The term "cellular membranes" comprises both intracellular membranes and (limiting) cell membranes. "Cellular" can be read as "biological," which in its turn means "nonartificial."

In this article two fields of research, namely, cellular membranes and vitamin E, will in the first instance be reviewed separately insofar as they are essential for the present subject. Some important contributions have not been reviewed because they are outside the scope of this article which aims to integrate both fields. A problem analysis will then be made, relevant to each of the two research topics. Finally, the experimental evidence will be assessed and discussed especially from the point of view of a cell biologist.

II. Cellular Membranes

A. Development of the Membrane Concept

As indicated above membranes in tissue cells are basic elements, on which attention is especially focused in modern cell biology. In the middle of the 19th century the classic cell theory was developed which established that the various organisms and tissues consisted of cells, each being a small clump of protoplasm containing a nucleus in its center. This cell theory, based on morphological studies with the light microscope, because of the relatively low resolving power of this instrument could not include a membrane concept. Such a concept emerged independently from two other fields of study—cell physiology and submicroscopic cytology in this order.

In the second half of the 19th century the idea of the existence of a diffusion barrier bordering cells, emerged from studies on their permeability (Pfeffer, 1875; Overton, 1895). Gorter and Grendel (1925) supposed the very nature of this barrier to be a limiting cell membrane, composed of two layers of lipid molecules. In 1935 Danielli and Davson summarized all experimental data and constructed the first hypothetical model for the architecture of the cell membrane. This model showed the membrane as a lipid bilayer with a hydrophobic center, strengthened by the apposition of electrostatically bound protein layers on both hydrophilic sides.

In fact, this nonmorphological postulate of a diffusion barrier was confirmed by the visualization of the cell membrane* with the electron microscope. However, more importantly the supreme resolving power of this instrument also disclosed the existence of a hitherto unexpected multitude of membranous elements in the cytoplasm surrounding the cell nucleus (Sjöstrand, 1953). Thus the cytoplasm turned out to be a space subdivided into compartments† by membrane systems, rather than one

---

* As a synonym for "cell membrane," many cell biologists use the term "plasma membrane." The latter will also be used in this paper.

† It should be mentioned that this definition of "compartment" is not necessarily identical with that used in some of the biochemical literature.

filled with a gel-like substance as had been supposed by generations of cytologists.*

B. BIOCHEMICAL CHARACTERISTICS

Cellular membranes divide tissues into cells and cells into compartments, each with its own micromilieu. Such a milieu is particularly determined and controlled by specific properties of the membrane concerned. Much biochemical information on the properties of these membranes has been obtained with the help of highly developed cell fractionation techniques (de Duve, 1971). The main characteristics of the lipid, protein, carbohydrate, and ribonucleic acid parts of isolated fractions of the plasma membrane and a series of intracellular membranes of *rat liver cells* will be partially summarized and compared here. It may be assumed that such a differentiation of membrane composition roughly exists in other organs of the rat and in tissues of other species as well. For detailed quantitative data the reader may refer to the literature cited.

1. *Lipids*

In all rat liver cellular membranes the lipid content is within the limits of 25–45% of the dry weight (Chapman and Leslie, 1970; Henning *et al.*, 1970; Skipski *et al.*, 1965; Spiro and McKibbin, 1956), the outer mitochondrial membrane having the highest percentage (Parsons *et al.*, 1967). The lipid composition of each class of cellular membranes of one and the same organ is markedly specific and constant under normal circumstances and any differences between analyses from the various laboratories for a given membrane can be ascribed largely to technical difficulties, rather than to real differences (Chapman and Leslie, 1970). Differences in composition between the various membranes are mainly found in the distribution of lipid classes (phospholipids, neutral lipids, and glycolipids) and their subclasses (sphingomyelin, cholesterol, etc.). The ratio of saturated to unsaturated fatty acids may differ with the type of membrane. Using the three above-mentioned criteria, important differences have been noted between intracellular membranes (inner- and outer mitochondrial membranes and endoplasmic reticular membranes) as a whole, on one hand, and the plasma membrane on the other hand.

First, the intracellular membrane total lipid has a very high phospholipid content (85–90%) and a minor neutral lipid content (5–15%) (Chapman and Leslie, 1970; Keenan and Morré, 1970). According to Skipski *et al.* (1965), the plasma membrane total lipid consists of phos-

* For a survey of the morphology and nomenclature of these membrane systems, e.g., endoplasmic reticulum, mitochondria, the reader may refer to the current textbooks.

pholipids (39%), neutral lipids (35%), and probably glycolipids (26%), whereas Keenan and Morré (1970) found only phospholipids (including glycolipids) (62%) and neutral lipids (38%).

Second, the intracellular membranes contain a high proportion of phospholipids such as phosphatidylcholine, phosphatidylethanolamine, and cardiolipin, the last one being present nearly exclusively in the inner mitochondrial membrane (Stoffel and Schiefer, 1968) with a high content of unsaturated fatty acid. The plasma membrane phospholipids contain a substantial amount of sphingomyelin in larger amounts than is found in any of the intracellular membranes (Skipski et al., 1965; Stoffel and Schiefer, 1968; Keenan and Morré, 1970). The molar ratio of cholesterol to phospholipids of plasma membranes amounts to 0.4 (Emmelot et al., 1964), whereas that of the intracellular membranes is much less at 0.07 for microsomes (Auliac, 1967) and outer mitochondrial membranes and 0.02 for inner mitochondrial membranes (Lévy and Sauner, 1968).

Third, the intracellular membranes tend to contain a considerable amount of polyunsaturated fatty acids (Fleischer and Rouser, 1965), whereas saturated and monounsaturated fatty acids (Skipski et al., 1965) predominate in lipids of plasma membranes. It is to be noted that microsomal lipids are the most unsaturated, followed by those of the inner mitochondrial membranes, whereas the outer mitochondrial membranes have the lowest degree of unsaturation (Huet et al., 1968). It can be concluded from these data that the plasma membrane takes up a special position as compared with microsomal and mitochondrial membranes. Its high content of cholesterol and of saturated and monounsaturated fatty acids all of which pack tightly in the lipid phase, make this type of membrane a more rigid structure than that of intracellular membranes, as has been stated by Benedetti and Emmelot (1968) and Colbeau et al. (1971).

As to other cellular membranes, it can be noted that lysosomal membrane lipids have many characteristics of the plasma membrane (Henning et al., 1970). Keenan and Morré (1970) also found that the lipids of the membranes of the Golgi- apparatus show a striking resemblance to those of the plasma membranes; nevertheless these authors suggest that the Golgi membrane could be partly derived from the endoplasmic reticulum.

2. Proteins

The protein content of nearly all membranes ranges from 55 to 75% of the dry weight and represents the total remaining weight after deduction of the lipid content mentioned in Section II, B, 1. The lowest value of about 55% is found in the outer mitochondrial membrane (Parsons et al., 1967). Some qualitative differences in the protein part of

cellular membranes apparently arise from the varied enzyme characteristics, and other differences may arise from structural protein components.
It is generally accepted that nearly every type of membrane has a rather
specific set of enzymes corresponding with its metabolic capacities. The
plasma membrane, for instance, is marked by the presence of Na-K-
ATPase and the endoplasmic reticulum membranes by $NADPH_2$-oxidase,
cytochromes P-450 and b_5, and glucose-6-phosphatase. Again the inner
mitochondrial membrane is marked by the enzymes of the respiratory
chain whereas the outer is characterized by monoaminooxidase (MAO).

3. Other Constituents

Carbohydrates such as hexoses, hexosamines, sialic acid, and N-
acetylneuraminic acid occur in bound form in the plasma membrane and
the lysosomal membrane as well (Benedetti and Emmelot, 1968; Henning et al., 1970), but there is no evidence yet in the literature that these
components occur in other cell membranes as well. Ribonucleic acid is
reported to be present in membranes of the endoplasmic reticulum in
small quantities, and a very low amount seems to be present in the
plasma membrane (Emmelot and Benedetti, 1967).

4. Summary

The main constituents of cellular membranes are lipids and proteins.
On the basis of lipid characteristics two main groups of cell membranes
can be distinguished: (a) plasma membranes, lysosomal membranes, and
membranes of the Golgi apparatus containing a large proportion of
sphingomyelin, cholesterol, and saturated and monounsaturated fatty
acids; (b) mitochondrial membranes and membranes of the endoplasmic
reticulum containing less sphingomyelin but having a very high content
of polyunsaturated fatty acids. Each type of membrane is also characterized by having a specific set of enzymes. Carbohydrates and ribonucleic
acids are minor constituents of plasma membranes and lysosomal
membranes.

C. ULTRASTRUCTURAL ASPECTS

1. Visualization of Membranes at the Molecular Level

Considering the biochemical constituents as surveyed in Section II, B,
the question arises: How are these molecules assembled in the membrane?
The problem of how to make the step from chemical composition to
chemical anatomy has puzzled many investigators for several decades.
The resolving power of the modern electron microscope is sufficiently
high that its use alone might answer this question if membranes could
be examined in their natural state. However, the visualization of the

membrane at the molecular level in this form is not possible since the current technique of electron microscopy requires the membrane to be subjected to various treatments before examination (see Section II, C, 2). Even the mildest of these procedures introduces factors that alter to some extent the interrelationship of the molecules within the membrane so that the electron micrograph obtained may not be a strictly true representation of the membrane before treatment. The procedures used generally involve chemical fixation and dehydration with organic solvents. Furthermore, metal staining or contrasting techniques do not show sufficient detail at the small molecule level because of the large size and arbitrary placement of metal deposits around the molecules to be visualized. These severe limitations prevent full use from being taken of the maximum resolving power of the microscope (Parsons, 1971).

Notwithstanding the apparent lack of direct information several membrane models have been proposed. The two main ones as applicable to all membranes are (i) the Danielli or laminar bilayer model in which the lipids are sandwiched between outer protein layers held to the lipid by electrostatic bonding and (ii) the so-called subunit model in which pockets of lipid micelles are interspersed in a matrix of proteins. Both are discussed in detail in a review by Stoeckenius and Engelman (1969). These models are based partly on experiments with artificial membranes, partly on biochemical analyses of isolated membrane systems and partly on conclusions drawn from electron micrographs of biological tissues or isolated tissue-fractions stained with heavy atoms. How far these models are relevant to natural cell membranes remains, however, to be determined. Consequently, owing to the impossibility of visualizing the membrane molecules *in situ* as mentioned above, the relative merits of these two models will not be discussed further in this article. It is more relevant to look into the staining mechanisms for membrane lipids and proteins. For these two major groups of substances constitute the major portion of the membrane (Sections II, B, 1 and 2) and provide the basis for the image obtained in the electron microscope. Until new electron microscopical techniques for observation of the membrane have been developed (Parsons, 1971), it is the principal way of getting morphological information in this field.

2. *Visualization of Membranes as Subcellular Constituents*

Membranes can be visualized in the electron microscope in two ways by means of the following routine methods. First, the tissue can be fixed by an aldehyde (mostly glutaraldehyde), postfixed with osmium tetroxide, dehydrated by alcohol or acetone, and embedded in plastic. Subsequently ultrathin sections are prepared, which are stained with solution containing lead or uranyl ions. The membranes are thus positively stained. Second, the tissue can be homogenized in media of appropriate osmotic strength, fractionated by differential or gradient centrifugation with various organelles, and the various membrane fractions can be negatively stained. In doing so, heavy atoms are grouped around membrane details, thus producing a negative image of the detail to be visualized.

a. *Membranes in Positive Contrast.* When membrane structures in electron micrographs of ultrathin sections have been visualized, they actually appear as electron dense regions, mainly because of their selective binding of the heavy atoms, osmium being the most widely used. Riemersma and Booy (1962) found in model experiments that the number of moles of osmium tetroxide bound per mole of lecithin is related stoichiometrically to the number of double bonds present. From these model experiments, however, only tentative conclusions can be drawn concerning the interaction between osmium tetroxide and lipids in tissue cells, especially those which have gone through the process of fixation. However, there is evidence that membranes which are rich in unsaturated fatty acids derive their contrast in "unstained" ultrathin sections of osmium tetroxide-fixed tissue largely from the double bonds (Riemersma, 1970). The subsequent staining with lead ions of ultrathin sections of osmium tetroxide-prefixed material as is generally done, must be considered as an "intensifying staining," i.e., the lead is attached to sites where osmium is already present (Daems and Persijn, 1962). Although the various classes of cellular membranes have different lipid compositions and also different degrees of unsaturation (see Section II, B, 1) their electron density on electron micrographs of ultrathin sections look approximately the same after fixation with osmium tetroxide. To what extent proteins, which are also thought to react with osmium tetroxide (Bahr, 1954), contribute to the electron densities, is still under discussion but it is considered to be moderate by most authors (Fleischer *et al.*, 1967; Hake, 1965; Riemersma, 1970). Carbohydrates and nucleic acids do not react with osmium tetroxide at all (Bahr, 1954).

Heavy metal staining of membranes as discussed above forms one of the main tools with which the electron microscopist can make his observations on the details of membranes. Robertson (1955, 1959) fixed tissue with potassium permanganate at high resolution and visualized a triple-layered structure, which could be observed in the plasma membrane and also in the intracytoplasmic membranes. This structure, showing two outer dark bands and one inner light band was called the unit membrane, because of its universal occurence. Its nature was explained by the lipid bilayer hypothesis. It was suggested that each type of cellular membrane is composed of a central bilayer about 35 Å thick in which phospholipid molecules are bound together by nonpolar bonds, while both protein layers are represented by the dense bands, each 20 Å thick.

Differences in membrane detail can form a morphological basis for membrane classification: high resolution measurements of the thickness of various intracellular membrane systems by Yamamoto (1963) and Sjöstrand (1963b) revealed different classes of unit membranes. According to Yamamoto, two distinct classes of unit membranes were observed after potassium permanganate fixation: (i) a thinner group including mitochondrial, nuclear membranes, Golgi lamellae and granulated endoplasmic reticular membranes and (ii) a thicker group including those of synaptic vesicles, vesicles and capsules of multivesicular bodies, and Golgi vesicles, and plasma membranes. Furthermore it was stated that the unit membrane structure of group (i) membranes was not so easily demonstrable as that of group (ii) membranes, especially after osmium tetroxide-fixation but also after potassium permanganate-fixation.

On the other hand, if very careful preparation methods are used, no unit membrane is seen at all. In tissue fixed with glutaraldehyde alone for a very short period and rapidly extracted with ethylene glycol, a procedure which highly preserves the conformation of protein molecules, the cytoplasmic and mitochondrial membranes, but not the plasma membrane appeared to consist of globular structures of about 40 Å (Sjöstrand, 1963a,b, 1971). These globular structures were assumed to be protein molecules or lipoprotein complexes. The absence of such globules in the unit membrane image was explained on the basis of artificial protein denaturation caused by conventional tissue fixation methods. The abovementioned biochemical and electron microscopy findings which conflict with the unit membrane theory led to a new concept as to the structural role of proteins in intracellular membranes. Protein rather than phospholipid would form the core of a membrane; this was also suggested by D. E. Green et al. (1961). Evidence that proteins alone can maintain membrane structure was presented by Fleischer et al. (1967) and Cunningham et al. (1967), who showed that the inner membrane of mitochondria was preserved even after 90% of the lipid was extracted (see also Section II, B, 2). Phospholipids, however, being secondary structural elements and locally arranged in the membrane according to the lipid bilayer model, could stick between the globular structures of either protein or lipoprotein complexes (Sjöstrand, 1968).

   b. *Membranes in Negative Contrast.* With the negative staining technique, several isolated membrane systems have been studied. It is well known that the inner membrane of the mitochondrion shows protrusions

80–100 Å in length, called "elementary particles" by Fernández-Morán (1962); the outer membrane does not have such subunits but shows an irregular pattern of alternate electron dense and electron lucent areas. Benedetti and Emmelot (1968) have demonstrated in rat liver plasma membranes a temperature-dependent hexagonal subunit pattern not shown by mitochondrial membranes or membranes of the endoplasmic reticulum. They also showed the presence of globular knobs 50–60 Å in diameter on certain areas of the membrane surface, distinct from the mitochondrial "elementary particles."

It has to be stressed that little is known on the mechanism of the negative staining process. Johnson and Horne (1970) come to the conclusion on the basis of drying experiments that some negative stains (e.g., phosphotungstic acid) set in a rigid "glass" and thus preserve the biological structures before the latter are completely dehydrated either in air or in the vacuum of the electron microscope. However, they produce no evidence for the rigidity of the dried heavy metal stain. Therefore it is to be doubted that the "morphology" of the dried stain, especially where it has penetrated into the interior of the biological structure, gives a true image of the structure to be depicted. Moreover, the preparation is subjected to the electron beam which interacts with material and stain, thus causing morphological changes.

3. Visualization of Membrane-Localized Enzyme Activity

One functional aspect of cellular membranes, i.e., the activities of some of their special enzymes, can be visualized by a combination of electron microscopy and of biochemical techniques, known as electron enzyme cytochemistry. Enzyme activity can be observed qualitatively within the cell or its organelles. The site of action of a phosphatase can be visualized after incubating the membrane preparation in a medium, containing lead ions, which precipitate when phosphate ions are liberated from a suitable substrate by the enzyme activity. In this way the latter has been shown to occur at sites adjacent to a series of cellular membrane systems. This, however, does not necessarily imply that the enzyme forms an integral part of the particular membrane. Only a combination of electron enzyme cytochemical methods and biochemical examination of isolated membrane fractions can provide evidence as to a localization of the enzyme in the membrane.

The distribution of some enzymes linked to membranes have been referred to in Section II, B, 2. Marchesi and Palade (1967) showed a Na-K-ATPase activity on the inner side of the plasma membrane of the erythrocyte ghost. Duodenal mucosal cells have an alkaline phosphatase activity localized adjacent to their plasma membrane as reported by Hugon and Borgers (1966). The endoplasmic reticulum and the nuclear envelope of rat liver parenchymal (Ericsson, 1966) and of intestinal epithelial cells (Hugon *et al.*, 1971) have been shown to possess glucose-6-phosphatase. The Golgi cisternae show nucleoside diphosphatase- and thiaminepyrophosphatase activity as found by Gold-fischer *et al.* (1971). Succinic dehydrogenase and cytochrome *c* oxidase activities are found adjacent to the inner mitochondrial membranes of heart, liver, and kidney, using the diaminobenzidine detection method (Seligman *et al.*, 1968).

4. *Summary*

Strong experimental evidence can be put forward that cellular membranes, which are rich in unsaturated fatty acids, derive the electron density seen in ultrathin sections of osmium tetroxide fixed tissue largely from the double bonds in the fatty acyl chains. Proteins do not contribute greatly to the formation of osmium deposits.

Evidence exists for a diversity in ultrastructure of cellular membrane systems, as was also presented in Section II, B with regard to their biochemical diversity. A functional diversity of cellular membranes can also be demonstrated by visualization of fixed products of membrane-bound enzyme activity with the method of electron enzyme cytochemistry.

III. CURRENT HYPOTHESES ON THE FUNCTION OF VITAMIN E RELEVANT TO CELLULAR MEMBRANES

As stated before, many aspects of the role of vitamin E in metabolism are still uncertain. Four major concepts will be successively reviewed.

A. VITAMIN E AS THE NONENZYMATIC BIOLOGICAL ANTIOXIDANT

This antioxidant theory of vitamin E action has found strong advocates in Tappel (1962, 1965) and Horwitt (1965). It states that vitamin E inhibits the peroxidation of unsaturated fatty acid moieties of lipid *in vivo* by molecular oxygen. The reaction is nonenzymatic and is analogous with some reactions in olefinic chemistry. The oxidative attack is random on free and membrane-bound unsaturated fatty acids and is inhibited by biological antioxidants. Vitamin E is supposed to be nature's lipid antioxidant of choice.

One argument put forward in support of this theory is that a relationship exists between the amount of unsaturated fatty acids given with the diet and the minimum amount of vitamin E required to prevent deficiency symptoms. The higher the degree of unsaturation of the dietary fat, the more vitamin E is needed (Alfin-Slater, 1965; Jager, 1968, 1969;

Jager and Houtsmuller, 1970). Recently, however, Jager (1972) analyzed linoleic acid intake versus vitamin E requirement in rats and in ducklings. It was found that an intake of lineolic acid of up to 7% of total calories did not increase their vitamin E requirement but that an intake of over 20% did increase it. This was thought to be due to increased destruction of the vitamin in the intestinal tract (Jager, 1969; Vogtmann and Prabucki, 1971).

Several authors tried to produce experimental evidence for the peroxidation of lipids *in vivo* by studying the suggested relation between vitamin E and lipids in tissues. Carpenter (1966) examined the effect of vitamin E deficiency on the lipids of rat testes. In the vitamin E-deficient rat testis compared with controls, no changes were found in total lipids, lipid phosphorus, cholesterol, cholesteryl esters, amino nitrogen, and total double bonds until the organs were very degenerate. At that stage the total lipid content decreased, the percentage composition, however, remained the same. As to the fatty acids, a relative decrease in the level of the docosenoic acid (C 22:5ω6)* was found rather than an increase with age as occurs normally. Since the content of C 20:4ω6 remained the same, a defect in its conversion to C 22:5ω6 was suggested in vitamin E deficiency. A decided decrease in the level of the latter, however, was observed in vitamin E-deficient rat testis by Lee and Barnes (1969), and more recently Carney and Walker (1971), using ^{14}C-labeled precursors, found that the formation of C 22:5ω6 from linoleate was blocked at the step between C 20:4ω6 and C 22:5ω6.

The liver of the rat seems to react similarly to vitamin E deficiency as demonstrated by Witting and Horwitt (1966). They found an increased incorporation of labeled acetate into the polyunsaturated fatty acids (PUFA). The total amount of PUFA, however, decreased in liver phospholipids of the vitamin E-deficient rat as the level of arachidonate increased. These results were interpreted as a homeostatic response to the increased peroxidative loss of higher PUFA including C 22:5ω6 in vitamin E deficiency, but the above-mentioned studies of Carpenter (1966) and Carney and Walker (1971) indicate that another interpretation, e.g., the inhibition of the enzyme system leading to formation of C 22:5ω6 from C 20:4ω6 is possible as well. It must be pointed out, however, that these results were obtained on different kinds of tissue. Gillian and McCay (1966) have carried out similar experiments with vitamin E-deficient chicks. A greater incorporation of acetate into arachidonate relative to palmitate and/or stearate was also found; the

* This nomenclature indicates successively: length of the carbon chain, number of double bonds, and site of the first double bond as counted from the terminal methyl group.

authors, however, did not report on specific activities of the individual polyunsaturated fatty acids.

In a more detailed study, Witting et al. (1967) produced evidence for an increased incorporation of acetate into both the tetraenoic and pentaplus hexaenoic acid fractions from rat liver lipids in contrast to the above-discussed results of Carney and Walker (1971) with rat testis. Moreover, it can be concluded from experiments by Harman et al. (1966) that the increase in arachidonic acid in vitamin E deficiency is only temporary and is followed by a phase of decreasing arachidonic acid content of liver lipids. No data on changes in total liver lipid have been reported. This conclusion can be drawn from their experiments in which rats were prefed diets high in PUFA with an adequate supply of vitamin E, and then linoleate and the latter were removed from the diet. About 100 days later, changes in vitamin E and in amounts of the tetra- and pentaenoic acids became apparent. The vitamin E content of fat dropped to about 25% of its initial value, as did linoleic acid as a percentage of total fatty acids. The arachidonate percentage, however, after an initial drop returned to the original level and then decreased again to about 50% of the initial value. When the rats were maintained on the deficient diet for a further period, the vitamin E level in the tissue gradually dropped to about 10% of the initial value. These experiments, however, are not completely conclusive because in addition to vitamin E deficiency, some essential fatty acid deficiency may also have been introduced. Lee and Barnes (1969) demonstrated a decrease in C 20:4ω6 of liver phospholipids in rats on a vitamin E-deficient, essential fatty acid-sufficient diet for 14 months.

Strong experimental evidence against the antioxidant theory has been produced by several authors, even resulting in a new hypothesis for the mode of action of vitamin E to which will be referred in Section III, D. J. Green et al. (1967) observed, using ^{14}C-labeled α-tocopherol, that whenever lipid autoxidation occurred in vitro there was always a concomitant destruction of tocopherol, whether a second antioxidant was present in the medium or not. This is presumably the same phenomenon as reported by McCay et al. (1969), who showed that this oxidation of lipids is of microsomal origin (see Section III, B). It should be mentioned, however, that the concomitant destruction of α-tocopherol was also observed by J. Green et al. (1967) in peroxidizing methyllinoleate. These in vitro findings contrasted strongly with the results obtained from in vivo studies because no difference in the rates of vitamin E depletion of tissues could be observed when rats were fed a vitamin E deficient diet supplemented with either the polyunsaturated linseed oil fatty acids or oleic acid.

As to the supposed formation of lipid peroxides in vivo, Bunyan et al.

(1967) demonstrated that no increase occurred in lipid peroxide content of liver, kidney, testis, or adipose tissue of rats during the onset of vitamin E deficiency. The values were also unaltered by a substantial change in the degree of unsaturation of the dietary fatty acids or by addition of vitamin E to the diet. Furthermore, addition of either N,N'-diphenyl-p-phenylenediamine or 6-ethoxy-1,2-dihydro-2,2,4-trimethyl-quinoline as an antioxidant to the diet did not alter the observed peroxide values. In other experiments, Glavind (1972) did not find an increased amount of lipid peroxides in parenchymal tissues of vitamin E-deficient rats. An exception was the adipose tissue, for which J. Green (1972) also found proof in later experiments.

Similarly the effects of vitamin E deficiency in the chick have been reported by Diplock et al. (1967). In the cerebellum and brain of chicks with incipient encephalomalacia the same tocopherol concentrations were found as in those of normal chicks. Also in this tissue Bunyan et al. (1967) could not show any difference in lipid peroxide content. According to these authors vitamin E could, however, delay the onset of encephalomalacia when the cerebellar concentration was about 0.2 μg per gram of lipid, a concentration well below the level for effective antioxidant action.

Another variable in vitamin E-lipid peroxidation relationship may be the oxygen pressure as originally described by Puig Moset and Val-dezasas (1946). Cawthorne et al. (1967), however, could not demonstrate an increased formation of lipid peroxides in rat brain after hyperbaric O_2 treatment. Likewise the metabolic destruction of ^{14}C-labeled α-tocopherol was not changed by this treatment.

In summary, the results of the studies mentioned in this section do not easily fit in with the proposed antioxidant mode of action of vitamin E in biological tissues for two main reasons. First, it is clear that despite many attempts no consensus of opinion could be attained as to the influence of vitamin E deficiency on the tissue concentrations of PUFA, in particular arachidonic acid. Second, dietary stress with PUFA supplements does not cause a decrease in vitamin E tissue levels and an increase in lipid peroxides as might be expected. Only refinement in experimental approach and theory could throw new light on the original concept that tocopherols protected lipids from peroxidation, as can be seen in the next Section.

B. VITAMIN E AS A FACTOR IN ENZYME-DEPENDENT
   LIPID PEROXIDATION

It has been shown that a membrane-bound enzyme system (NADPH$_2$-oxidase) in microsomes which involves transport of electrons from this substrate to oxygen, promotes simultaneously the peroxidation of the

β-position of arachidonic acid (May and McCay, 1968a) *in vitro*. The C 22:6ω3 and C 18:2ω6 acids were also oxidized, the former even to a higher percentage than C 20:4ω6 (May and McCay, 1968b). The saponi-fication values of the microsomal lipids did not decrease during this oxidation, indicating that the polyunsaturated fatty acid moiety was oxidized *in situ*. The structure of the microsomal membranes underwent physical change during this oxidation of PUFA, as a significant decrease in light scattering concomitant with a decrease in C 20:4ω6, was observed (McCay *et al.*, 1971). During this reaction, 90% of the microsomal α-tocopherol was converted to tocopherylquinone and other oxidation products (McCay *et al.*, 1969) without vitamin E activity (Boguth, 1969).

In normal liver, the cytoplasmic NADP:NADPH$_2$ ratio is about 0.01 (Krebs and Veech, 1970); this could be sufficient to maintain this type of oxidation *in vivo*. Inorganic ferric or ferrous ions are an obligatory requirement for the reaction (McCay *et al.*, 1971), and the K_m for iron has been determined at $1.6 \times 10^{-6} M$ (Poyer and McCay, 1971). The concentration of inorganic iron in tissues generally is unknown, but the total concentration of iron in liver for instance is about 40 μM of which roughly half can be found in the cytoplasm (Long, 1968). There would appear to be sufficient iron for the above reaction to take place although it is not known in which form inorganic iron occurs in the liver, except for ferritin where it is bound.

This type of lipid peroxidation does not occur through a lack of vitamin E but takes place in the presence of the vitamin. Again, it is not prevented by the addition of α-tocopherol to the assay system *in vitro*. This distinguishes it from the previously observed nonenzymatic lipid peroxidation which can occur in tissues *in vitro* and is prevented by adding vitamin E. It is the more remarkable, however, that vitamin E given with the diet for 2 days prior to assay induces a lag phase before peroxidation starts (McCay *et al.*, 1971). The length of this lag phase depends on the amount of vitamin E given with the diet, and this phenomenon has been explained as follows. As vitamin E is converted to tocopherylquinone and other oxidation products, the vitamin E content of the membrane rapidly falls. When a certain level is reached, PUFA peroxidation then proceeds uninhibited (McCay *et al.*, 1971). If this explanation is correct, vitamin E given with the diet is available to the microsomal membrane in a different phase and apparently more liable to oxidation than vitamin E added *in vitro*. This means that vitamin E reaches the functional site on the microsomal membrane only if the vitamin is provided with the diet. The transfer of the vitamin to its functional site in the membrane, when added *in vitro* is probably a relatively slow process. However, data on the fate of vitamin E during the lag phase are not available. Such studies would resolve the apparent contradiction with the observed concomitant oxidation of vitamin E and PUFA.

Summarizing, a new antioxidant concept has been suggested for vitamin E. It relates to a specific microsomal oxidase system capable of initiating peroxidation of membrane-bound polyunsaturated fatty acids *in vitro* where the vitamin E is thought to exert its effect within the membrane rather than nonspecifically. Whether such a reaction also occurs *in vivo* is probably dependent on the concentration of free iron in the tissues.

C. Vitamin E as a Factor in Biological Oxidations or Oxidative Phosphorylation

The role of vitamin E in mitochondrial oxidations is still unclear. To unravel this, one could use three criteria (Slater, 1958) which have to be fulfilled before a compound can be accepted as a member of the respiratory chain. First, it must be present in the enzyme preparation in amounts commensurate with the proposed enzyme activity. The recent analyses by Oliveira et al. (1969) have shown that, at least in heart mitochondria, the amount of α-tocopherol is of the same order as that of the cytochromes. These analyses have furthermore shown that the vitamin E is predominantly localized in the inner mitochondrial membrane, the membrane where the other members of the respiratory chain are also localized. The first criterion seems therefore to be fulfilled. Second, its removal from the enzyme preparation must result in an inactivation, while the activity can be restored by addition of the compound. Such an experiment has never been reported for vitamin E. This does not mean, however, that vitamin E deficiency cannot cause changes in the rate of oxidation of some mitochondrial substrates, which will be discussed below. No experimental evidence is therefore available for the second criterion. Third, it must undergo redox cycles during the enzymatic reaction at a rate in agreement with the overall enzymatic activity. Again no experimental evidence is available for this criterion.

Whether α-tocopherol is a member of the respiratory chain is therefore questionable. It does, however, have a profound effect on some membrane-bound oxidative functions. Corwin (1965) studied the regulation of succinate oxidation by vitamin E and concluded that vitamin E may have a function in site I phosphorylation. In vitamin E-deficient mitochondria an accumulation of oxaloacetate was observed during succinate oxidation, which could be prevented by addition of vitamin E to the mitochondria. This was interpreted as being due to reduction of oxaloacetate by $NADH_2$, generated energy-linked during succinate oxidation. Interference with oxidative phosphorylation has also been suggested by Naito et al. (1966). It was found that methyllinoleate hydroperoxide decreased the P:O ratio in succinate and β-hydroxybutyrate oxidation, which could be restored by the addition of α-tocopherol. It was furthermore demonstrated that methyllinoleate hydroperoxide inhibited soluble mitochondrial ATPase. This is a necessary condition for an antioxidant mode of action of vitamin E in these mitochondrial processes, but it is not sufficient. It has not been demonstrated that the observed decrease in P:O ratio in succinate and β-hydroxybutyrate oxidation is indeed due to an increased concentration of methyllinoleate hydroperoxide in the vitamin E-deficient mitochondria. Moreover, a decrease in the P:O ratio points to uncoupling of oxidative phosphorylation which may not necessarily be due to inhibition of the mitochondrial ATPase.

Carabello et al. (1971) have shown that the P:O ratio of citrate oxidation by liver mitochondria of vitamin E-deficient guinea pigs was 22% lower than in controls. This phenomenon could be completely abolished by injection of vitamin E into the vena portae of the deficient animal prior to sacrifice. N,N'-diphenyl-p-phenylenediamine could not replace vitamin E, nor did methyllinoleate hydroperoxide lower the P:O ratio of the control [in contrast to the results reported by Naito et al. (1966)]. The effect seems therefore not to be related to the nonenzymatic antioxidant capacity of vitamin E. Carabello et al. (1971) ascribed the effect to a metabolic product of vitamin E. The effect of vitamin E deficiency seemed to be limited to the first segment of the respiratory chain, as it was found that the P:O ratio observed in ascorbate plus tetramethyl paraphenylenediamine oxidation was not affected, while the P:O ratio of β-hydroxybutyrate oxidation was lowered like that observed in citrate oxidation. These results are consistent with those of Corwin (1965).

The microsomal oxidative system is equally sensitive to vitamin E deficiency. Gram and Fouts (1966) observed an inactivation of drug metabolizing enzymes in liver microsomes of vitamin E-deficient rats in vitro, which could not be restored by addition of vitamin E, although in vitro lipid peroxidation was inhibited by the addition of vitamin E. This has been confirmed by Carpenter (1967), who furthermore observed that the specific activity of the oxidative demethylation of codein and aminopyrine, which in deficient rats was only one-third the level in controls, could be restored within 48 hours after administration of vitamin E to deficient rats. The increase was prevented by simultaneous administration of actinomycin D. It was concluded that vitamin E may have a regulatory function at the level of synthesis or structural organization of the endoplasmic reticulum. McCay (1966) reached a similar conclusion on the role of vitamin E in microsomal membranes in his studies on the inhibition of gulunolactone oxidation by a microsomal phospholipid fraction. This inhibition is totally reversed by α-tocopherol added in vitro, although not specifically, because Mn^{2+}, Co^{2+}, and EDTA showed the same effect. It is suggestive, however, for a role of vitamin E in the stabilization of enzyme–phospholipid interactions in membranes of the endoplasmic reticulum, which may also be taken over by Mn^{2+}, Co^{2+}, or EDTA.

In conclusion, it seems unlikely that vitamin E is a member of the respiratory chain. However, there is evidence for a profound effect on some membrane-bound oxidative functions in mitochondria and endoplasmic reticulum. A direct or indirect influence of vitamin E deficiency on the oxidative phosphorylation at site I, however, is not unlikely.

D. VITAMIN E AS A MEMBRANE STABILIZER WITH REDOX CAPACITIES

The hypothesis developed by Diplock, Baum, and Lucy states that vitamin E may function on the one hand as a membrane stabilizer, on the other hand as a membrane-bound redox substance. Diplock (1972) and Lucy (1972) have jointly suggested from model building experiments that the hydrophobic side chain of the α-tocopherol molecule is aligned alongside the arachidonic acid and fits remarkably with its hydrocarbon chain (see Fig. 1). The methyl group at C-4 of the phytol side chain fits into a pocket provided by the cis double bond nearest to the carboxyl group of arachidonic acid. Similarly, the methylgroup at C-8 of α-tocopherol can interact with the third cis double bond of arachidonic acid. The chromanol ring of α-tocopherol and the polar groups of arachidonic acid-containing phospholipids are then all the same end of the complex, where they can interact at the polar surface of the lipid bilayer-structured regions of the membrane regions. It is postulated that the association of the phytol side chain of α-tocopherol with arachidonic acid contributes significantly to the stability of the membrane.

The redox function localized in the hydrophilic chromanol ring structure, is thought to be directed toward oxidative sensitive centers of membrane-associated proteins, containing either sulfur or selenium, or both (Diplock et al., 1971a). The nonheme iron proteins are likely candidates as substrates for the proposed redox function of α-tocopherol, because these proteins contain sulfide at the active center; selenide-containing nonheme iron proteins are not known, however, although an exchange between sulfide and selenide can be achieved in a nonheme iron protein in vitro (Tsibris et al., 1968).

Before this challenging hypothesis can be accepted, several criteria

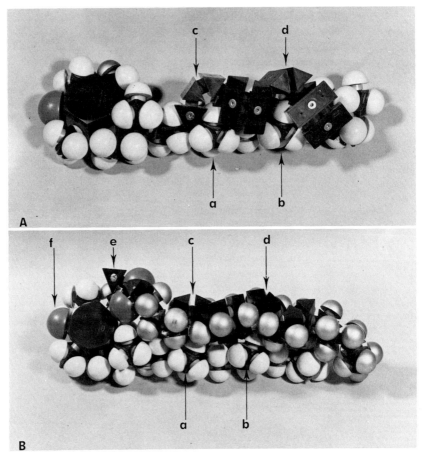

Fig. 1. Space-filling molecular models illustrating the way in which it is proposed that a phospholipid molecule containing an arachidonyl residue may interact with α-tocopherol in a biological membrane. (A) Model of part of the carbon skeleton of arachidonic acid (from C-4 to C-16) aligned with a model of α-tocopherol to allow the methyl groups at C-4, and C-8, of the vitamin (arrowed: a and b) to fit into pockets created, respectively, by the Δ^5 and Δ^{11} cis double bonds of the fatty acid (arrowed: c and d). The quasi-helical conformation of the unsaturated archidonyl chain that is required for the formation of the "complex" between the two molecules is clearly apparent. (B) A similar model (reproduced at a slightly lower magnification) in which the complete unsaturated chain of an arachidonyl phospholipid, with its hydrogen atoms, is shown interacting with α-tocopherol. The methyl groups of α-tocopherol, and the arachidonyl double bonds, are labeled as before. The carbon skeleton of the glycerol moiety of the phospholipid (arrowed: e), and the hydroxyl group of α-tocopherol (arrowed: f) lie at the same end of the complex. (By courtesy of Professor J. A. Lucy and Dr. A. T. Diplock.)

must be fulfilled. First, vitamin E deficiency should result in a higher oxidation state of membrane-bound sulfur and selenium. This has indeed been observed for selenide in rat liver (Diplock et al., 1971a). Addition of vitamin E to the diet reversed this effect. Similar studies for sulfur have not been reported in the literature. In another study, the effect of vitamin E on the intracellular distribution of selenium in rat livers was reported (Caygill et al., 1971). It was found that in livers of rats fed a diet sufficient in vitamin E and selenium, selenide was particularly associated with mitochondria whereas little selenide was found in liver mitochondria of vitamin E-deficient, selenium-sufficient rats. In addition to its location in mitochondria, selenide was also found in the smooth endoplasmic reticulum of livers of rats fed a diet sufficient in vitamin E and selenium. Vitamin E deficiency resulted in a decreased incorporation of labeled selenium as selenide in this fraction of liver. Addition of vitamin E to the diet restored to normal the incorporation of selenium as selenide in both fractions.

Second, vitamin E deficiency should result in a lower specific activity of nonheme iron protein-dependent reactions as far as these catalysts are rate-limiting or become so upon vitamin E deficiency. Nonheme iron proteins have been implicated in phosphorylation at site I of the mitochondrial respiratory chain (Ragan et al., 1970). They may function at site II as well (cf. Van Dam and Meyer, 1971). Definite proof for such a participation of nonheme iron proteins in oxidative phosphorylation is, however, lacking. Carabello et al. (1971) have indeed shown, as cited earlier in Section III, C, that the P:O ratio for citrate oxidation by liver mitochondria of vitamin E-deficient guinea pigs was lower than that of controls. They could furthermore show that the effect was limited to the first segment of the respiratory chain. Electron spin resonance studies should be carried out to determine whether a nonheme iron protein signal is involved in this phenomenon (cf. Slater et al., 1972).

Participation of nonheme iron proteins in adrenal cortex microsomal mixed function oxidase reactions has been demonstrated by Omura et al. (1965): a reconstituted system was found to be completely dependent on the addition of nonheme iron protein.

Carpenter (1967) has shown that vitamin E deficiency leads to a decrease in specific activity of oxidative demethylation of codeine and aminopyrine by liver microsomes, which could be prevented by addition of vitamin E to the diet 48 hours prior to sacrifice of the animals. Subsequent studies (Carpenter, 1968) revealed that induction in liver of microsomal hydroxylation reactions with phenobarbital in vitamin E-deficient rats resulted in a larger induction than in controls. The decay of the induced activity was, however, also faster. Diplock et al. (1971b) demonstrated that this induction by phenobarbital is associated with an increased incorporation of selenium as selenide in the microsomal membrane. Vitamin E deficiency decreased this incorporation. If, however, vitamin E deficiency decreases the incorporation of selenium as selenide in the presence of inducing barbiturates, but on the other hand the specific activity of hydroxylation reactions increases under these conditions, the participation of selenium as selenide in this type of reaction becomes unlikely, unless it is assumed that the selenide was not rate limiting in these experiments.

There is furthermore the problem whether a nonheme iron protein is involved in liver microsomal hydroxylation reactions at all. Mason et al. (1965) and Miyake et al. (1967) have failed to give conclusive evidence for or against the participation of nonheme iron proteins in liver hydroxylations. Here again ESR studies are badly needed to correlate vitamin E deficiency with the proposed mode of action of vitamin E on sulfur or selenium of nonheme iron protein.

Third, it should be demonstrated that redox changes of the chromanol ring structure of α-tocopherol are opposite in sign to that of sulfur or selenium of nonheme iron proteins. Such a direct link has not been shown, and it probably will be very difficult to show this experimentally.

Summarizing, up to now the evidence for this hypothesis is based only upon the existence of selenium in a reduced form as selenide in mitochondrial and microsomal fractions. Like the value of all hypotheses, that of this one is entirely determined by the new line of experiments that can be built upon it. As such, the hypothesis advanced by Diplock et al. (1971a) is a challenging one.

IV. Problem Analysis

Analyzing the relationship between vitamin E and cellular membranes, it has to be stated first that in vitamin E research, and consequently in this review, attention is focused especially on vitamin E deficiency as the major tool for studies on the function of vitamin E. Studies on the deficiency of a given factor can be very operative in gaining valuable information about the morphological and biochemical consequences of the absence of that particular factor for the organism and its tissues, cells, and organelles. Evidence may then be produced for a relation between this factor and the organism or its parts. It must be noted, however, that this kind of experiment must fail to produce a complete and clear insight into the functional mechanism of the factor under study in cellular metabolism of a "healthy" organism. Nevertheless, the changes introduced in the membrane by vitamin E withdrawal could become manifest in two basic properties of the membrane: its form and its function. In the term "form" is comprised its ultrastructure and the underlying biochemical composition. The term "function" relates to its permeability and enzymatic activities.

The question as put above can now be reformulated as follows: (i) Does vitamin E deficiency influence the ultrastructure and biochemical composition of cellular membranes? (ii) Does the permeability and membrane-bound enzyme activity also change; if so, is there a causal relationship between the ultrastructural and compositional alterations? (iii) Are the four current hypotheses on the function of vitamin E (see Section III) adequate to explain the results of the experiments bearing on the questions (i) and (ii)? (iv) Which experiments are needed for a better understanding of the function of vitamin E? These four questions will successively be discussed in the next section.

V. DISCUSSION

(i) Evidence will be presented for an effect of vitamin E deficiency on the ultrastructure and chemical composition of cellular membranes. First of all, it was found that vitamin E has a positive effect of the ultrastructure of membranes in vitamin E-deficient patients. Molenaar *et al.* (1968) reported on two patients with abetalipoproteinemia, a disease in which the absorption of fats is disturbed and with it also that of fat-soluble vitamins, e.g., vitamin E. Investigations with the electron microscope of jejunal biopsies of these vitamin E deficient-patients disclosed that membranes could not be visualized with the routine preparation methods including postfixation with osmium tetroxide (see Section II, C, 2), at least not in positive contrast. Ribosomes, arranged in the same way as to be expected in normal cells (e.g., in linear array) were seen, but without visible membranes (see Figs. 2 and 3). Four months' treatment of the patients with vitamin E resulted in a dramatic change in the electron optical image: a completely normal cellular ultrastructure could be observed (see Fig. 4).

This relation between vitamin E and membrane contrast could also be demonstrated, but in reverse, in jejunal epithelial cells of Pekin ducklings with experimental vitamin E deficiency (Molenaar *et al.*, 1970). In these experiments the loss of positive contrast was less evident than in the above-mentioned patients before vitamin E medication. The mitochondrial membranes, rough endoplasmic reticular membranes and nuclear outer membranes lost a great deal of their positive contrast (Fig. 5). The outer mitochondrial membrane had less contrast than the inner one, was mostly thinner and not always continuous (Figs. 6 and

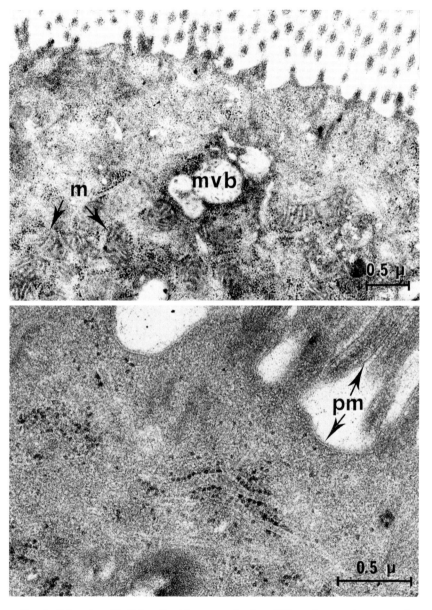

FIG. 2. Jejunal epithelial cell with parts of microvilli at the top from a patient with abetalipoproteinemia resulting in hypovitaminosis E. Note the lack of membranes in general. Multivesicular bodies (*mvb*) are visible. Mitochondria (*m*) show their matrix, but lack positively contrasted membranes (× 25,000). From Molenaar *et al.* (1968), by permission of the National Academy of Sciences, Washington, D. C.

FIG. 3. Jejunal epithelial cell of the same patient. Ribosomes are present in linear array, but without membranes in positive contrast. Only on the microvilli is a weakly stained plasma membrane (*pm*) visible. × 40,000. From Molenaar *et al.* (1968), by permission of the National Academy of Sciences. Washington, D. C.

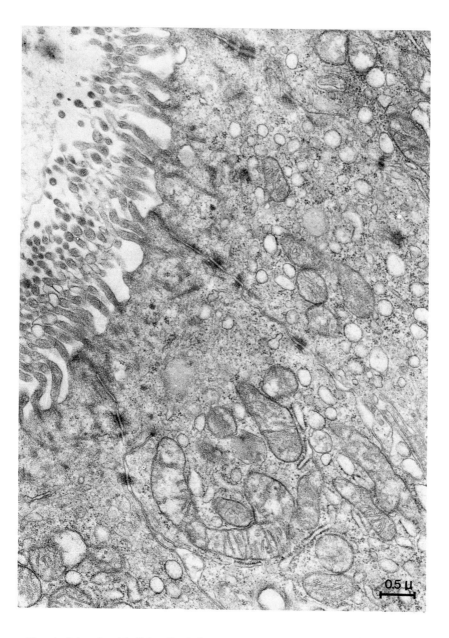

Fig. 4. Jejunal epithelial cell of the same patient after 4 months of vitamin E medication. The cells have a normal ultrastructural aspect; apart from a rather large number of vacuoles, membranes are visible in normal contrast. × 20,000. From Molenaar et al. (1968), by permission of the National Academy of Sciences, Washington, D. C.

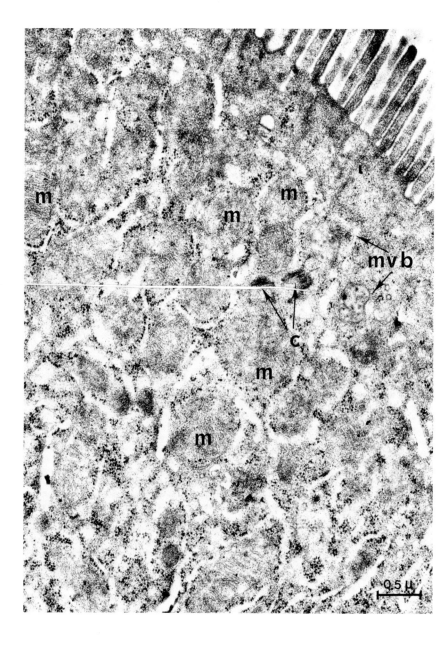

Fig. 5. Vitamin E-deficient duckling; jejunal epithelial cell. Note the poor membrane contrast, especially in the mitochondria (*m*). Multivesicular bodies (*mvb*) and centrioles (*c*) are visible. × 10,800. From Molenaar, I., Vos, J., Jager, F. C., and Hommes, F. A. (1970). The influence of vitamin E deficiency on biological membranes. *Nutr. Metab.* **12,** 361, 362.

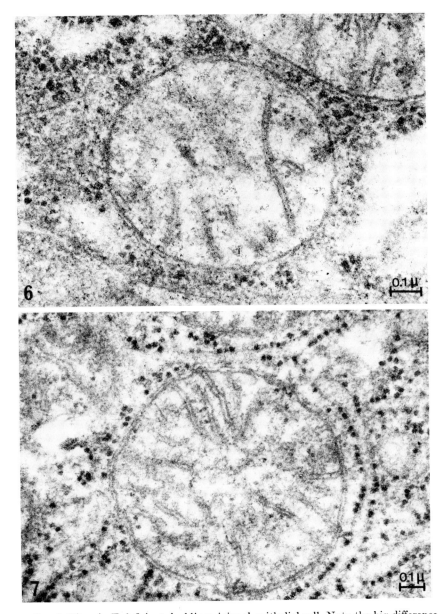

Fig. 6. Vitamin E-deficient duckling; jejunal epithelial cell. Note the big difference in contrast between inner and outer mitochondrial membrane; compare with Fig. 7. × 90,000. From Molenaar, I., Vos, J., Jager, F. C., and Hommes, F. A. (1970). The influence of vitamin E deficiency on biological membranes. *Nutr. Metab.* **12,** 361, 362.

Fig. 7. Non-vitamin E-deficient duckling; jejunal epithelial cell. The electron density of both mitochondrial membranes is almost alike. Compare with Fig. 6. × 70,000. From Molenaar, I., Vos, J., Jager, F. C., and Hommes, F. A. (1970). The influence of vitamin E deficiency on biological membranes. *Nutr. Metab.* **12,** 361, 362.

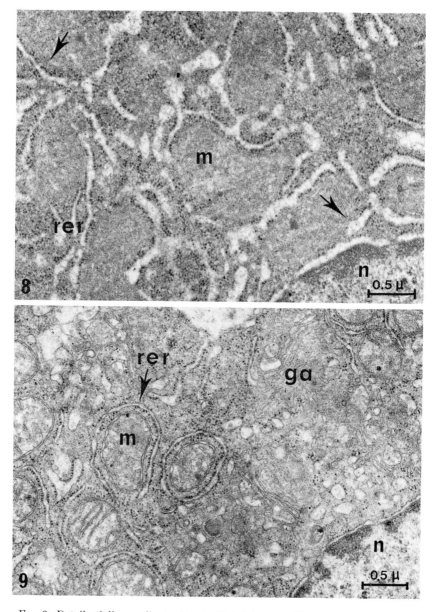

Fig. 8. Detail of liver cell of vitamin E-deficient duckling. Both mitochondrial membranes (→) and the membranes of the rough endoplasmic reticulum (*rer*) are only just visible as very thin lines in positive contrast. *m*, mitochondrion; *n*, nucleus. Compare with Fig. 9. × 26,000.

Fig. 9. Detail of liver cell of control duckling. Cellular membranes of different type are clearly visible in positive contrast. *n*, Nucleus; *ga*, Golgi apparatus; *rer*, rough endoplasmic reticulum; *m*, mitochondrion. Compare with Fig. 8. × 26,000.

7). The inner mitochondrial membranes, plasma membranes and the membranes of Golgi lamellae and vesicles did not show such a loss of contrast. The difference in contrast between the outer and inner membranes of mitochondria in deficient animals indicated a selective loss of contrast within these organelles. The same studies demonstrated a relation between the degree of vitamin E deficiency—as judged from the degree of myopathy—and the number of mitochondria with outer membranes less electron dense than normally.

In subsequent studies, samples of the two mitochondrial membranes, showing the above described selective loss of contrast, and of microsomal membranes were chosen for biochemical investigation in order to obtain quantitative data on the fatty acid composition of membranes in vitamin E deficiency. Liver mitochondria were studied in this case since the previously mentioned loss of membrane contrast had also been observed in liver tissue (Vos, 1972) (Figs. 8 and 9), and the preparation of intestinal mucosal mitochondrial membranes proved to be rather difficult because of the high contamination with mucus. The fatty acid analyses of outer and inner mitochondrial membranes and microsomal membranes of livers of vitamin E-deficient ducklings showed a specific loss of arachidonic acid. The outer mitochondrial membranes showed an especially marked decrease in arachidonic acid content of 67% while the decreases for the inner mitochondrial and microsomal membranes were less at 43 and 13%, respectively. An analogous decrease was observed in linoleic acid content of outer mitochondrial membranes (44%), but not in inner mitochondrial and microsomal membranes (<10%). These relative decreases were found to be balanced by increases in palmitoleic and oleic acids in outer and inner mitochondrial membranes and by an increase in content of stearic acid in microsomal membranes (Vos et al., 1972b; Vos, 1972). These results are summarized in Table I.

Vitamin E deficiency thus decreases the polyunsaturated fatty acid content in those membranes where a decrease in osmium contrast has been observed. As has been reviewed in Section II, C, 2, a, binding of osmium to membranes occurs presumably at the double bonds of the fatty acid moieties of membrane phospholipids. A decreased contrast of certain membranes as observed in vitamin E deficiency is therefore to a high degree consistent with the observed decrease in membrane-bound polyunsaturated fatty acids.

However, the partial discrepancy between the fatty acid analysis of *microsomal* membranes and their positive contrast in osmium tetroxide-fixed tissue is to be noted (compare Table I and Figs. 8 and 9). Starting from the assumption that the decrease in positive membrane contrast is explained only as a result of a critical loss of double bonds in vitamin

I. MOLENAAR, J. VOS, AND F. A. HOMMES

TABLE I

FATTY ACID COMPOSITION OF INNER AND OUTER MITOCHONDRIAL MEMBRANES
AND MICROSOMES FROM VITAMIN E-DEFICIENT DUCKLING
LIVERS (D) AND CONTROLS (C)

	Content (wt % of total fatty acids)					
	Inner mitochondrial membrane[a]		Outer mitochondrial membrane[b]		Microsomes[c]	
Fatty acid	C	D	C	D	C	D
C 16:0	20.4	24.1	29.6	27.2	25.6	23.9
C 16:1ω7	1.9	3.3	1.9	3.4	1.6	1.6
C 18:0	25.0	22.1	25.3	26.4	18.2	20.9
C 18:1ω9	20.9	25.3	21.9	25.2	21.6	20.5
C 18:2ω6	13.3	12.2	6.8	3.6	4.5	4.7
C 22:0	1.1	0.2	+	+	0.4	1.2
C 20:4ω6	13.3	7.6	9.4	3.3	16.9	14.7
C 24:0	+	+	0.7	+	1.6	2.2
C 22:6ω3	1.6	1.0	1.2	2.0	2.0	3.4
Unidentified	2.5	4.0	3.2	8.9	7.6	6.9
Total saturated	46.5	46.4	55.6	53.6	45.8	48.2
C 16:1ω7 + C 18:1ω9	22.8	28.8	23.8	28.6	23.2	22.1
C 18:2ω6 + C 20:4ω6	26.6	19.8	16.2	6.9	21.4	19.4

[a] Average of 4 determinations, 10 control and 10 deficient animals.
[b] Determination of 3 combined fractions, 8 control and 8 deficient animals.
[c] Average of 3 determinations, 8 control and 9 deficient animals.

E deficiency, the membranes of the endoplasmic reticulum could not be expected to lose contrast, on the basis of the biochemical results.

However, other factors, for instance the effect of preparation methods, can explain the apparently controversial results in this type of membrane. Roozemond (1969) found a differential loss of lipids from tissues during fixation with glutaraldehyde, depending on the structural properties of these lipids. It would be very well possible that the absence of α-tocopherol molecules lessens the stability of cellular membranes (Lucy, 1972), resulting in a relatively great loss of membrane lipids during fixation. This could also be valid for the extraction of lipids after fixation with osmium tetroxide and before embedding in plastic during dehydration of tissue in an alcohol, or acetone, series. For normal tissue, it is known that during this dehydration only a small part of the membrane-bound phospholipids is extracted, due to the fixing action of osmium tetroxide (Korn, 1966; Silva et al., 1968).

In addition to the above mentioned decrease in membrane contrast the second striking effect to be observed was the diversity in behavior with regard to the changes in electron density of membrane systems in general and the two mitochondrial membranes in particular in vitamin E deficiency (Molenaar et al., 1968, 1970). The plasma membrane holds a special position: both in patients and duckling experiments its contrast did not change very much. In this connection it is interesting to note that on the basis of lipid characteristics and membrane thickness measurements two main groups of cellular membranes can be distinguished (see Sections II, B, 4, and II, C, 2, respectively). It is tempting to assume that the difference in content of polyunsaturated fatty acids in both groups of membranes causes a different reaction pattern in ultrastructural and biochemical terms after vitamin E supplementation or depletion.

As yet no changes in the ultrastructure of membranes have been reported at the high resolution level with negative staining techniques. Vos et al. (1972a,b) could only show that isolated outer mitochondrial membranes from vitamin E-deficient duckling livers were fractured to a higher degree than those of control animals (Fig. 10). This finding points to a higher fragility and corresponds with the electron image of this group of membranes in ultrathin sections (Molenaar et al., 1970).

(ii) Permeability is an important aspect of membrane function. As far as we know no studies have been reported on the permeability of membranes in vitamin E deficiency. Scarpa and de Gier (1971) have demonstrated that the permeability for cations of artificial membranes (liposomes) is to a large degree dependent on the chemical composition of the lecithins used for the preparation of these liposomes. To mention one example, a significant increase in K^+ permeability could be demonstrated with increasing unsaturation of the lecithin fatty acids, while the concomitant increase in Na^+ permeability was less than that for K^+. In other words, besides a change in permeability, an increasing capacity to discriminate between ions was introduced by the higher degree of unsaturation. These studies have given some insight into the relation between the chemical composition of the apolar part of a lipid bilayer system and permeability properties.

Such changes in the apolar part of membranes can also take place in vitamin E deficiency. Indeed McCay et al. (1971) have demonstrated that the oxidative loss of particularly arachidonate from microsomal membranes results in increased swelling of the endoplasmic reticular vesicles (microsomes) in vitro. The studies of Lee and Barnes (1969) on tissue total phospholipids and the experiments of Vos et al. (1972a,b) and Vos (1972) on isolated membranes yielded evidence for a decreased content of unsaturated fatty acids induced by vitamin E deficiency. It

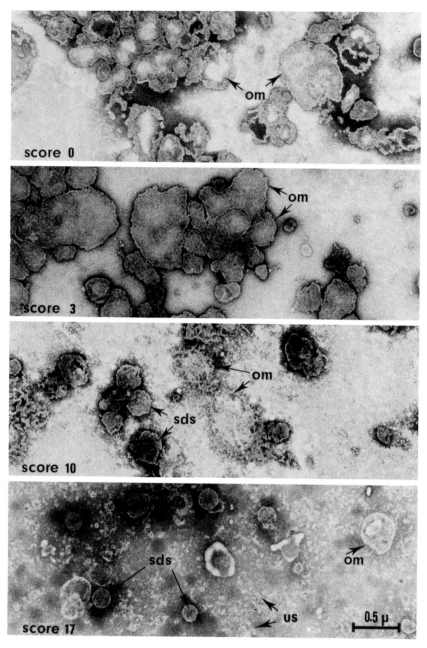

FIG. 10. Variation in ultrastructural aspect of outer mitochondrial membrane fraction from groups of ducklings with different degrees of vitamin E deficiency as judged by myopathy scores (0–17). Note the gradual deterioration of outer membrane (*om*) integrity and the increase in number of unidentified structures (*us*). Small dense sacs (*sds*) are not derived from outer membranes. × 26,000.

can therefore be expected that such changes will affect the permeability properties of various cell organelles, although detailed studies are lacking. Such studies may be very useful for a better understanding of the many pathological effects which are associated with vitamin E deficiency. The theory of Diplock et al. (1971a) may have special significance in this respect. Scarpa and de Gier (1971) have also demonstrated that increased incorporation of cholesterol into liposomes decreases the permeability for cations. A similar role could be ascribed to the arachidonic acid-α-tocopherol adduct as proposed by Diplock et al. (1971a). Vitamin E deficiency would then lead to an increased permeability for cations. The concentration of vitamin E in membranes seems, however, to be relatively low. The data on vitamin E content of the inner mitochondrial membranes given by Oliveira et al. (1969), for instance, permit a rough estimation of 1 mole of α-tocopherol per 50 moles of arachidonic acid. Further studies are therefore needed to investigate the suggested influence of vitamin E deficiency on membrane permeability.

When changes in permeability become profound, then also macromolecules will leak through the membranes. This could result in serious damage to the cellular ultrastructure when lysosomal membranes are involved and hydrolytic enzymes are released. On the basis of time-scale studies on the development of muscular dystrophy in vitamin E-deficient rabbits, Zalkin et al. (1962) concluded that a primary injury of lysosomal membranes was responsible for the disease. This conclusion is opposite to that of Cheville (1966) and Van Vleet et al. (1968), who deny a primary role of lysosomes in vitamin E deficiency. Therefore it is still controversial whether vitamin E deficiency causes specific lesions of the lysosomal membranes only, resulting in a leakage of hydrolytic enzymes. Molenaar et al. (1970) found that the lysosomal membranes lost contrast, just like some other cellular membranes. This points to a nonpreferential lysosomal membrane lesion.

Another function of cellular membranes is to provide a suitable supporting site for enzymes. As to this function Machado et al. (1971) report on a progressive decrease in the activity of Na-K-ATPase and 5'-nucleotidase in the plasma membrane of rat liver cells, studied with electron enzyme cytochemical and biochemical methods. These changes were found before the development of specific vitamin E deficiency symptoms. The rats in these experiments were however fed a diet deficient not only in vitamin E, but also in selenium. The biochemical evidence for the decrease in Na-K-ATPase of isolated plasma membranes is impressive, in contrast to that for the decrease in 5'-nucleotidase, which does not seem to be significant. It has not been established

whether the ATPase activity demonstrated by electron enzyme cytochemistry is indeed the Na-K-ATPase. It is not clear in this study
whether the observed decrease in Na-K-ATPase is due to a change in
the plasma membrane or due to a decrease of the enzyme activity per se.
Machado *et al.* (1971) favor the first-mentioned alternative.

(iii) In Section III the current hypotheses on the function of vitamin
E have been reviewed. The question arises now whether any of these
theories can explain the effects of vitamin E deficiency on cellular
membranes.

Such an effect is the decreased membrane contrast in vitamin E deficiency (Molenaar *et al.*, 1968, 1970). This is most distinctly observed
in the outer mitochondrial membrane, having the largest decrease in
arachidonate (Table I). Oliveira *et al.* (1969) have further shown
that the mitochondrial α-tocopherol is exclusively localized in the inner
mitochondrial membrane. No vitamin E could be demonstrated to be
present in the outer membrane. These experiments were carried out with
beef heart mitochondria. It is questionable whether the results can be
applied to the mitochondria of Pekin duckling liver and jejunum. If this
happens to be the case, which could be experimentally verified for liver,
then the following problem arises. If a non-vitamin E-deficient outer
mitochondrial membrane does not contain vitamin E, it cannot protect
the arachidonate of this membrane from lipid peroxidation as defined
by Tappel (1962, 1965), nor can vitamin E stabilize that membrane as
advanced by Diplock *et al.* (1971a,b). It is not clear why polyunsaturated
fatty acid moieties of a non-vitamin E-containing membrane are more
susceptible to peroxidation in a vitamin E-deficient state of the animal
than in a vitamin E-sufficient state, unless it is assumed that the steady
state concentration of free radicals involved in lipid peroxidation is
higher in a vitamin E-deficient organ. Such an assumption would, however, have as a consequence a higher steady state level of peroxides,
which, for liver at least, has not been observed (Glavind, 1972; J. Green,
1972). Both the nonenzymatic biological antioxidant role of vitamin E
and the theory of vitamin E as a membrane stabilizer can therefore not
apply to the outer mitochondrial membrane.

The results of Vos *et al.* do not exclude a role of vitamin E as a factor
in enzyme-dependent lipid peroxidation as suggested by McCay *et al.*
(1971) and summarized in Section II, B. At the same time they cannot
be regarded as proof for such a role. It should be mentioned that the
decrease in the C 20:4ω6 acid observed in the microsomal membranes
was less than that for mitochondrial membranes, especially the outer
mitochondrial membrane where such a NADPH$_2$-oxidation dependent
generation of free radicals has as yet not been demonstrated.

Considering the above-mentioned facts and arguments, we propose the following modes of action of vitamin E. α-Tocopherol, if present in a given membrane is probably located within it according to the model of Diplock *et al.* (1971a). This location is especially suited for one function of the α-tocopherol molecule: decreasing enzyme-dependent peroxidation of membrane-bound polyunsaturated fatty acids *in vivo* according to McCay *et al.* (1971). Peroxidation according to Tappel (1962, 1965) in vitamin E deficiency is only found in adipose tissue (cf. Glavind, 1972), where fat is stored as large droplets in the vacuoles of the fat cells. This fat has no structure and is not situated in the direct neighborhood of membranes, which possibly have a lowered content of vitamin E.

(iv) The analyses of fatty acids of some membrane systems of organs of vitamin E-deficient animals as compared to those of controls make it desirable to extend these studies to other cellular membranes as well. A correlation should then be made between membrane contrast as seen in the electron microscope, fatty acid analysis, and vitamin E content of the membranes.

Permeability studies on liposomes, prepared with known, but varying, ratios of vitamin E to arachidonic acid, may throw some light on the alleged changes in permeability in vitamin E deficiency. Such studies could also be carried out with mitochondria isolated from vitamin E-deficient organs.

The hypothesis concerning the role of vitamin E as a membrane stabilizer with redox capacity needs further studies directed toward the state of iron in nonheme iron proteins of membranes. The electron spin resonance technique seems to be most appropriate for this purpose.

Vitamin E as a factor in enzyme-dependent lipid peroxidation may not necessarily be restricted to microsomes. The process may, in principle at least, occur wherever free radicals are generated in membrane-bound enzyme reactions. The inner mitochondrial membrane is then a likely candidate.

It seems promising to use the careful preparation technique as suggested by Sjöstrand (1971) and to improve electron-enzyme cytochemical methods. Thus more reliable observations on changes in membrane ultrastructure and enzyme localization can be obtained. Furthermore, it will be of great value to study the membrane and its alterations with advanced methods of electron microscopy. Phase contrast-, dark field-, and high-voltage electron microscopy will enable the investigator to study the membrane in the natural form (Parsons, 1971).

VI. CONCLUDING REMARKS

The main effects of vitamin E deficiency on cellular membranes seem to be reflected in the lipid moiety more than in the protein part. It can furthermore be stated that these effects differ for various cellular membranes. This diversity in reaction pattern might, at higher levels of structural organization, be correlated with the characteristic course of vitamin E deficiency: a gradual, but unmistakable worsening in the general condition is followed by a relatively sudden death of the animal concerned. It is very well conceivable that the first period of the illness is determined by an altered membrane function based upon the proven changes in membrane composition. This problem of permeability seems to be of paramount importance for the maintenance of cellular compartmentalization and cell metabolism. Further research will be needed to clarify this point. The second phase of the illness, a phase in which the animals die suddenly, may coincide with a deterioration of lysosomal membranes. Research in composition and integrity of these lysosomal membranes with and without vitamin E deficiency are therefore highly desirable.

It is well known that vitamin E deficiency affects species differently, and within one species a marked tissue specificity in susceptibility to vitamin E deficiency can be observed. Among the very susceptible tissues are muscle, testis, liver, and adrenal cortex. It would be interesting to analyze, in terms of membranes, the general common factor of these susceptible tissues and cells, which furthermore occurs in higher amounts in these tissues and cells as compared with others. It is to be noted that especially the smooth endoplasmic reticulum is abundant in these tissues. If the membranes of this organelle are the most sensitive to vitamin E deficiency, the impairment of their function could explain many results reported so far. However, such a simple solution for this problem would certainly underestimate the long way research had and probably has to go in investigating this vitamin. Nevertheless, it seems to be warranted that, at least in the case of vitamin E deficiency, the "cellular pathology" of Rudolf Virchow can be read in terms of "membrane pathology."

ACKNOWLEDGMENT
The authors thank Dr. C. E. Hulstaert for critical and helpful discussion.

REFERENCES

Alfin-Slater, R. B. (1965). *Fed. Proc., Fed. Amer. Soc. Exp. Biol.* **24,** 622.
Auliac, P. B. (1967). Thesis, University of Paris (as cited by Moulé, 1968).
Bahr, G. F. (1954). *Exp. Cell. Res.* **7,** 457.
Benedetti, E. L., and Emmelot, P. (1968). *In* "The Membranes" (A. J. Dalton and F. Haguenau, eds.), pp. 95–99. Academic Press, New York.
Boguth, W. (1969). *Vitam. Horm. (New York)* **27,** 1.

Bunyan, J., Murrell, E. A., Green, J., and Diplock, A. T. (1967). *Brit. J. Nutr.* **21,** 475.

Carabello, T., Lien, F., Canes, C., and Bird, J. (1971). *Fed. Proc., Fed. Amer. Soc. Exp. Biol.* **30,** 639 (abstr.).

Carney, J. A., and Walker, B. L. (1971). *Fed. Proc., Fed. Amer. Soc. Exp. Biol.* **30,** 639 (abstr.).

Carpenter, M. P. (1966). *Fed. Proc., Fed. Amer. Soc. Exp. Biol.* **25,** 764.

Carpenter, M. P. (1967). *Fed. Proc., Fed. Amer. Soc. Exp. Biol.* **26,** 475.

Carpenter, M. P. (1968). *Fed. Proc., Fed. Amer. Soc. Exp. Biol.* **27,** 677.

Cawthorne, M. A., Diplock, A. T., Muthy, J. R., Bunyan, J., Murrell, E. A., and Green, J. (1967). *Brit. J. Nutr.* **21,** 671.

Caygill, C. P. J., Lucy, J. A., and Diplock, A. T. (1971). *Biochem. J.* **125,** 407.

Chapman, D., and Leslie, R. B. (1970). *In* "Membranes of Mitochondria and Chloroplasts" (E. Racker, ed.), p. 95. Van Nostrand-Reinhold, Princeton, New Jersey.

Cheville, N. F. (1966). *Pathol. Vet.* **3,** 208.

Colbeau, A., Nachbaur, J., and Vignais, P. M. (1971). *Biochem. Biophys. Acta* **49,** 462.

Corwin, L. M. (1965). *J. Biol. Chem.* **240,** 34.

Cunningham, W. P., Prezbindowsky, K. S., and Crane, F. L. (1967). *Biochim. Biophys. Acta* **135,** 614.

Daems, W. T., and Persijn, J. P. (1962). *Histochemie* **3,** 79.

Danielli, J. F., and Davson, H. (1935). *J. Cell. Comp. Physiol.* **5,** 495.

De Duve, C. (1971). *J. Cell Biol.* **50,** 20D.

Diplock, A. T. (1972). *Acta Agr. Scand.* (in press).

Diplock, A. T., Bunyan, J., McHale, D., and Green, J. (1967). *Brit. J. Nutr.* **21,** 103.

Diplock, A. T., Baum, H., and Lucy, J. A. (1971a). *Biochem. J.* **123,** 721.

Diplock, A. T., Jeffery, E. H., and Caygill, C. P. J. (1971b). *Abstr. Commun., 7th Meet., Eur. Biochem. Soc., 1971* p. 247.

Emmelot, P., and Benedetti, E. L. (1967). *In* "Carcinogenesis: A Broad Critique," (Anderson Hosp., Texas), pp. 471–533. Williams & Wilkins, Baltimore, Maryland.

Emmelot, P., Bos, C. J., Benedetti, E. L., and Rümke, P. (1964). *Biochim. Biophys. Acta* **90,** 126.

Ericsson, J. L. E. (1966). *J. Histochem. Cytochem.* **14,** 361.

Fernández-Morán, H. (1962). *Circulation* **26,** 1039.

Fitch, C. D. (1968). *Vitam. Horm. (New York)* **26,** 501.

Fleischer, S., and Rouser, G. (1965). *J. Amer. Oil Chem. Soc.* **42,** 588.

Fleischer, S., Fleischer, B., and Stoeckenius, W. (1967). *J. Cell Biol.* **32,** 193.

Gillian, J. M., and McCay, P. B. (1966). *Fed. Proc., Fed. Amer. Soc. Exp. Biol.* **25,** 241.

Glavind, J. (1972). *Acta Agr. Scand.* (in press).

Goldfischer, S. G., Essner, E., and Schiller, B. (1971). *J. Histochem. Cytochem.* **19,** 349.

Gorter, E., and Grendel, F. (1925). *J. Exp. Med.* **41,** 439.

Gram, T. E., and Fouts, J. R. (1966). *Arch. Biochem. Biophys.* **114,** 331.

Green, D. E., Tisdale, H. D., Griddle, R. S., Chen, P. Y., and Bock, R. M. (1961). *Biochem. Biophys. Res. Commun.* **5,** 109.

Green, J. (1972). *Ann. N. Y. Acad. Sci.* (in press).

Green, J., Diplock, A. T., Bunyan, J., McHale, D., and Muthy, J. R. (1967). *Brit. J. Nutr.* **21,** 69.

Hake, T. (1965). *Lab. Invest.* **14,** 470.

Harman, E. M., Witting, L. A., and Horwitt, M. K. (1966). *Amer. J. Clin. Nutr.* **18**, 243.

Henning, R., Kaulen, H. D., and Stoffel, W. (1970). *Hoppe-Seyler's Z. Physiol. Chem.* **351**, 1191.

Herting, D. C. (1971). *Lipids* **6**, 238.

Horwitt, M. K. (1965). *Fed. Proc., Fed. Amer. Soc. Exp. Biol.* **24**, 68.

Horwitt, M. K., Harvey, C. C., and Harman, E. M. (1968). *Vitam. Horm.* (*New York*) **26**, 487.

Huet, C., Lévy, M., and Pascaud, M. (1968). *Biochim. Biophys. Acta* **150**, 521.

Hugon, J., and Borgers, M. (1966). *J. Histochem. Cytochem.* **14**, 429.

Hugon, J. S., Maestracci, D., and Ménard, D. (1971). *J. Histochem. Cytochem.* **19**, 515.

Jager, F. C. (1968). *Nutr. Dieta* **10**, 215.

Jager, F. C. (1969). *Nutr. Dieta* **11**, 270.

Jager, F. C. (1972). *Ann. N. Y. Acad. Sci.* (in press).

Jager, F. C., and Houtsmuller, A. M. T. (1970). *Nutr. Metab.* **12**, 3.

Johnson, M. W., and Horne, R. W. (1970). *J. Roy. Microsc. Soc.* [3] **91**, 197.

Keenan, T. W., and Morré, D. (1970). *Biochemistry* **9**, 19.

Korn, E. D. (1966). *Biochim. Biophys. Acta* **116**, 309.

Krebs, H. A., and Veech, R. L. (1970). *In* "Pyridine Nucleotide Dependent Dehydrogenases" (H. Sund, ed.), p. 413. Springer-Verlag, Berlin and New York.

Lee, D. J. W., and Barnes, M. Mc. (1969). *Brit. J. Nutr.* **23**, 289.

Lévy, M., and Sauner, M. T. (1968). *Chem. Phys. Lipids* **2**, 291.

Long, C. (1968). "Biochemical Handbook," p. 817. Spon, London.

Lucy, J. A. (1964). *Nature* (*London*) **204**, 156.

Lucy, J. A. (1972). *Ann. N. Y. Acad. Sci.* (in press).

McCay, P. B. (1966). *J. Biol. Chem.* **241**, 2333.

McCay, P. B., Stipe, B., and Shealy, S. (1969). *Fed. Proc., Fed. Amer. Soc. Exp. Biol.* **28**, 757.

McCay, P. B., Poyer, J. L., Pfeiffer, P. M., May, H. E., and Gillian, J. M. (1971). *Lipids* **6**, 297.

Machado, E. A., Porta, E. A., Hartroft, W. S., and Hamilton, F. (1971). *Lab. Invest.* **24**, 13.

Marchesi, V. T., and Palade, G. E. (1967). *J. Cell Biol.* **35**, 385.

Mason, H. S., North, J. C., and Vonneste, M. (1965). *Fed. Proc., Fed. Amer. Soc. Exp. Biol.* **24**, 1172.

May, H. E., and McCay, P. B. (1968a). *J. Biol. Chem.* **243**, 2288.

May, H. E., and McCay, P. B. (1968b). *J. Biol. Chem.* **243**, 2296.

Miyake, Y., Mason, H. S., and Landgraf, W. (1967). *J. Biol. Chem.* **242**, 393.

Molenaar, I., Hommes, F. A., Braams, W. G., and Polman, H. A. (1968). *Proc. Nat. Acad. Sci. U. S.* **61**, 982.

Molenaar, I., Vos, J., Jager, F. C., and Hommes, F. A. (1970). *Nutr. Metab.* **12**, 358.

Moulé, Y. (1968). *In* "Structure and Function of the Endoplasmic Reticulum in Animal Cells" (F. C. Gran, ed.), p. 9. Academic Press, New York.

Naito, H., Johnson, B., and Johnson, B. C. (1966). *Proc. Soc. Exp. Biol. Med.* **122**, 545.

Oliveira, M. M., Weglicki, W. B., Nason, A., and Nair, P. P. (1969). *Biochim. Biophys. Acta* **180**, 98.

Omura, T., Sato, R., Cooper, D. Y., Rosenthal, O., and Estabrook, R. W. (1965). *Fed. Proc., Fed. Amer. Soc. Exp. Biol.* **24**, 1181.

Overton, E. (1895). *Vierteljahresschr. Naturforsch. Ges. Zuerich* **40**, 159.

Parsons, D. F. (1971). *In* "Cell Membranes" (G. W. Richter and D. G. Scarpelli, eds.), pp. 30–37. Williams & Wilkins, Baltimore, Maryland.

Parsons, D. F., Williams, G. R., Thompson, W., Wilson, D., and Chance, B. (1967). *In* "Round Table Discussion on Mitochondrial Structure and Compartmentation" (E. Quagliarello *et al.*, eds.), pp. 29–73. Adriatica Editrice, Bari.

Pfeffer, W. (1875). "Osmotische Untersuchungen," p. 121, Leipzig.

Poyer, J. L., and McCay, P. B. (1971). *J. Biol. Chem.* **246**, 263.

Puig Moset, P., and Valdezasas, F. G. (1946). *Trab. Inst. Nac. Cienc. Med., Madrid* **6**, 389.

Ragan, C. I., Clegg, R. A., Haddock, B. A., Light, P. A., and Garland, P. B. (1970). *FEBS Lett.* **8**, 333.

Riemersma, J. C. (1970). *In* "Biological Techniques in Electron Microscopy" (D. F. Parsons, ed.), pp. 75–87. Academic Press, New York.

Riemersma, J. C., and Booy, H. L. (1962). *J. Histochem. Cytochem.* **10**, 89.

Robertson, J. D. (1955). *J. Biophys. Biochem. Cytol.* **1**, 271.

Robertson, J. D. (1959). *Biochem. Soc. Symp.* **16**, 3.

Roozemond, R. C. (1969). *J. Histochem. Cytochem.* **17**, 482.

Scarpa, A., and de Gier, J. (1971). *Biochim. Biophys. Acta* **241**, 789.

Seligman, A. M., Karnovsky, M. J., Wasserkrug, H. L., and Hanker, J. S. (1968). *J. Cell Biol.* **38**, 1.

Silva, M. T., Carvalho Guerra, F., and Magalhaes, M. M. (1968). *Experientia* **24**, 1074.

Sjöstrand, F. S. (1953). *Nature (London)* **171**, 31.

Sjöstrand, F. S. (1963a). *J. Ultrastruct. Res.* **9**, 340.

Sjöstrand, F. S. (1963b). *J. Ultrastruct. Res.* **9**, 561.

Sjöstrand, F. S. (1968). *In* "Regulatory Functions of Biological Membranes" (J. Järnefelt, ed.), pp. 1–20. Elsevier, Amsterdam.

Sjöstrand, F. S. (1971). *In* "Cell Membranes" (G. W. Richter and D. G. Scarpelli, eds.), pp. 1–29. Williams & Wilkins Co., Baltimore, Maryland.

Skipski, V. P., Barclay, M., Archibald, F. M., Erebus-Kekisch, O., Reichman, E. S., and Good, J. J. (1965). *Life Sci.* **4**, 1673.

Slater, E. C. (1958). *Advan. Enzymol.* **20**, 147.

Slater, E. C., Lee, I. V., Van Gelder, B. F., Albracht, S. P. J., and Berden, J. A. (1972). *Biochim. Biophys. Acta* **256**, 14.

Spiro, M. J., and McKibbin, J. M. (1956). *J. Biol. Chem.* **219**, 643.

Stoeckenius, W., and Engleman, D. M. (1969). *J. Cell Biol.* **42**, 613.

Stoffel, W., and Schiefer, H. G. (1968). *Hoppe-Seyler's Z. Physiol. Chem.* **349**, 1017.

Tappel, A. L. (1962). *Vitam. Horm. (New York)* **20**, 493.

Tappel, A. L. (1965). *Fed. Proc., Fed. Amer. Soc. Exp. Biol.* **24**, 73.

Tsibris, J. C. M., Namtredt, M. J., and Gunsalus, I. C. (1968). *Biochem. Biophys. Res. Commun.* **30**, 323.

Van Dam, K., and Meyer, A. J. (1971). *Annu. Rev. Biochem.* **40**, 115.

Van Vleet, J. F., Hall, B. V., and Simon, J. (1968). *Amer. J. Pathol.* **52**, 1067.

Vogtmann, H., and Prabucki, A. L. (1971). *Int. Z. Vitaminforsch.* **41**, 33.

Vos, J. (1972). Thesis, University of Groningen.

Vos, J., Molenaar, I., Searle-van Leeuwen, M., and Hommes, F. A. (1972a). *Acta Agr. Scand.* (in press).

Vos, J., Molenaar, I., Searle-van Leeuwen, M., and Hommes, F. A. (1972b). *Ann. N. Y. Acad. Sci.* (in press).

Witting, L. A., and Horwitt, M. K. (1966). *Fed. Proc., Fed. Amer. Soc. Exp. Biol.* **25**, 241.

Witting, L. A., Theran, J. J., and Horwitt, M. K. (1967). *Lipids* **2**, 97.
Yamamoto, T. (1963). *J. Cell Biol.* **17**, 413.
Zalkin, H., Tappel, A. L., Caldwell, K. A., Shibko, S., Desai, I. D., and Holliday, T. A. (1962). *J. Biol. Chem.* **237**, 2678.

FSH-Releasing Hormone and LH-Releasing Hormone*†

A. V. SCHALLY, A. J. KASTIN, AND A. ARIMURA

Endocrine and Polypeptide Laboratories and Endocrinology Section of the Medical Service, Veterans Administration Hospital, New Orleans, Louisiana, and Department of Medicine, Tulane University School of Medicine, New Orleans, Louisiana

*Some original studies originating in this laboratory and described in this review were supported by grants from VA, U. S. Public Health Service AM-07467 and AM-09094 and The Population Council, New York, New York.

†This chapter is dedicated to the memory of Geoffrey W. Harris, C. B. E., F. R. S., Dr. Lee's Professor of Anatomy in the University of Oxford, who established the basic theories of hypothalamic control of the pituitary gland. A few months before his untimely passing he had the satisfaction of seeing his brilliant concepts and life's work confirmed.

83

I. GENERAL INTRODUCTION

Observations on the deleterious effects of castration on reproductive functions date back to antiquity. Extensive work in the 1920s and the 1930s resulted in the physiological and chemical characterization of the testicular and ovarian steroid hormones.

It had also been observed for centuries that seasonal and emotional factors influence reproduction, but the perplexing nature of the hypothalamopituitary–gonadal axis hindered significant advances until the demonstration of specific gonad-stimulating hormones in the anterior pituitary lobe (P. E. Smith, 1926; Zondek and Aschheim, 1926, 1927;

P. E. Smith and Engle, 1927). Systematic investigations of the relationship between the central nervous system (CNS) and the secretion of pituitary gonadotropins began in the early 1930s. Experiments utilizing the techniques of stimulation, ablation, and transplantation established the hypothesis of the hypothalamic control of the secretion of gonadotropins (Harris, 1937, 1948a, 1955). It was postulated that this control is exercised through the hypophyseal portal blood supply and mediated by neurohumoral substances originating in the median eminence area of the hypothalamus. Other factors, among them environmental stimuli (F. H. A. Marshall, 1936, 1956) and gonadal steroids (Moore and Price, 1932; Hohlweg and Junkmann, 1932), were also shown to influence hypophyseal gonadotropin secretion. Their actions were thought to be mediated at least in part by the hypothalamus.

Since then, the involvement of the CNS in the control of gonadotropic secretion has been demonstrated in a number of ways: pharmacological activation and inhibition of release of pituitary gonadotropin by centrally acting drugs (Markee et al., 1948, 1952; Everett and Sawyer, 1949, 1950, 1953; Sawyer et al., 1949, 1950, 1951), pituitary inhibition by the intrahypothalamic implantation of gonadal steroids and by the recording of changes in the electrical activity of the brain associated with pituitary stimulation. These phenomena have been reviewed recently by Everett (1969), Sawyer (1969a, 1970, 1971), and Flerko (1971). However, it was not until the demonstration of LH-releasing activity in hypothalamic extracts of rats and domestic animals (McCann et al., 1960; Harris, 1961; Courrier et al., 1963; Schally and Bowers, 1964a) that the concept of hypothalamic control of LH secretion was really firmly established. A few years later, the presence of FSH-releasing activity in hypothalamic extracts was reported (Igarashi and McCann, 1964b; Mittler and Meites, 1964; Kuroshima et al., 1965). About a decade after the first demonstration of LH-releasing activity in the hypothalamus, came the isolation, the determination of structure, and the synthesis of LH-releasing hormone (LH-RH) (Schally et al., 1971a,b,c,d,e,f,g,h,i; Matsuo et al., 1971a,b; Baba et al., 1971a; Nair and Schally, 1972). Simultaneously, based on the FSH-releasing activity of LH-RH, we put forward the concept that a single hypothalamic hormone controls the secretion of both LH and FSH from the pituitary gland (Schally et al., 1971a,b,c,d,e,g,i). Although many questions still remain unanswered, determination of the structure and synthesis of hypothalamic LH-RH/FSH-RH should have far-reaching consequences (apart from its practical clinical value), and will enable further crucial basic investigation to proceed. This chapter is written (if an excuse is required) in the belief that a review at this time of some of the work accomplished in this area may be of heuristic value and could be of help in unraveling the complex mechanism of the interactions of sex steroids with hypothalamic LH-RH/FSH-RH. Our present view is that these interactions, both at the hypothalamic and pituitary level, are responsible for the final regulation of LH and FSH secretion.

II. The Role of FSH and LH in Reproductive Processes

Involvement of the anterior pituitary in processes of reproduction can be said to have begun with the discovery of gonadotropic activity in the pituitary. P. E. Smith (1926), Zondek and Aschheim (1926, 1927), P. E. Smith and Engle (1927), and Fevold et al. (1933) demonstrated that hypophyseal extracts and implants produced precocious sexual development in immature female and male rats. Enlargement of ovarian follicles and corpus luteum formation were reported after injection of pituitary extracts into immature rats or mice.

It was also observed that in the young animal hypophysectomy will cause a failure of the gonads to mature with a resulting lack of sexual development and sterility. In mature animals, such an operation is followed by atrophy of the gonads and other parts of the reproductive system. Thus, in man, after hypophysectomy, there is secondary testicular atrophy characterized by loss of the germinal elements, atrophy of the germinal epithelium and fibrosis of the seminiferous tubules. In women, the ovaries atrophy so that no follicular developments beyond the antrum stage occurs; menstruation of course, ceases. Hypophysectomy early in the pregnancy of dogs, cats, and rabbits will induce abortion.

Fevold, Hisaw, and Leonard (see Fevold et al., 1931, 1933, 1940; Fevold, 1943) were the first to recognize the dual nature of the pituitary gonadotropic secretion and separated these extracts into two active fractions, follicle-stimulating hormone (FSH) and luteinizing hormone (LH). Another name used for LH, particularly in reference to male animals, is interstitial cell-stimulating hormone (ICSH). Later pure FSH and LH preparations were made from sheep and hog hypophyses (Li et al., 1940, 1949; Li, 1949). They were found to be glycoproteins. Important contributions on the chemistry of LH and FSH have been made recently by Ward et al. (1968), Reichert et al. (1969), Sherwood et al. (1970), Papkoff and Ekblad, 1970, and Papkoff et al. (1971).

FSH stimulates the growth of the ovarian follicle by promoting mitotic proliferation of the granulosa cells. The response to FSH is demonstrable by the presence of follicles in all stages of development, initiation of antrum formation, and increase in ovarian weight. FSH is a gametogenic hormone in the male; it affects the function and structure of seminiferous tubules and production of spermatozoa. In the hypophysectomized rat as well as in hypophysectomized humans, FSH, given together with LH, stimulates spermatogenesis (Lostroh, 1969; Mancini *et al.*, 1969). The presence of androgens seems to be necessary for full spermatogenesis. On the other hand, FSH has no effect on interstitial tissue (Hamburger, 1957) and very pure FSH preparations failed to stimulate steroidogenesis by mouse ovary (Eshkol and Lunenfeld, 1967).

LH is now well accepted to be responsible for stimulation of steroidogenesis in the ovarian follicle and for ovulation in the ovary previously stimulated by FSH, as well as the transformation of the graafian follicles into corpora lutea (Keyes, 1969). When ovulation is to take place, the events mediated by LH include expansion and maturation of the graafian follicle until the ovarian wall ruptures, releasing the ovum together with some viscous follicular fluid and cells. The exact mechanism for the release of the ovum is still unknown. The follicles which have not ovulated undergo regressive changes. After ovulation, under the influence of LH, some granulosa cells increase in size and undergo the process of luteinization. There are differences between species as to the regulation of the secretory function of the corpus luteum (Greep, 1961). In some species the luteotropic agent is LH, while in other species such as the rat this function is assumed by prolactin (Meites and Nicoll, 1966).

In the male animal, LH stimulates maturation of the testicular interstitial tissue (the cells of Leydig) causing secretion of androgen and some estrogen (Hamburger, 1957). The androgen, in turn, exerts an effect on the seminiferous tubules and other structures, but a direct effect of LH on the tubules cannot be ruled out at present.

III. Development of the Concept of Hypothalamic Control of Pituitary Gland

A. Anatomical Considerations

A detailed description of the anatomy of this region is beyond the scope of this chapter; for this the reader is referred to the book by Harris (1955). It will suffice to say that the hypothalamus is part of the diencephalon, lies at the base of the brain, ventral to the thalamus, and forms the floor and part of the lateral wall of the third ventricle. The funnel-shaped median eminence at the "bottom" of the hypothalamus is attached at its lower end to the pituitary gland by a stalk.

The development of modern ideas on neurohumoral control of the anterior pituitary gland may have begun with the theory of Hinsey and Markee (1933) that hypothalamic stimuli activated the posterior lobe of the pituitary, which in turn influenced the anterior lobe by hormonal pathways. In the same period, the work of F. H. A. Marshall (1936, 1942) indicated that the central nervous system was involved in the control of secretion of gonadotropic hormones from the anterior pituitary gland. Marshall emphasized the importance of environmental stimuli, acting through the nervous system and anterior pituitary gland, in regulating reproductive rhythms and cycles. Since an adequate nerve supply to the cells of the anterior lobe was lacking, attention was concentrated on the blood vessels connecting the median eminence area of the tuber cinereum with the anterior pituitary gland. This system of hypophyseal portal vessels occurs in many mammalian species and was first discovered by Popa and Fielding (1930, 1935). Green and Harris (1947) demonstrated clearly that the direction of the blood flow was from the hypothalamus to the pituitary gland. These findings enabled Green and Harris (1947) to postulate that the hypothalamus controls anterior pituitary function by a neurohumoral mechanism. According to this hypothesis, nerve fibers from the hypothalamus were said to liberate neurohormonal materials into the capillaries of the primary plexus of the portal vessels in the median eminence. These neurohumors were then supposed to be carried by the portal veins of the hypophyseal stalk into the sinusoids of the anterior pituitary gland, where they were assumed to influence the secretion of various pituitary hormones. This view received indirect support from the neurosecretory theory of Bargman (1949) and Scharrer and Scharrer (1954, 1963). These investigators suggested that the posterior pituitary hormones, oxytocin and vasopressin, were formed within the neurosecretory cells of the paraventricular and supraoptic nuclei of the hypothalamus. The hormones were said then to be transported down the axons of the hypothalamohypophyseal tract to nerve endings in the neural lobe which served as their storage and release center. The possible role of neurosecretory neurons in the hypothalamus in the control of pituitary gonadotropic function has been reviewed by Jorgensen (1965). In summary, the neurohumoral theory of the control of LH and FSH secretion assumed that the nerve terminals of hypothalamic nerve fibers liberated humoral transmitters into the capillaries in the median eminence which, after reaching the anterior pituitary, regulated its gonadotropic function.

Physiological and anatomical evidence supporting this view and establishing the importance of the hypophyseal portal vessels in the regulation of anterior pituitary activity (Green and Harris, 1947) accumulated in the years that followed.

B. EFFECT OF STALK SECTION ON LH AND FSH SECRETION

Early evidence based on the techniques of stalk section supported the contention that the hypothalamus controls the gonadotropic function of the pituitary; it has been summarized by Harris (1948b, 1955) and, more recently, by Donovan (1971). Some of the newer results will be briefly discussed below. Where it contributes to the understanding of this recent work, some selected older work also will be reviewed.

Gonadal atrophy has been shown to occur after stalk section in the rat and in the rabbit (Westman and Jacobsohn, 1938, 1940). Earlier experiments involving transection of the pituitary stalk did not always lead to consistent results (Harris, 1955; Everett, 1964). It was stated that since the portal vessels appear to regenerate quickly, the cut ends of the pituitary stalk must be kept apart by artificial barriers of waxed paper or metal foil. Nikitovitch-Winer (1960) repeated the experiments of Westman and Jacobsohn (1938, 1940). After cutting the stalk in adult estrous rats and preventing regeneration of the portal vessels, she found persistent corpora lutea together with atrophy of other sections of the ovaries in rats. This demonstrated diminished secretion of FSH and LH by the pituitary gland separated from the influence of the hypothalamus, although the release of adequate quantities of prolactin continued.

Some of the early literature has been contradictory, but where normal gonadal function was observed after stalk section, it could be explained by regeneration of portal vessels. Greep and Barnett (1951) stated that gonadal atrophy after stalk section could be due in part to the interference with the total blood supply to the pituitary. But Benoit and Assenmacher (1953) showed that section of the portal vessels in the drake abolished the response to light (increase in size of the testes and increased spermatogenesis), even though the anterior lobe was supplied with adequate blood from other sources. This supported the view that the neurosecretory influence of the hypothalamus transmitted via the portal vessels maintains the pituitary secretion of FSH and LH. Donovan and Harris (1954) showed that the hypophyseal portal vessels in the ferret are part of the pathway by which light stimulates anterior pituitary secretion and induces estrous behavior. Although Thomson and Zuckerman (1953) came to diametrically opposed conclusions, their results can be explained by the regeneration of hypophyseal portal vessels. The experiment of Donovan and Harris (1954) clearly indicated that the connecting link for optic impulses from the brain to the pituitary gland involved the hypophyseal portal vessels (Harris, 1955). Thus, it must be concluded that the return of ovarian function after pituitary stalk section in several species is thus directly related to the regeneration of hypophyseal portal vessels (Harris, 1955).

C. Effect of Lesions of the Brain on the FSH and LH Secretion

This subject was also reviewed extensively by Harris (1955) and more recently by Davidson (1966). Electrolytic lesions involving the median eminence and adjacent areas of the basal tuberal-posterior region of the hypothalamus may result in gonadal atrophy in rats, guinea pigs, rabbits, cats, and dogs (Dey *et al.*, 1940; Dey, 1941, 1943; Bogdanove, 1957; Sawyer, 1959; Flerko, 1963). Following such median eminence hypothalamic lesions, pituitaries of male rats have been found to contain decreased amounts of total gonadotropin (Bogdanove *et al.*, 1955; Bogdanove, 1957). Similarly, in dogs with hypothalamic lesions, pituitary content of both LH and FSH was depressed (Davidson *et al.*, 1960). Hypothalamic lesions prevent the normal rise in plasma LH that occurs after ovariectomy in the rat (Taleisnik and McCann, 1961). Disturbances of the cycle, such as the syndrome of persistent vaginal diestrus (characterized by atrophic ovaries and uteri and the persistence of corpora lutea), may also result in rats after median eminence lesions (Dey *et al.*, 1940; Hillarp, 1949). Gorski and Barraclough (1962) reported that destruction of the anterior hypothalamus in androgen-sterilized rats inhibits the release of FSH.

Halasz and Gorski (1967) studied gonadotropin secretion in female rats after partial or total interruption of neural connections to the medial basal hypothalamus by transection with a special knife. They concluded that neural afferents which reach the medial basal hypothalamus are required for ovulation and that the nervous structures responsible for the cyclic release of gonadotropin-releasing hormones are located outside the medial basal hypothalamus, but that they influence the pituitary through it.

D. EFFECT OF ELECTRICAL STIMULATION OF THE HYPOTHALAMUS
   ON THE SECRETION OF LH AND FSH

Early experiments by F. H. A. Marshall and Verney (1936) showed that electrical stimulation applied to the head may result in ovulation and pseudopregnancy in the rabbits. More sophisticated techniques were used by later workers. Electrical stimulation of different regions of the hypothalamus was found to result in the discharge of LH (Harris, 1937; Haterius and Derbyshire, 1937). Harris used the remote control method of stimulation in the unanesthetized rabbit for the localization of the neural structure involved in LH release (Harris, 1948a). The stimulating electrodes were placed in contact with the hypothalamus and other parts of the CNS. In a preliminary operation he implanted a small secondary coil beneath the scalp of the animal, with the electrode penetrating through the skull to the site investigated. The stimulation was produced by placing the head of the animal in an electromagnetic field. Harris (1948a) found that the stimuli applied to the tuber cinereum region of the hypothalamus would cause ovulation. In contrast, the stimuli applied to the pituitary or to the stalk had no effect. That electrical stimulation of the hypothalamus was effective in causing ovulation, but that direct stimulation of the pituitary gland was not, was also demonstrated by Markee *et al.* (1946) in the rabbit.

Critchlow (1958) induced ovulation by hypothalamic stimulation in the pentobarbital-anesthetized rat in proestrus. Everett (1964) discussed differences in the stimulation experiments and pointed out the need to separate results induced by a true electrical stimulation from those caused by indirect irritative stimulation due to electrolytic deposits from the stainless steel electrodes. Everett (1964) also demonstrated that rats in proestrus may release enough LH to induce ovulation within 45 minutes of the stimulation, whereas rats in diestrus required more time.

Quinn (1961) showed that stimulation of the preoptic area of the hypothalamus will increase the release of LH in male as well as in female rats. Barraclough (1963) reported that electrical stimulation of the ventromedial–arcuate region in the progesterone-primed, androgen-sterilized constant-estrus rats reduced the content of LH from 1.2 μg/mg to 0.8 μg/mg and at the same time induced ovulation. Recently Quinn (1969) induced ovulation in guinea pigs by electrical stimulation in various hypothalamic regions. The areas that responded to the stimulation were the same as in the rat, that is the preoptic area, anterior hypothalamus, and the arcuate–nuclear region. On the basis of experiments involving electrochemical stimulation of the hypothalamus, Kalra *et al.* (1971) claimed that there are different loci (sites) controlling the release of LH and FSH. The conditions for induction of ovulation by preoptic stimulation in rats recently were evaluated by Everett *et al.* (1970) and Holsinger and Everett (1970). Sawyer (1970) recently has further reviewed the electrophysiological correlates of the release of pituitary gonadotropins.

Sawyer and Kawakami (1959, 1961) investigated electrical activity and electrical excitability of rabbit brain after coitus or vaginal stimulation. They described a specific sequence of changes in electroencephalographic activity (EEG) after coitus in rabbits.

E. EFFECT OF PITUITARY TRANSPLANTATION ON LH AND FSH SECRETION

It is well established that the secretion of FSH and LH is greatly reduced by transplantation of the pituitary gland to a site remote from hypothalamus. Early experiments of Greep (1936), who hypophysectomized rats and transplanted the pituitaries into the sella turcica, showed that the pituitaries transplanted to their original site, in contrast to those transplanted to other sites, supported sexual functions. Harris and Jacobsohn (1952) grafted rat pituitaries directly into the median eminence. These pituitaries supported cyclical reproductive function. In contrast, pituitaries grafted to the temporal lobe of the brain failed to maintain the gonads. Everett (1956a) and Nikitovitch-Winer and Everett (1957, 1958, 1959) showed that pituitary glands transplanted from the sella turcica to the kidney capsule apparently secreted little FSH and LH and failed to support ovarian functions. In a subsequent operation, after a few weeks had elapsed, the pituitaries were regrafted from the kidney into the median eminence. The gonadotropic function of such retransplanted pituitaries was reinitiated, as demonstrated by the return of the animals to normal estrous cycles and to reproductive capacity. Recently, Piacsek et al. (1969) showed that FSH secretion by transplanted pituitaries could be stimulated by light, but the presence of an intact medial basal hypothalamus was essential for this response. An experiment of Knigge (1962) with neonatal pituitaries showed that by transmitting neurohumors from the median eminence, portal vessels ensure not only normal gonadotropic function but also are capable of inducing maturation of the pituitaries glands grafted nearby. It must be said that the degree of ovarian atrophy seen in rats with a few pituitary grafts in the kidney is not so severe as after complete hypophysectomy. Furthermore, as many as 30 remote pituitary grafts can cause maturation of ovarian follicles and formation of corpora lutea (Gittes and Kastin, 1966). Consequently, the transplanted pituitary secretes some gonadotropin (Hertz, 1960). Some hypothalamic gonadotropin-releasing hormone may in fact reach the transplanted pituitary through the systemic circulation, as suggested by Gittes and Kastin (1966). The recent work of Beddow and McCann (1969) also supports this view. These authors showed that hypothalamic lesions reduced testicular weight in hypophysectomized rats with pituitary transplants.

F. EFFECT OF EXTERNAL ENVIRONMENTAL FACTORS ON LH
   AND FSH SECRETION

Observations on the effect of external environmental factors on the secretion of gonadotropins have been facilitated by the fact that many animals undergo so-called reproductive cycles or rhythms. The onset of reproductive cycles involves the process of maturation of the CNS. Once sexual maturity is achieved in the female of certain species, the reproductive cycles can be affected by many exteroceptive factors.

The seasonal breeding observed in birds and domestic animals can be influenced by various external environmental stimuli. Rowan (1925, 1928) was the first to demonstrate that light exerts a major influence on the reproductive functions of birds. He showed that by artificially increasing the length of the day (light) in late fall and winter it was possible to induce premature sexual activity in migrating birds. Baker and Ranson (1932) and Bissonnette (1932) extended these observations to mammals. In classical studies, F. H. A. Marshall (1936, 1942, 1956) showed that in addition to light the sexual rhythm of mammals is influenced by factors such as temperature and food supply.

Changes in illumination may result in disturbances in the estrous cycle in rats (Critchlow, 1963; Everett, 1964). Thus, continuous lighting may cause persistent estrus in rats. Light acts primarily through the eye and optic nerve, which relay the impulses to the hypothalamus (Wolfson, 1963). It has been shown in several species including the rat that the effects of light on gonadal function require the presence of an intact pituitary (Hill and Parkes, 1933; Benoit, 1935). Fiske (1941) showed that light affects the storage and release of FSH and LH in the rat.

The transmission of optic impulses from the eye to the pituitary involves hypophyseal portal vessels. Benoit and Assenmacher (1951, 1953) and Donovan and Harris (1954, 1956) showed in the duck and in the ferret that intact hypophyseal portal vessels are required to elicit the response to light.

In the Japanese quail, gonadal development is controlled photoperiodically (Mather and Wilson, 1964; Follett and Farner, 1966), as in other birds (Farner, 1965). Recent studies showed that the physiological basis of the photoperiodic response in the quail depends upon a circadian rhythm of "photosensitivity"; thus gonadotropin release occurs only when there is coincidence between light and photosensitive phase of the rhythm (Follett and Sharp, 1969). At least two discrete regions within the quail hypothalamus are essential for gonadotropin secretion to occur. Both are located in the posterior hypothalamus, one in the ventral region around the tuberal (infundibular) nucleus, the other more dorsally in the area of the posterior medial hypothalamic nucleus (Sharp and Follett, 1969; Follett, 1970).

Studies using reflex ovulators, such as rabbits, cats, and ferrets, which ovulate after copulation or genital stimulation, also indicate that LH release and ovulation are controlled by the brain. The stimuli received from the reproductive tract as well as the emotional state of the animal may result in an activation of the anterior pituitary and a discharge of LH (Harris, 1955; Everett, 1964). The effect of light on the ovarian cycle in the rat was recently reviewed by Everett (1970) and in birds by Farner and Follett (1966).

It is also well known that alterations can occur in human reproductive cycles after emotional disturbances. Emotional upsets or electroshock therapy have been reported to cause serious disturbances in the menstrual cycle (Reichlin, 1963; Fuerstner, 1944). Disturbances in gonadotropic function of the pituitary in central nervous system disease were recently reviewed by Peake and Daughaday (1968) and Reichlin (1968).

G. EFFECT OF PHARMACOLOGICAL AGENTS ON LH AND FSH SECRETION

Pioneer studies by Sawyer, Markee, and Everett proved that the release of LH and ovulation depend upon neural stimuli that can be affected by various drugs and steroids. These investigators, and others, studied a wide variety of drugs for their effect on the release of gonadotropins from the pituitary gland, both in spontaneously ovulating species like the rat and in reflex ovulators like the rabbit (Everett et al., 1949; Sawyer et al., 1949, 1950, 1951; Markee et al., 1948, 1952; Everett, 1956b; Everett and Sawyer, 1949, 1950, 1953). These studies demonstrated that both a cholinergic and adrenergic component, acting in sequence, were involved in the neurohumoral mechanism of LH release. These studies will not be summarized here; the reader is referred to the reviews of Everett (1964), Markee et al. (1948, 1952), Harris (1955), and Sawyer (1963, 1965, 1969a). However, the studies on the capacity of certain drugs and pharmacological blocking agents to inhibit the release of pituitary gonadotropins will be briefly described.

A wide variety of drugs—antiadrenergic, anticholinergic, anesthetic, analgesic, and tranquilizing agents—can block the release of pituitary gonadotropin (Sawyer, 1963). After the demonstration that catecholamines could induce ovulation in the rabbit, Sawyer et al. (1951) discovered that a quick postcoital injection of adrenergic blocking agents prevented the release of LH normally discharged by stimulus of copulation. The ovulation blocking activities of these agents, dibenamine and SKF-501, [N-(9-fluorenyl)-N-ethyl-β-chlorethylamine, HCl], were proportional to their adrenergic blocking activities (Sawyer et al., 1950). Anticholinergic agents, atropine (Sawyer et al., 1949), and Banthine (methanthaline) (Sawyer et al., 1951) could cause a similar blockade of copulation-induced ovulation in the rabbit. Atropine and dibenamine could also block the release of pituitary gonadotropin and ovulation in the rat (Sawyer et al., 1949; Everett et al., 1949; Everett, 1951, 1956b; Everett and Sawyer, 1949). To be effective, the blocking agent had to be injected prior to 2 PM on the day of natural or steroid-induced proestrus (Everett, 1956b; Sawyer, 1963). It also was found that simple anesthesia of the rats with ether or barbiturates, or administration of chlorpromazine or reserpine during this critical period (2:00–4:00 PM) on the day of proestrus would block the stimulus and delay ovulation for 24 hours (Everett and Sawyer, 1950; Barraclough and Sawyer, 1957).

Inhibition of cyclic release of pituitary gonadotropin by pharmacological agents has also been observed in other spontaneously ovulating species, such as the hen and cow (Sawyer, 1963). In conclusion, most drugs that block the release of pituitary LH and FSH exert their effects indirectly via the central nervous system (Sawyer, 1963, 1965, 1969a).

H. SUMMARY

The concept of hypothalamic regulation of the secretion of gonadotropins from the anterior pituitary gland was established by experiments involving lesions and electrical stimulation of the hypothalamus, interruption of the blood vessels between the hypothalamus and the pituitary by sectioning the pituitary stalk, and transplantation of the pituitary to various sites. The experiments revealed that regulation of secretion of LH and FSH from the pituitary may be dependent on the integrity of its hypophyseal portal blood supply (Harris, 1955). It was assumed that these portal vessels carried neurohumoral agent(s), now known as releasing hormone(s), whose function was to stimulate the secretion of LH and FSH from the anterior pituitary. Procedures such as hypothalamic lesions, pituitary stalk section and transplantation of the pituitary, which interfered with the production or distribution of hypothalamic hormone(s) controlling gonadotropins release resulted in deprivation of anterior lobe of the hormone(s) (Halasz, 1962; Bogdanove, 1964) and in the ensuing gonadal deficiency or failure. Other studies (Sawyer, 1963) also clearly implicated the CNS in the control of release of gonadotropins.

IV. CHEMISTRY AND PHYSIOLOGY OF LH-RELEASING HORMONE (LH-RH) AND FSH-RELEASING HORMONE (FSH-RH)

A. DEMONSTRATION OF HYPOTHALAMIC LH-RH AND FSH-RH

The work summarized in the preceding section, based on anatomical and physiological evidence, suggested that the CNS and hypothalamus control gonadotropic function of the anterior pituitary gland through a neurohumoral mechanism. However, direct evidence for the specific chemotransmitter involved in the release of LH and FSH was lacking. Demonstration of the existence of corticotropin-releasing factor in posterior pituitary and hypothalamic materials (Saffran and Schally, 1955; Saffran et al., 1955; Schally et al., 1958) opened the way for the investigation of the presence of other regulators of anterior pituitary function.

The first direct evidence for the existence of a hypothalamic neurohumor regulating LH release was provided independently by McCann et al. (1960) and by G. W. Harris and his group (Harris, 1961; Campbell et al., 1961). That hypothalamic extracts of at least 7 animal species are capable of stimulating LH release was subsequently demonstrated by several groups of investigators (Courrier *et al.*, 1961; Nikitovitch-Winer, 1962; Guillemin *et al.*, 1963a; Schally and Bowers, 1964a,b; Campbell *et al.*, 1964; McCann *et al.*, 1965; Fawcett *et al.*, 1965; Endroczi and Hilliard, 1965; Schally *et al.*, 1965a, 1967a; Piacsek and Meites, 1966).

In the same period, hypothalamic extracts or highly purified substances obtained from them were also shown to be capable of stimulating the release of thyrotropin (Schreiber *et al.*, 1962; Guillemin *et al.*, 1963b; Bowers *et al.*, 1964), growth hormone (Deuben and Meites, 1964; Schally *et al.*, 1965c), and FSH (Mittler and Meites, 1964; Igarashi and Mc-Cann, 1964b; Kuroshima *et al.*, 1965) and of inhibiting the release of prolactin (Talwalker *et al.*, 1963; Schally *et al.*, 1965b) and melanocyte-stimulating hormone (Kastin and Schally, 1966). Thus, in about a decade after the demonstration of the first hypothalamic hormone (Saffran and Schally, 1955), the presence of at least six other activities in the hypothalamus was clearly established.

B. FSH-RH ACTIVITY IN HYPOTHALAMIC EXTRACTS OF VARIOUS
   SPECIES AND EARLY METHODS FOR ITS DETECTION

Meites and Mittler used tissue cultures of rat pituitaries and showed that pituitary tissue cultured with rat cerebral cortical extract did not release much FSH, whereas pituitaries cultured with rat hypothalamic extract released highly significant amounts of FSH (Mittler and Meites, 1964) as measured by the specific Steelman and Pohley assay (1953).

Igarashi and McCann (1964b) also used crude rat hypothalamic extracts and demonstrated that 10 minutes after the intravenous injection of a crude acidic extract of 2 rat stalk–median eminences, a significant elevation in plasma FSH occurred in the ovariectomized, estrogen, progesterone-blocked rats, whereas cerebral cortical extract was without effect. Stalk–median eminence extract also increased FSH activity in the plasma of ovariectomized rats in which release of FSH had been blocked by hypothalamic lesions, whereas cortical extract was ineffective under these conditions. They concluded that an FSH-releasing activity resides in hypothalamic tissue. However, the measurement of FSH activity in blood was performed by the controversial method of Igarashi and Mc-Cann (1964a), which is based on the increase in uterine weight in mice. This method was later criticized by deReviers and Mauleon (1965) and Lamond and Bindon (1966) as being nonspecific. Gellert *et al.* (1964) used crude beef hypothalamic extracts and showed an induction of precocious vaginal opening in immature female rats through the release of pituitary FSH.

Our laboratory used boiled acid extracts of stalk–median eminence tissue of ovine, bovine, and porcine origin to demonstrate elevations of plasma FSH levels in ovariectomized rats pretreated with estrogen and progesterone as well as accelerated FSH release *in vitro* (Kuroshima *et al.*, 1964, 1965; Schally *et al.*, 1965a). The incubation medium and plasma were assayed for FSH by the Steelman–Pohley (1953) and the Igarashi–McCann (1964a) methods. Later, we developed test systems for FSH-RH activity based on depletion of pituitary FSH content in ovariectomized rats with or without pretreatment with estrogen and progesterone (Kuroshima *et al.*, 1966) and in castrated male rats pretreated with testosterone propionate (Schally *et al.*, 1966b, 1967d; Saito *et al.*, 1967a). We have also utilized the Corbin and Story (1966) modification of the test of David *et al.* (1965a), which is based on depletion of pituitary FSH content in normal male rats. Using the Steelman–Pohley method for assays of pituitary FSH, it was demonstrated that rat, pig, beef, and human stalk–median eminence extracts depleted pituitary FSH content in recipient rats. A rise in plasma FSH in castrated male rats pretreated with testosterone or ovariectomized female rats pretreated with estrogen and progesterone, was found by the Igarashi–McCann method (1964b) to occur simultaneously with the depletion of pituitary FSH content (Kuroshima *et al.*, 1966; Saito *et al.*, 1967a). The possible nonspecificity of these pituitary depletion methods later became apparent.

C. LH-RH ACTIVITY IN HYPOTHALAMIC EXTRACTS OF VARIOUS SPECIES AND EARLY METHODS FOR ITS DETECTION

Some of the early studies on LH-releasing activity, although elegant, were carried out with crude extracts that contained LH and vasopressin. Others were performed with only partially purified LH-RH preparations. Some groups utilized assays for LH-RH based directly on ovarian ascorbic acid depletion in immature rats pretreated with gonadotropin (McCann and Taleisnik, 1962), whereas others used the induction of ovulation in rats or rabbits (Campbell *et al.*, 1961, 1964; Nikitovitch-Winer, 1962).

Our laboratory was the first to demonstrate LH-RH activity in purified fractions of hypothalamic extracts both on the basis of *in vitro* and of *in vivo* assays (Schally and Bowers, 1964a). Before defining a substance as a hypothalamic hormone, such as LH-RH, it should be shown to be active *in vitro*, since *in vitro* tests are based on incubation of isolated rat pituitary tissue and involve complete disruption of hypothalamohypophyseal connections. Thus, an *in vitro* test can prove that the neurohumor acts directly on pituitary tissue.

The group of McCann carried out physiological studies with crude rat hypothalamic extract and should be credited with providing solid physiological evidence for the existence of LH-RH. The most frequently used techniques in this early work are listed below:

1. *Ovarian Ascorbic Acid Depletion in Immature Test Rats*

McCann and Taleisnik (1962) prepared crude hydrochloric acid extracts of rat stalk–median eminence tissue and injected them intravenously into immature female rats, which had been pretreated with gonadotrophins as in the assay for LH of Parlow (1961). Immediately prior to injection, an ovary was removed to obtain a control concentration of ovarian ascorbic acid. One hour after injection of extracts, the second ovary was removed and the depletion of ovarian ascorbic acid could thereby by calculated. McCann and Taleisnik found that stalk-median eminence extracts evoked an ovarian ascorbic acid depletion and elicited a dose response curve, even though the pituitaries of these rats were low in LH. They concluded that this crude hypothalamic extract evoked LH release from the hypophysis (McCann and Taleisnik, 1962).

2. *Elevation of Plasma LH in Donor Animals*

Ten minutes after intravenous injection of hypothalamic preparations into suitably prepared rats, blood was collected from these donor animals and plasma was assayed for LH by the Parlow method (Parlow, 1961).

a. McCann and Ramirez (1964) found that significant elevation in plasma LH activity was produced by the hypothalamic extract within 10 minutes of its injection into female rats in which the plasma LH had been lowered by the prior destruction of the median eminence region of the hypothalamus.

b. A consistent elevation of plasma LH after the injection of hypothalamic extracts was also found to occur in chronically ovariectomized rats pretreated 72 hours previously with subcutaneous injections of estradiol benzoate plus progesterone. This treatment with steroids lowered plasma LH below the elevated levels found in the ovariectomized animal, and the effect of hypothalamic extract in elevating plasma LH could be easily demonstrated (McCann and Taleisnik, 1962; McCann *et al.*, 1961; Ramirez and McCann, 1963b).

3. *Induction of Ovulation in Rabbits*

Harris (1961) and Campbell *et al.* (1961, 1964) infused beef hypothalamic extract into the anterior pituitary of estrous female rabbits and consistently caused ovulation in most animals. Infusion of control substances (including other brain extracts) rarely caused ovulation in the animals tested. Since ovulation in rabbits is attributable to the action of a sudden surge of luteinizing hormone from the pituitary, they used this technique as a bioassay for the purification of LH releasing activity from beef and sheep hypothalamic tissue.

4. *In Vitro Release of LH*

The *in vitro* pituitary incubation system of Saffran and Schally (1955) was modified by Schally and Bowers (1964a) for the study of stimulation of luteinizing hormone (LH) secretion. The modification consisted of the use of pituitaries from chronically ovariectomized and estrogen-progesterone-treated rats. The basal rate of LH secretion *in vitro* was established. Purified preparations of LH-releasing hormone of bovine and ovine origin (free of LH) were shown to effect significant stimulation of LH release *in vitro*. These preparations were also active *in vivo* in depleting ovarian ascorbic acid in immature rats pretreated with gonadotropins and in increasing plasma LH levels in rats chronically ovariectomized and estrogen-progesterone-pretreated rats by the method of Ramirez and McCann (1963b). Thus, the results of the *in vitro* experiments were in agreement with those from the *in vivo* studies (Schally and Bowers, 1964a).

5. *Induction of Ovulation in Rats*

The method by Nikitovitch-Winer (1962) for measuring LH-releasing activity was based on the induction of ovulation in pentobarbital-treated proestrus rats.

6. *Other Methods*

Increased release of LH after administration of hypothalamic extracts could also be measured in rabbits by progestin secretion from ovaries of pregnant or pseudopregnant rabbits (Endroczi and Hilliard, 1965).

The methods described above and their variations were utilized for demonstrating the presence of LH-RH activity in extracts of hypothalamus from rats (Courrier *et al.*, 1961; Nikitovitch-Winer, 1962; Piacsek and Meites, 1966; Stevens *et al.*, 1968), rabbits (Campbell *et al.*, 1961, 1964; Endroczi and Hilliard, 1965), guinea pigs (Barry *et al.*, 1967), dogs (Endroczi and Hilliard, 1965), sheep (Guillemin *et al.*, 1963a; Schally and Bowers, 1964a; McCann *et al.*, 1965), cattle (Nikitovitch-Winer, 1962; Schally and Bowers, 1964b; Fawcett *et al.*, 1965; Schally *et al.*, 1965a, 1968a), monkeys (Campbell *et al.*, 1964), pigs (Schally *et al.*, 1967a), and man (Schally *et al.*, 1967e). Recently, gonadotropin-releasing activity was similarly found in quail hypothalamus (Follett, 1970).

D. Purification of FSH-RH Activity from Hypothalamic Extracts of Domestic Animals

1. Bovine FSH-RH

Acetic acid extracts of beef hypothalami were subjected to gel filtration on columns of Sephadex G-25 in 0.1 M pyridine acetate (Schally et al., 1966b). Subsequently, the zone with FSH-releasing activity was concentrated by phenol extraction and then chromatographed on columns of carboxymethyl cellulose. This step separated FSH-releasing activity from TRH. The FSH-releasing substance thus purified was able to deplete pituitary FSH content in vivo at the doses of 10 μg dry weight, equivalent to 0.2 hypothalamus (Schally et al., 1966b), but some doubt remains whether these materials represented polyamines or FSH-RH.

2. Ovine FSH-RH

Dhariwal et al. (1965b) claimed the purification of ovine FSH-RH and its separation from LH-RH. The purification steps included gel filtration on Sephadex and CMC chromatography. As in the case of beef FSH-releasing activity, considerable uncertainty exists as to the true FSH-RH nature of these concentrates. Jutisz and De La Llosa (1967) also reported the purification of ovine FSH-RH by gel filtration on Sephadex and ion-exchange chromatography.

3. Porcine FSH-RH

FSH-releasing activity in lyophilized acetic acid extracts of hypothalamic tissue of porcine origin was concentrated by reextraction with glacial acetic acid and then subjected to purification by several successive methods. The fractionation procedure consisted of gel filtration on Sephadex G-25, concentration by phenol extraction, chromatography and rechromatography on carboxymethyl cellulose, and column electrophoresis. FSH-RH activity was measured by depletion of pituitary FSH content in castrated male rats pretreated with testosterone as well as in normal male rats. In these tests, highly purified FSH-RH was active in vivo at doses of the order of 10 ng. Since these fractions also released FSH from isolated rat pituitaries incubated in vitro, they must have contained some true FSH-RH. It was also stated that, after purification by column electrophoresis, FSH-RH was freed of LH-RH (Schally et al., 1967d), but now this does not appear to be correct.

In subsequent work, White et al. (1968) isolated five polyamine substances from porcine hypothalamic extracts. They stated that together these substances accounted for most of the FSH-depleting activity in crude hypothalamic extracts when tested by the depletion of pituitary FSH levels in normal and in castrated, testosterone-pretreated male rats. Of the substances isolated, histamine was present in the highest amount. However, in the assay method used, histamine was active only in microgram doses, whereas putrescine, which occurred in smaller amounts, was active in doses of a few nanograms. Spermidine, spermine, and lysine, which have also been identified, were active in the pituitary depletion test at intermediate dose levels (White et al., 1968). Although it was not stated that these polyamines represented FSH-RH, a strong implication of this was conveyed nevertheless.

Subsequent work by Schally et al. (1970d) showed that low concentrations of putrescine, cadaverine, spermine, spermidine, and agmatine did not enhance the release of FSH from anterior pituitaries of male rats incubated in vitro. All the polyamines tested were equally ineffective when incubated with pituitaries in the presence of hypothalamic tissue. In contrast, highly purified porcine FSH-releasing hormone (FSH-RH), in a dose 1000 times lower than the dose of putrescine tested, significantly stimulated FSH release in vitro by pituitaries from normal intact male rats, ovariectomized rats pretreated with estrogen and progesterone, and castrated rats pretreated with testosterone propionate. The results clearly demonstrated that the polyamine substances tested did not represent the true FSH-RH (Schally et al., 1968a, 1970d). Kamberi and McCann (1969) reached the same conclusion.

Although the separation of FSH-RH activity from LH-RH was claimed, it appears now that the electrophoretic experiments in question (Schally et al., 1967d; White et al., 1968) separated from LH-RH only putrescine and other polyamines found in hypothalamic extracts. These polyamines were said to have FSH-RH activity on the basis of depletion of pituitary FSH content in vivo (Schally et al., 1966b, 1967d, 1968a; White et al., 1968). However, the depletion of pituitary FSH content may not be a specific test for FSH-RH activity. As stated above, it is now well established on the basis of specific in vitro assays, that these polyamines do not represent the primary physiological FSH-RH which acts directly on the pituitary gland (Schally et al., 1968a, 1970d). However, another amine, dopamine, may be involved not in the release of FSH, but of FSH-RH (Kamberi et al., 1970b) (see Section XI).

The claims of the separation of FSH-RH from LH-RH, described in the sections above, may only be of historical significance, since recent studies established with a high degree of probability that, at least in the pig, LH-RH is identical with FSH-RH (see below).

E. PURIFICATION OF LH-RH ACTIVITY FROM HYPOTHALAMIC EXTRACTS

1. Bovine LH-RH

Schally and Bowers (1964b) extracted hypothalamic tissue of bovine origin with $2 N$ acetic acid at 8°C. The acetic acid extracts were lyophilized and subjected to gel filtration on Sephadex columns. LH-RH activity was followed by *in vivo* and *in vitro* tests. Emerging from Sephadex before arginine vasopressin, LH-RH was then further purified by chromatography on carboxymethyl cellulose. The purified LH-RH was active *in vivo* in doses of 5 μg. The amino acids found in the hydrolyzates of purified LH-RH indicated that LH-RH might be a basic polypeptide different from oxytocin and vasopressin (Schally and Bowers, 1964b).

Fawcett *et al.* (1968) also used beef median eminence tissue as a source of LH-RH for small-scale experiments to explore methods for its isolation. Its presence was detected by the ovulation response in rabbits after intrapituitary infusion of the extract. Gel filtration was found to be suitable for the purification of these extracts. Fawcett *et al.* concluded that LH-RH appeared to be a basic peptide of molecular weight in the range 1200–2500.

2. Purification of Porcine LH-RH

Schally *et al.* (1967a) concentrated LH-RH activity in acetic acid extracts of pig hypothalamic tissue by a precipitation-extraction procedure and then subjected it to purification by several successive techniques. The purification procedure consisted of gel filtration on Sephadex G-25, concentration by phenol extraction, chromatography and rechromatography on carboxymethyl cellulose, and column electrophoresis (Schally *et al.*, 1967a). Although it was said that column electrophoresis freed LH-RH of FSH-RH activity, this may have been due only to removal of some polyamines which were active in the FSH depletion tests. Later, using specific assays, it was found that, during the fractionation of pig hypothalamic extracts, the location of FSH-RH activity always coincided with that of LH-RH (Schally *et al.*, 1971b, 1972d) (see below).

3. The Hypothesis of a Common Releasing Hormone for LH and FSH

Initially, it was thought that two different substances were responsible for stimulating release of LH and FSH (McCann and Ramirez, 1964; McCann *et al.*, 1965; Schally *et al.*, 1968a; Harris and Naftolin, 1970). However, it became necessary to question this when porcine LH-RH, obtained in a high state of purity, stimulated release of both LH and

FSH in rats, chimpanzees, and human beings (White, 1970a,b; Schally *et al.*, 1970b, 1971d,e; Kastin *et al.*, 1969, 1970a). Furthermore, after the addition of highly purified porcine LH-RH to rat pituitaries incubated *in vitro*, LH and FSH were released simultaneously with superimposable time courses (White, 1970a).

It was not clear at first whether this FSH-releasing activity of porcine LH-RH was an intrinsic property of its molecule or whether it was due to a contamination with FSH-RH. Chemical and enzymatic inactivation of LH-RH was always accompanied by loss of FSH-releasing activity (White, 1970a,b; Schally *et al.*, 1970b, 1971d,e). Moreover, the LH-RH activity could not be separated from FSH-RH by the use of the most advanced fractionation techniques (Schally *et al.*, 1971e). This dilemma was solved after the isolation, elucidation of structure and synthesis of porcine LH-RH when it was found that natural and synthetic materials stimulated the release of both LH and FSH (see section below).

4. *Isolation of Pig LH-RH*

The isolation of pig LH-RH was achieved by two different methods (Schally *et al.*, 1971i).

a. The first method (Schally *et al.*, 1971b) was initially utilized for concentration of extracts from 160,000 pig hypothalami; the procedure is described under Section IV-E-2: (1) gel filtration on Sephadex G-25, (2) phenol extraction and (3) chromatography, and (4) rechromatography on carboxymethyl cellulose columns. The first isolation of porcine LH-RH, was then carried out by the following steps: (5) free-flow electrophoresis (FFE) in pyridine acetate buffer, (6) countercurrent distribution (CCD) in a system of 0.1% acetic acid:1-butanol:pyridine = 11:5:3 (v/v) for 500 transfers, (7) partition chromatography on a column of Sephadex G-25, using a solvent system which consisted of 1-butanol:acetic acid:water:benzene = 4:1:5:0.33, (8) column partition chromatography using a solvent system consisting of 1-butanol:ethanol:water:acetic acid:pyridine:benzene = 25:7:30:2:1:10, and (9) high voltage zone electrophoresis in pyridine acetate buffer, pH 6.3, on a vertical column packed with cellulose powder (Porath, 1957).

LH-RH thus obtained was apparently homogeneous by chromatography and electrophoresis. The isolated LH-RH stimulated the release of FSH and LH *in vivo* and *in vitro* in doses of a few nanograms (Schally *et al.*, 1971b). FSH-RH activity appeared to be intrinsic to LH-RH. The amino acid composition of this LH-RH as determined on acid hydrolyzates was: His 1, Arg 1, Ser 1, Glu 1, Pro 1, Gly 2, Leu 1, and Tyr 1 (Schally *et al.*, 1971b). Subsequent acid hydrolyses by the method of Matsubara and Sasaki (1969) in the presence of thioglycolate revealed the additional presence of the residue of tryptophan (Matsuo *et al.*, 1971b).

b. Another method which led to the isolation of LH-RH in a very high yield from extracts of 250,000 pig hypothalami was based mainly on countercurrent distribution (CCD) and was simpler and more elegant (Schally *et al.*, 1971h,i). The steps in this procedure were as follows: (1) preparative gel filtration of pig hypothalamic extracts on a large column of Sephadex G-25 using 1 *M* acetic acid as a solvent, (2) concentration and desalting by phenol extraction, (3) preparative CCD in a system of 0.1% acetic acid:1-butanol:pyridine, 11:5:3, by the single withdrawal method for 250 transfers, (4) chromatography on a carboxymethyl cellulose column, using ammonium acetate buffers, (5) countercurrent distribution in a system of 0.1% acetic acid:1-butanol: pyridine = 11:5:3 (v/v) for 800 transfers with recycling, (6) countercurrent distribution in a system of 1-butanol:acetic acid:water = 4:1:5 (v/v) for 900 transfers.

The yield from 240,000 porcine hypothalami was 11.4 mg. Thin-layer chromatography and electrophoresis showed that the material was homogeneous. The amino acid analysis showed, as before, the presence of 2 residues of glycine and one residue each of histidine, arginine, tryptophan, serine glutamic acid, proline, leucine, and tyrosine. The decapeptide stimulated release of both LH and FSH *in vivo* as well as *in vitro* in doses less than 1 ng (Schally *et al.*, 1971i).

5. *Purification of Ovine LH-RH*

Several groups of investigators used sheep hypothalamic extracts for the purification of LH-RH.

a. In early studies Guillemin *et al.* (1963a) purified LH-RH by gel filtration on Sephadex followed by ion-exchange chromatography on carboxymethyl cellulose. Dhariwal *et al.* (1965a) used the same methods.

b. Jutisz *et al.* (1967) obtained a highly purified ovine LH-RH by fractionation of hypothalamic extract on a Sephadex G-25 column, chromatography on Dowex 50 and on Amberlite CG-4B. After the last step of this method, which consisted of chromatography on a carboxymethyl cellulose column, a material about 1600 times more potent than the crude extract was obtained.

c. Fawcett *et al.* (1968) used an extract of sheep hypothalamic tissue to establish a multistage isolation procedure that resulted in a great purification of LH-RH. The purification process consisted of: (1) two cycles of gel filtration, (2) anion-exchange chromatography, (3) gel filtration in a partially organic medium, and (4) thin-layer chromatography on cellulose. The LH-RH thus prepared contained only five or six peptide components, but the small amounts obtained were insufficient for full characterization (Fawcett *et al.*, 1968).

d. In subsequent studies, many modifications in the purification procedures for sheep LH-RH were introduced by the group of Burgus and Guillemin. In 1966, Guillemin and his associates suggested that TRH and LH-RH may not be polypeptides (Guillemin *et al.*, 1966; Guillemin, 1967a,b). This wrong hypothesis caused much confusion, which was only partially reversed by the demonstration of 3 amino acids in the TRH molecule (Schally *et al.*, 1966a). Guillemin *et al.* (1966) also criticized the use of CCD for the purification of TRH and LH-RH. In 1971, Amoss *et al.* reported the purification of ovine LH-RH from lyophilized ovine hypothalami by the steps of (1) alcohol–chloroform extraction, (2) ultrafiltration through Diaflo Membranes (UM-05), (3) gel filtration on Sephadex G-25 in 0.5 *M* acetic acid, (4) ion-exchange chromatography on CMC, (5) column electrophoresis, (6) partition chromatography in 0.1% acetic acid:1-butanol:acetic acid:water, 4:1:5. The amino acids found in ovine LH-RH were similar to those already reported by Schally *et al.* (1971b) and Matsuo *et al.* (1971b), but tryptophan was not detected or mentioned. It was also reported that the ovine material stimulated the release of FSH concomitantly with LH (Amoss *et al.*, 1971).

6. *Purification of Human LH-RH and FSH-RH*

Acetic acid extracts of more than 300 defatted human hypothalami were concentrated and then subjected to separation by several successive steps in order to purify and characterize human FSH-releasing hormone and LH-releasing hormone. LH-RH was measured by elevation of plasma LH in rats and FSH-RH was assayed by stimulation of FSH release *in vitro*. FSH and LH in plasma or the incubation medium were measured by bioassay and radioimmunoassay. Gel filtration on Sephadex G-25 separated TRH, LH-RH, and FSH-RH activity from GH-RH. LH-RH and FSH-RH activity was concentrated by phenol extraction and then chromatographed on carboxymethyl cellulose. This procedure separated TRH from LH-RH and FSH-RH. It was found that the behavior of human LH-RH and FSH-RH on Sephadex and carboxymethyl cellulose was identical with that of LH-RH and FSH-RH of porcine and bovine origin. The amount of material available did not permit the comparison of human and porcine LH-RH in other physicochemical systems. LH-RH fractions were always associated with considerable FSH-RH activity. It appeared that this FSH-RH releasing activity was intrinsic to human LH-RH rather than due to contamination with FSH-RH. It was concluded that hypothalamic releasing hormones were present in man and that their chemical characteristics (molecular weights, isoelectric points, etc.) were very similar to those of domestic animals (Schally *et al.*, 1970a).

F. CHEMICAL PROPERTIES OF LH-RH AND FSH-RH

At the 1969 NIH workshop conference on hypothalamic hormones, Fawcett reviewed the existing evidence and concluded that the chemical properties of LH-RH and FSH-RH were so poorly defined that there was much disagreement as to their chemical nature as well as their stability to chemical and enzymatic treatments (Fawcett, 1970). The results of these early experiments will not be repeated here.

Schally and his associates established the first clear evidence for the peptide nature of LH- and FSH-releasing hormone. They studied the effects of several enzymatic and chemical treatments on the biological activity of highly purified porcine LH-RH and FSH-RH (Schally *et al.*, 1971d,e,f; Baba *et al.*, 1971a,b,c). The conclusions were that LH-RH and FSH-RH activity were not affected by trypsin, pepsin, neuraminidase, carboxypeptidase A and B, leucine aminopeptidase, and aminopeptidase M. However, incubation with endopeptidases, such as chymotrypsin, subtilisin, and papain, abolished the LH-RH/FSH-RH activity (Table I).

In the initial experiments, aminopeptidase M and leucine aminopeptidase were reported to inactivate LH-RH (Schally *et al.*, 1971d). However, better preparation of these enzymes were later shown not to affect LH-RH activity (Baba *et al.*, 1971c; Schally *et al.*, 1971b) (Table I). Inactivation of LH-RH of ovine origin by pyrrolidone carboxylyl (PCA) peptidase from *Bacillus subtilis* was reported by Amoss *et al.* (1970). However, a significant contamination of such preparations by endopeptidases is known (Baba *et al.*, 1971a). Consequently, Baba *et al.* (1971b,c) carried out experiments with this enzyme using an A-25 preparation of PCA-peptidase (Doolittle and Armentrout, 1968), the action of which was confined more specifically to the pyroglutamyl linkage. After this treatment, about 80% of the LH-RH activity was destroyed (Baba *et al.*, 1971c) (Table I). The presence of an N-terminal pyroglutamyl residue in LH-RH explained the lack of inactivation by several exopeptidases and by Edman degradation. The resistence to trypsin was later explained by the presence of the Arg-Pro bond.

Before the structure of LH-RH was elucidated, the substance was also examined for the presence of sugar moieties because of the possible similarity of LH-RH to the glycoproteins LH and FSH. No evidence for the presence of a sugar moiety in the LH-RH molecule was found by structural analysis. Neuraminidase did not affect LH-RH activity, and periodate caused only a partial inactivation which was explained by

TABLE I

EFFECT OF VARIOUS PROTEOLYTIC ENZYMES ON THE BIOLOGICAL ACTIVITY OF
LH-RH AND FSH-RH[a,b]

Treatment	LH-RH activity	FSH-RH activity
pH 8.1 buffer	No effect	No effect
pH 2 buffer	No effect	No effect
pH 5.1 buffer	No effect	No effect
Trypsin	No effect	No effect
Pepsin	No effect	No effect
Chymotrypsin	Inactivation	Inactivation
Subtilisin	Inactivation	Inactivation
Papain	Inactivation	Inactivation
Aminopeptidase M	No effect	No effect
Leucine aminopeptidase	No effect	No effect
PCA-peptidase[c]	Inactivation	Inactivation
Carboxypeptidase A	No effect	No effect
Carboxypeptidase B	No effect	No effect
Carboxypeptidases A and B	No effect	No effect

[a] Revised from Schally et al. (1971d). Courtesy of Biochem. Biophys. Res. Commun. and Academic Press, New York.

[b] E:S = 1:10 for all enzymes except PCA peptidase. Incubated at 37°C for 20 hours, except for carboxypeptidases A and B, which was 48 hours. When inactivation was denoted, it was essentially complete.

[c] PCA peptidase = pyrrolidone carboxylyl peptidase.

oxidation of the tryptophan residue (Schally et al., 1971d; Baba et al., 1971c). To check for the possible presence of a glycosidic linkage between a sugar moiety and the hydroxyl group of serine, LH-RH was treated with 0.5 N NaOH for 3 days. The activity was completely abolished. No amino acid contained in this peptide was significantly decomposed under these conditions. However, dansylation of the product resulting from the treatment of LH-RH with 0.5 N NaOH revealed that partial cleavage of several peptide bonds as well as the opening of the pyrrolidone ring in the pyroglutamyl residue had occurred under these conditions.

LH-RH preparations were also treated with various other chemical reagents which are known to specifically modify certain amino acids (Table II). The inactivation which occurred after treatment with N-Bromosuccinimide is in agreement with the presence of tyrosine, tryptophan, and histidine. The importance of tyrosine and/or histidine residues for the biological activity of LH-RH was also demonstrated by the inactivation after treatment with diazotized sulfanilic acid (Pauly's reagent). The reaction with acetic anhydride was tried in two kinds of media. Acetylation in pyridine abolished the LH-RH activity, whereas

TABLE II
EFFECT OF VARIOUS CHEMICAL TREATMENTS ON BIOLOGICAL ACTIVITY OF
LH-RH AND FSH-RH[a]

Treatment	LH-RH	FSH-RH
HCl 0.9 M, 60 minutes, 100°C	Inactivation	Inactivation
N-Bromosuccinimide	Inactivation	Inactivation
Diazotized sulfanilic acid	Inactivation	Inactivation
Sodium carbonate, 5%	No effect	No effect
Nitrous acid	No effect	No effect
2-Hydroxy-5-nitrobenzyl bromide	Inactivation	Inactivation
Sodium periodate	Partial inactivation	Partial inactivation
0.5 N NaOH	Inactivation	Inactivation
Glyoxal	Inactivation	Inactivation

[a] Revised from Schally et al. (1971d). Courtesy of Biochem. Biophys. Res. Commun. and Academic Press, New York.

that in aqueous sodium bicarbonate caused only a partial inactivation. The hydroxyl groups of both the serine and tyrosine residue would be acetylated in pyridine, but only the tyrosine residue is affected by acetylation in aqueous sodium bicarbonate. These results suggest that the hydroxyl group of serine is essential for the LH-RH activity, but that the phenolic hydroxyl group of tyrosine might not be. Lack of inactivation by nitrous acid was explained by the absence of lysine and of free N-terminal group (Baba et al., 1971c).

Glyoxal abolished the LH-RH activity completely, demonstrating the essential character of the guanidyl group in the arginine residue. The effect of 2-hydroxy-5-nitrobenzyl bromide on the biological activity of a preparation of pure porcine LH- and FSH-releasing hormone (LH-RH/FSH-RH) was also investigated. Since this treatment, as well as performic acid and incubation with anhydrous trifluoroacetic acid, caused a complete inactivation of LH-RH and FSH-RH, the tryptophan residue was deemed to be essential for the biological activity of this polypeptide (Baba et al., 1971b; Bogentoft et al., 1971). In all these experiments, the patterns of the inactivation of FSH-RH activity completely paralleled those of LH-RH activity (Schally et al., 1971e). The structure–activity relationship for LH-RH/FSH-RH was recently reviewed by Baba et al. (1971c).

G. DETERMINATION OF THE STRUCTURE OF
    PORCINE LH-RH/FSH-RH

The amino acid sequence of porcine LH-RH was first provisionally determined by Matsuo et al. (1971b) by the use on a microscale of the combined Edman-dansyl procedure (Gray, 1967; Hartley, 1970), coupled with the selective tritiation method for C-terminal analysis (Matsuo et al., 1966; Matsubara and Sasaki, 1969). These procedures were used directly after digestion of LH-RH with chymotrypsin and thermolysin, without separation of the fragments. Additional data were provided by high-resolution mass spectral fragmentation of LH-RH. On the basis of these results, the following decapeptide sequence for LH-RH was proposed: (pyro)Glu-His-Trp-Ser-Tyr-Gly-Leu-Arg-Pro-Gly-NH₂ (Matsuo et al., 1971b).

This proposed amino acid sequence of porcine LH-RH was reinvestigated (Baba et al., 1971a) by Edman–dansyl degradation after cleavage of the N-terminal pyroglutamyl residue by pyrrolidonecarboxylyl (PCA) peptidase (Doolittle and Armentrout, 1968). The G-200 preparation of this enzyme was found to be unsatisfactory because of probable contamination with endopeptidases. A more purified A-25 preparation of PCA-peptidase was then used. Digestion of LH-RH by this enzyme, followed by Edman–dansyl degradation, first revealed DNS-histidine. This confirmed the (pyro)Glue-His linkage, previously unproved. When Edman-dansyl degradation was continued until the ninth step, the amino acid sequence His-Trp-Ser-Tyr-Gly-Leu-Arg-Pro-Gly was clearly confirmed.

Other experiments revealed that a C-terminal fragment from the chymotryptic digest of LH-RH was identical with synthetic Gly-Leu-Arg-Pro-Gly-NH₂. The results indicated that the structure provisionally proposed was correct. The amino acid sequence of porcine LH-RH/FSH-RH was thus confirmed as (pyro)Glu-His-Trp-Ser-Tyr-Gly-Leu-Arg-Pro-Gly-NH₂ (Baba et al., 1971a).

The structure of porcine LH-RH (Fig. 1) was also reconfirmed by mass spectroscopy (Nair and Schally, 1972). LH-RH was subjected to high and low resolution mass spectral fragmentation before and after formation of derivatives by ¹⁴C-acetylation, methanolysis, and ¹⁴C-permethylation. The di- and triketopiperazines revealed in the mass spectra of free LH-RH, together with the sequential fragmentation pattern of the ¹⁴C-

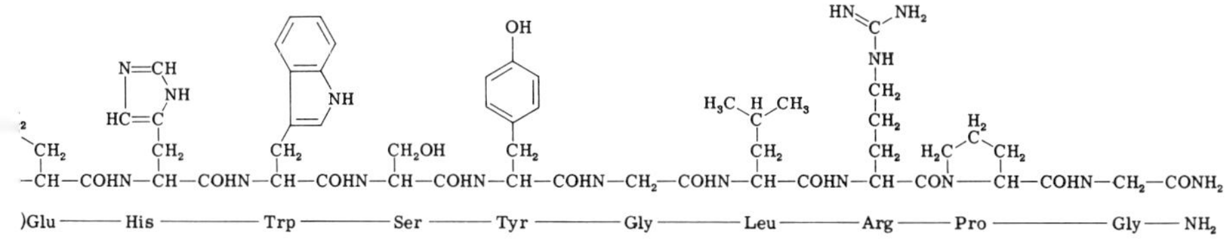

Fig. 1. Molecular structure of porcine LH- and FSH-releasing hormone (LH-RH/FSH-RH).

acetylated and permethylated LH-RH, showed the amino acid sequence to be (pyro)Glu-His-Trp-Ser-Tyr-Gly-Leu-Arg-Pro-Gly-NH₂. This structure was in agreement with our sequential work by methods described above.

H. SYNTHESIS OF LH-RH

Synthetic work further confirmed that the structure established for LH-RH was correct. The synthesis of LH-RH (Matsuo *et al.*, 1971a) was carried out by the solid phase method (Stewart and Young, 1969; Merrifield, 1967).

The protected decapeptide resin ester (Boc-Gln-His-Trp-(O-Bzl-Ser)-(O-Bzl-Tyr)-Gly-Leu-(NO₂-Arg)-Pro-Gly-resin ester), corresponding to the amino acid sequence of LH-RH/FSH-RH, was synthesized starting with the Boc-Gly resin ester. The *tert*-butyloxycarbonyl (Boc) group was used for protecting the α-amino group of all amino acids including the following derivatives: Gln(O Np), O-Bzl-Ser, O-Bzl-Tyr, and NO₂-Arg. Coupling was achieved with dicyclohexylcarbodiimide (DCCI), except that glutamine was coupled by means of its *p*-nitrophenyl ester. Stepwise synthesis was carried out in methylene chloride and/or dimethyl formamide. Removal of the Boc-group in the first seven steps was performed by treatment with 50% trifluoroacetic acid in methylene chloride for 20 minutes, as suggested by Li and Yamashiro (1970). After the incorporation of the tryptophan residue, 1 N HCl in acetic acid containing 1% of 2-mercaptoethanol was used for removal of the Boc group, as described by G. R. Marshall (1968). Neutralization was carried out by shaking with 10% triethylamine in chloroform. Nitrophenyl ester coupling of Boc-Gln was performed with 10 equivalents of the active ester for 5 hours, followed by an additional treatment for 5 hours in the presence of 5 equivalents of imidazole (Li and Yamashiro, 1970; Wieland *et al.*, 1963). In order to achieve cyclization of the N-terminal glutaminyl group to the pyroglutamyl ring, the Boc-glutaminyl-peptide resin ester was treated with 1 N HCl in acetic acid, containing 1% of 2-mercaptoethanol (Manning, 1968). For the cleavage of the solid support, the peptide resin ester was submitted to ammonolysis. Removal of all protecting groups from the decapeptide amide was carried out by treatment with hydrogen fluoride (Stewart and Young, 1969; Sakakibara *et al.*, 1967). Repurification of synthetic LH-RH was effected by the use of countercurrent distribution, free flow electrophoresis, and CMC.

On the basis of its behavior on CCD, paper chromatography and electrophoresis, TLC and TLE, as well as biological results (see Section VIII), it was concluded that this synthetic product was identical with the natural porcine LH-RH/FSH-RH (Matsuo *et al.*, 1971a).

Other syntheses of LH-RH reported by Flouret *et al.* (1972) at Abbott

Laboratories and Monahan *et al.* (1971) were also based on the Merrifield solid phase method. On the other hand, Geiger *et al.* (1971) at Farbwerke Hoechst synthesized LH-RH by using classical methods of peptide synthesis. The Abbott and Hoechst materials had biological activity equivalent to natural porcine LH-RH (Schally *et al.*, 1972c) (see Section VIII). Synthesis of LH-RH in Japan by classical methods was also very recently reported by Kimura *et al.* (1971) and Yanaihara *et al.* (1971). All these syntheses of LH-RH/FSH-RH (Geiger *et al.*, 1971; Flouret *et al.*, 1972; Monahan *et al.*, 1971; Kimura *et al.*, 1971; Yanaihara *et al.*, 1971) were based on the decapeptide sequence of porcine LH-RH/FSH-RH established by us (Matsuo *et al.*, 1971b; Baba *et al.*, 1971a; Schally *et al.*, 1971a) and previously confirmed by our own synthesis (Matsuo *et al.*, 1971a,b).

I. OTHER MATERIALS WITH LH-RH ACTIVITY

While it is interesting theoretically that this tetrapeptide (which does not correspond to any amino acid sequence of LH-RH) has some LH-RH activity (as well as FSH-RH), Chang *et al.* (1971) and Bowers *et al.* (1971) reported the synthesis of a tetrapeptide, *p*-Glu-Tyr-Arg-Trp amide, which had some LH-RH activity at extremely high doses. However, this material is about 10,000 times weaker *in vivo* than natural LH-RH. While it is interesting theoretically that this tetrapeptide (which does not correspond to any amino acid sequence of LH-RH) has some LH-RH activity (as well as FSH-RH activity), the degree of activity is so low that it should preclude its use in clinical or veterinary work. Another synthetic tripeptide with LH-RH activity, (pyro)Glu-Gln-Ala-NH$_2$, has been reported by Igarashi (1971), but again it is at least 100,000 times weaker *in vivo* than natural LH-RH. Fawcett and McCann (1971) also reported that the synthetic tripeptides, pyroGlu-Ser-Val-NH$_2$ and/or pyro-Glu-Val-Ser-NH$_2$ may have some LH-RH activity *in vivo* and *in vitro*. They said that these peptides may be present in sheep hypothalamic extracts. However, our recent tests and further work by Fawcett and McCann (1972) indicate that the degree of LH-RH activity *in vivo* of these two peptides is very low (if any), since neither we, nor these authors could find any rise in plasma LH levels in ovariectomized, estrogen- and progesterone-pretreated rats when doses as high as 5 μg of crystalline (pyro)Glu-Val-Ser-NH$_2$ or (pyro)Glu-Ser-Val-NH$_2$ were used (Schally *et al.*, 1972a). Natural or synthetic (pyro)Glu-His-Trp-Ser-Tyr-Gly-Leu-Arg-Pro-Gly-NH$_2$ is active in this test at doses of 0.2 ng. Thus the LH-RH activity, if any, of these tripeptides is at least 25,000 times lower than that of LH-RH decapeptide. It is likely that the presence of the complete amino acid sequence of this decapeptide is necessary for maximal LH-RH and FSH-RH activity *in vivo*.

J. The Relationship of Prolactin Release-Inhibiting Factor
to LH-RH

The demonstration of a hypothalamic agent inhibiting prolactin secretion (Pasteels, 1962; Talwalker *et al.*, 1963; Schally *et al.*, 1965b) raised the old question whether this hormone might be the same as LH-RH (Everett, 1956a; Haun and Sawyer, 1960). However, Rothchild (1960) demonstrated that the secretion of prolactin and LH can occur together. Everett and Quinn (1966) showed that neural mechanisms initiating pseudopregnancy were distinct from mechanisms controlling ovulation. Moreover, partially purified LH-RH preparations did not inhibit prolactin release *in vivo* or *in vitro* (Schally *et al.*, 1964; Arimura *et al.*, 1967a).

Recently, we showed that a single injection of purified natural or synthetic LH-RH had no effect on prolactin levels in rats and in sheep (Debeljuk *et al.*, 1972c). This indicates that prolactin release-inhibiting factor and LH-RH are not the same. However, chronic treatment of hypophysectomized rats with pituitary grafts under the kidney capsule with synthetic LH-RH increased the number of LH cells and decreased prolactin cells (Arimura *et al.*, 1971b).

K. Summary

About ten years after the detection of LH-RH activity in hypothalamic extracts of rats, the isolation of LH-RH was achieved from pig hypothalami.

Pure natural LH-RH of porcine origin was found to stimulate the release of both FSH and LH from the pituitary gland of several species of animals, including man. The structure of this decapeptide, redesignated LH- and FSH-releasing hormone (LH-RH/FSH-RH), was determined to be (pyro)Glu-His-Trp-Ser-Tyr-Gly-Leu-Arg-Pro-Gly-NH$_2$. Its synthesis was also achieved by us, and subsequently by several other laboratories, thus confirming the correctness of the structure proposed by us. Synthetic (pyro)Glu-His-Trp-Ser-Tyr-Gly-Leu-Arg-Pro-Gly-NH$_2$ had the same LH-RH and FSH-RH activity as the pure natural material.

V. The Role of Sex Steroids in the Regulation of Secretion
of LH and FSH

A. Introduction

The subject of the influence of gonadal steroids on the hypothalamic–hypophyseal system has been the subject of many excellent reviews (Greep and Chester-Jones, 1950; Flerko, 1963; Bogdanove, 1964; Everett,

1964; Rothchild, 1965; Sawyer, 1969a,b; Davidson, 1969). Most of the views expressed in them appear to be essentially correct. We shall try to reconcile these concepts with the most recent results. Current investigations of the regulation of secretion of LH and FSH confirm what has been suspected for a long time, that is, the influence of gonadal steroids on the release of gonadotropins may be both stimulatory and inhibitory, in part direct and exerted on the pituitary and in large part indirect and exerted via the hypothalamus.

B. POSITIVE FEEDBACK OF STEROIDS ON FSH AND LH SECRETION

The facilitating effect of estrogen on LH release was first proposed by Holweg and Junkmann (1932) and Fevold et al. (1937). There are indeed certain events in the female sexual cycle during which a rise in estrogen secretion is followed by increased release of pituitary gonadotropins. This creates a situation of "positive" or "stimulatory" feedback. Recently, it has been demonstrated that the rise in urinary estrogens and plasma estradiol during the menstrual period in the human female precedes the usual mid-cycle ovulatory peak of plasma LH (Burger et al., 1968; Korenman et al., 1969; Corker et al., 1969; Goebelsman et al., 1969). Similar findings have been reported in the monkey (Hotchkiss et al., 1971). In rats, the peak in plasma estradiol occurs on the morning of proestrus, before the ovulatory surge of LH (Brown-Grant et al., 1970). Ramirez and Sawyer (1965b, 1966) found that intracarotid administration of small doses of estrogen to immature female rats advances the onset of puberty and causes a decrease in pituitary LH and a rise in plasma LH levels. These effects of estrogen may be mediated by the release of hypothalamic LH-RH since the levels of LH-RH in the median eminence were found to be reduced on the day of normal vaginal opening (Ramirez and Sawyer, 1966). Callantine et al. (1966) observed that subcutaneous injections of 17β-estradiol for 7 days to adult intact rats decreased pituitary LH and increased plasma LH concentrations.

The sites of the positive feedback have not been clearly determined. Palka et al. (1966) reported marked increases in rat plasma LH concentrations 4–5 days after median eminence (ME) implants of estrogen. Similarly, Motta et al. (1968) showed that implantation of estradiol into the median eminence of 26-day-old rats induced premature vaginal opening, ovulation, and increase in plasma LH levels. On the other hand, Docke and Dorner (1965) and Weick and Davidson (1970) concluded that the anterior pituitary is the main site of action of the positive feedback of estrogen.

Recent results of Arimura and Schally (1971) and Reeves et al. (1971b) strongly suggest that estrogen may potentiate the responses to

LH-RH in rats and sheep at the pituitary level (see Section IX). These results are in agreement with those of Weick et al. (1971), who argued that estrogen decreases the pituitary threshold to LH-RH.

In summary, small doses of estrogen may facilitate LH-release and increase the responsiveness to LH-RH. A hypothesis about the effects of positive and negative feedbacks on LH synthesis, storage, and release was recently presented by Barraclough and Haller (1970). The results of Corbin and Daniels (1969) indicate that estrogen can also activate the FSH-RH/FSH complex at puberty, since rats going through natural puberty and rats in which puberty was advanced by estrogen treatment showed a fall in pituitary FSH and hypothalamic FSH-RH content (see Section VI, B).

Progesterone can either stimulate or inhibit the release of LH that leads to ovulation, depending upon the time of administration during the estrous cycle (Everett, 1961, 1964; Sawyer and Everett, 1959; Lisk, 1969). It has long been known that progesterone administered to a 5-day cyclic rat on the third day of diestrus advances ovulation by 24 hours (Everett, 1948). Progesterone administered in proestrus will increase plasma LH levels (Nallar et al., 1966). This facilitating action of progesterone with respect to LH release is dependent on previous exposure to estrogen (Brown-Grant, 1969). Recently, Caligaris et al. (1968) also showed that progesterone has a biphasic effect, first stimulating and then inhibiting the release of LH. It has been suggested that progesterone may facilitate LH release in rats by lowering the hypothalamic activation threshold to neural stimuli (Docke and Dorner, 1969). Docke and Dorner (1965) also suggested, on the basis of their lesion and implantation experiments, that the positive feedback of estrogen and progesterone may also involve the anterior hypothalamic region. The information about the localization of stimulatory feedback receptors for estrogen and other sex steroids was reviewed by Davidson (1969).

C. NEGATIVE FEEDBACK OF SEX STEROIDS

1. *Introduction*

The negative feedback theory of regulation of pituitary LH and FSH secretion has been known for about 40 years. According to the view of Moore and Price (1932) and Meyer et al. (1932), the adenohypophysis and the ovary were linked in a rigid system of hormonal interactions, and sex steroids acted by directly suppressing the secretion of gonadotropins from the pituitary gland. This direct action of steroids on the pituitary was challenged by Holweg and Junkmann (1932), who proposed the existence of a hypothalamic sex center (or another sex center located in other regions of the CNS) where such feedback would be exerted. At any rate, the outcome of this "negative feedback" is that the steroid hormones, secreted by the gonads under the influence of pituitary gonadotropins, reduce further secretion of LH and FSH from the hypophysis. The LH and FSH secretion is thus held in a reciprocal relationship with sex steroid secretion. When sex steroid secretion is reduced (e.g., by castration), secretion of LH and FSH is increased. The cytological changes in the rat pituitary, which constitute the well known castration reaction, can be prevented by administration of exogenous sex steroids (Purves, 1961).

Flerko and Szentágothai (1957) carried out the first direct attempts to find the sites at which gonadal steroids exert a negative feedback on gonadotropin secretion. They found that implantation of ovarian fragments into the hypothalamus near the paraventricular nucleus inhibited gonadotropic function in the rat. They concluded that estrogen feedback requires hypothalamic mediation. This approach has also been pursued by other investigators (Davidson and Sawyer, 1961a,b; Lisk, 1960, 1962a,b, 1967; Lisk and Newlon, 1963; Kanematsu and Sawyer, 1963a,b; Bogdanove, 1963; Ramirez et al., 1964).

Bogdanove found that the appearance of castration cells can be prevented by pituitary or intrahypothalamic implants of estrogen (Bogdanove, 1963). Similar results were reported in the rabbit (Kanematsu and Sawyer, 1963b), but intrahypothalamic implants of estradiol were more effective in preventing changes in gonadotropic cells than intrapituitary implants. On the basis of their work, Kanematsu and Sawyer (1963b) concluded that the basal tuberal region of the hypothalamus contains nervous elements sensitive to the negative feedback of sex steroids. Conclusions, such as these, drawn from implantation experiments, have been criticized by Bogdanove (1964); he stated that the pituitary gland might be transfused by the steroid better by the intrahypothalamic implants than by intrapituitary implants.

2. Estrogens

That estrogen, even in small doses, can inhibit the release of both LH and FSH in the rat was shown long ago (Hertz and Meyer, 1937) and confirmed more recently (Byrnes and Meyer, 1951; Gans, 1959).

Large doses or chronic administration of estrogen are even more effective in this respect (Bogdanove, 1964). Lisk (1960) and Davidson and Sawyer (1961b) showed that implants of estradiol into the basal tuberal region will inhibit gonadotropin secretion in rats and rabbits. On the other hand, Faure et al. (1966) and Motta et al. (1968), using the same approach, suggested that the receptors sensitive to the negative feedback of estrogen are located in the habenular region of the thalamus.

Since enhancement of LH release and synthesis following castration is not inhibited in rats with suprachiasmatic lesions (Antunes-Rodrigues and McCann, 1967), they concluded that its site of action of negative feedback probably resides more caudally in the hypothalamus. However, the evidence for a medial basal tuberal hypothalamic site appears stronger (Davidson, 1969).

These proposed hypothalamic sites of negative feedback of estrogen are at variance with work which indicates an action on the pituitary. Ramirez et al. (1964) demonstrated that implants of estradiol located in the anterior pituitary as well as in the median eminence region prevented the rise of plasma LH which occurs after castration. Bogdanove (1963) also showed that estrogen can inhibit the development of castration cells by a direct action on the pituitary. Palka et al. (1966) similarly suggested that estrogen acts in part directly on the pituitary cells.

Estrogen by itself can inhibit LH release in castrated rats (McCann, 1963; McCann and Taleisnik, 1961; Ramirez and McCann, 1963b; Schally et al., 1969). However, the combination of estrogen with progesterone appears to be more effective. Thus, it has been repeatedly demonstrated that in castrated male and female rats, administration of estradiol benzoate plus progesterone lowers plasma levels of LH and FSH (Igarashi and McCann, 1964b; Ramirez and McCann, 1963b; Kuroshima et al., 1965; Gay and Bogdanove, 1969). From the estimation of pituitary LH and FSH levels, Gay and Bogdanove (1969) concluded that in the castrated rat treatment with estrogen and progesterone reduces LH release and impairs both the release and synthesis of FSH.

In conclusion, most of the evidence obtained in vivo suggests that the negative feedback of estrogen on LH secretion is exerted principally on the hypothalamus rather than the hypophysis (Lisk and Newlon, 1963), but some effect on the pituitary is also indicated (Bogdanove, 1963; Palka et al., 1966). Clear-cut suppression by estrogen of the stimulatory effect of LH-RH/FSH-RH on the release of FSH and LH in vitro from isolated rat pituitaries (Schally et al., 1972c) demonstrates that a part of the negative feedback of estrogen on LH and FSH secretion is exerted directly at the pituitary gland.

3. Progesterone

The inhibitory effects of progesterone are less spectacular than those of estrogen. The complex effects of progesterone on LH release were recently discussed by Lisk (1969). Rothchild (1965) suggested that progesterone can suppress the ovulatory surge of LH release, but not the basal LH secretion. In ovariectomized rats, progesterone, even in very large doses, is a poor inhibitor of LH release (Nallar et al., 1966; McCann, 1963;

Schally *et al.*, 1969). However, together with estrogen, progesterone can readily suppress LH and FSH release (McCann, 1963; Ramirez and McCann, 1963b; Igarashi and McCann, 1964b; Kuroshima *et al.*, 1965; Schally *et al.*, 1969; Gay and Bogdanove, 1969). The work with synthetic progestogens suggested that the site of negative feedback of progestational steroids may be principally in the hypothalamus (Harris and Sherratt, 1969; Schally *et al.*, 1968b, 1970e) (see Section V, C, 5). Recently, Davidson (1969) discussed in a review article his previously unpublished implantation experiments which indicate that progesterone acts on the hypothalamus to inhibit LH, but not FSH, release. However, the recent evidence of Arimura and Schally (1970) and Hilliard *et al.* (1971) indicates that in rats and rabbits progesterone exerts some of its inhibitory effects directly on the pituitary.

4. Androgens

Testosterone can inhibit the release and synthesis of LH and release of FSH in castrated male and female rats, but it is much less effective than estrogen (Bogdanove, 1964, 1967; Schally *et al.*, 1967b). Nevertheless, Bogdanove (1967) and Steinberger and Duckett (1968) observed that the marked drop of pituitary FSH levels, associated with an elevation of plasma FSH levels in orchiectomized rats, can be prevented by administration of testosterone. These results were interpreted as supporting the hypothesis that testosterone has an inhibitory effect on the release of FSH from the pituitary gland. When the treatment with androgen is discontinued, plasma levels of LH and FSH rise (Bogdanove and Gay, 1967). The rise in plasma LH seen after the castration may be due to increased synthesis of LH (Yamamoto *et al.*, 1970). Testosterone was also reported to inhibit LH synthesis in the castrated ram (J. Pelletier, 1970).

The negative feedback centers sensitive to testosterone appear to be located in the hypothalamus as well as in the pituitary. Davidson and Sawyer (1961a) demonstrated that implantation of testosterone in the median eminence led to gonadal atrophy in dogs. Lisk (1962b) clearly showed that implants of testosterone in the median eminence region but not in the pituitary, will cause testicular inhibition in rats. E. R. Smith and Davidson (1967) also showed that testosterone implants in the median eminence will inhibit gonadotropin secretion in rats which had been hypophysectomized and then had pituitaries transplanted beneath the kidney capsule. It is established that the basal medial hypothalamic region is one of the probable sites of negative feedback of androgens (Davidson, 1969). Other evidence indicates that androgen also exerts some negative effect directly on the pituitary gland (Kingsley and Bogdanove, 1971; McEwen *et al.*, 1970; Debeljuk *et al.*, 1972c).

5. Oral Contraceptive Steroids

Since we reviewed this subject recently (Schally and Kastin, 1970), only a relatively few comments will suffice. Hilliard *et al.* (1966) reported that pretreatment of rabbits with norethindrone suppressed ovulation induced by intrapituitary infusion of crude hypothalamic extracts. Pretreatment with estrogen partially overcame this blockade. The authors concluded that the blockade of LH release by norethindrone was due to its ability to block estrogen receptors in the pituitary and median eminence. Spies *et al.* (1969) in the same laboratory, also concluded that chlormadinone blocks ovulation in the rabbit by an action exerted directly on the pituitary gland. However, the hypothalamic extracts they used were weak in LH-RH activity, so that only marginally effective doses were used.

The results of Spies *et al.* (1969), Hilliard *et al.* (1966), and Docke *et al.* (1968) were at variance with the data obtained by Exley *et al.* (1968), Harris and Sherratt (1969), and Schally *et al.* (1968b, 1970e). Exley *et al.* (1968) and Harris and Sherratt (1969) showed that administration of large doses of chlormadinone acetate did not block the ovulatory response in rabbits after electrical stimulation of the hypothalamus or intrapituitary infusion of hypothalamic extracts. Schally *et al.* (1968b, 1970e) demonstrated that the highly stimulatory effect of LH-RH on LH release in ovariectomized rats could not be blocked by pretreatment of these rats with massive doses of 12 different contraceptive preparations and suggested that the hypothalamus is the principal site of negative feedback of these steroids.

These results were clarified by the work of Arimura and Schally (1970), Hilliard *et al.* (1971), and Debeljuk *et al.* (1972b), who showed in rats and rabbits that the release of LH in response to threshold doses, but not larger doses of LH-RH, was inhibited by progesterone. Thus, both views are probably correct and the negative feedback of contraceptive steroids appear to be exerted both at the hypothalamic and the pituitary level. In this connection, it should also be mentioned that the observations of Minaguchi and Meites (1967) and Ectors and Pasteels (1967) suggest that the inhibition of LH and FSH release by contraceptive steroids is mediated by their suppressive action on the synthesis and release of FSH-RH and LH-RH.

D. HYPOTHALAMIC AND PITUITARY RECEPTORS FOR SEX STEROIDS

Much recent work supports the concept of the existence of hypothalamic and pituitary receptors sensitive to the action of estrogen. This view is based in part on the accumulation in *in vivo* and *in vitro* studies of labeled 17-β-^{3}H estradiol in the hypothalamus and the pituitary (Eisenfeld and Axelrod, 1965; Kato and Villee, 1967; Stumpf, 1968; McGuire and Lisk, 1969; Pfaff, 1968b; Leavitt et al., 1969; Kato, 1970). These receptors may participate in the discrimination of the circulating levels of estrogen and regulation of LH release. The action of estrogen in the control of hypothalamic or pituitary function may be mediated through an effect on RNA synthesis (Leavitt et al., 1969; Schally et al., 1969). Recently testosterone-^{3}H has also been shown to be concentrated in the hypothalamus (Pfaff, 1968a; S. K. Roy and Laumas, 1966) as well as the pituitary (McEwen et al., 1970). Similarly, labeled progesterone is selectively concentrated by the brain, especially by the posterior hypothalamic tissue (Laumas and Faroog, 1966; Seiki et al., 1968).

E. Steroids and Metabolism of the Hypothalamus

Differences in oxidative metabolism of the hypothalamus among male rats, diestrous rats, and persistent-estrus rats may be due to sex steroids (Libertun et al., 1969; Scacchi et al., 1971). Polypeptide metabolism of the hypothalamus is affected by estrogen, an increase in peptidase activity being noted after estradiol administration (Hooper, 1968). Protein metabolism is also affected by sex steroids (Moguilevsky et al., 1971).

Since actinomycin D, which is a inhibitor of messenger RNA synthesis (and consequently of RNA-dependent protein synthesis), nullifies the inhibitory effect of estrogen on the castration-induced rise in plasma LH (Schally et al., 1969), it was suggested that the suppressing effect of estrogen and progesterone on LH release may require normal RNA synthesis. Thus, estrogens may induce the synthesis of a blocking substance (nucleic acid or protein) in the hypothalamus, and this substance somehow leads to blockade of LH secretion.

F. "Short Feedback" Control of LH and FSH Release

Much evidence from several laboratories indicates that, in addition to the two main mechanisms for the control of LH and FSH (hypothalamic releasing hormones and sex steroids), another type of control exists in which the inhibitory impulse is provided by LH and FSH themselves. For this feedback the name of "short," "internal," or "auto" feedback has been proposed (Martini et al., 1968).

Over 13 years ago, Kawakami and Sawyer (1959) showed that injection of pituitary gonadotropic preparations into normal or castrated rabbits affected their electroencephalographic (EEG) patterns. This EEG afterreaction was first observed in female rabbits (normal as well as castrated) after mating. Kawakami and Sawyer (1959) suggested that this EEG "afterreaction" was due to the action on the brain of gonadotropic hormones released by coitus. Later it was shown by David *et al.* (1966) and Corbin and Cohen (1966) that implantation of LH into the median eminence results in a decrease in pituitary LH levels in normal and castrated male and female rats. Similarly, Corbin and Story (1967) and Martini *et al.* (1968) demonstrated that implants of FSH in the median eminence lower pituitary FSH levels and hypothalamic FSH-RH content in rats. Arai and Gorski (1968) showed that implants of FSH in the median eminence inhibit the ovarian compensatory hypertrophy in rats. This indicates that high plasma levels of FSH and LH may reduce the secretion of further amounts of FSH and LH through inhibition of release of FSH-RH/LH-RH. The existence of both negative and positive short feedback mechanisms was recently suggested by Ojeda and Ramirez (1969). Elevation of circulating LH and FSH levels in menopausal women or in castrated animals does not support a primary role for the short feedback mechanism. The physiological importance of the short feedback mechanisms has not yet been ascertained.

VI. LH-RH and FSH-RH Levels in Hypothalamus and Blood

A. Localization of FSH-RH

Watanabe and McCann (1968) cut frozen sections in 3 planes through the rat hypothalamus to determine the localization of FSH-RH. They found most activity in the medial basal tuberal region, an area which includes the median eminence and arcuate nucleus, less activity in the pituitary stalk, and none in the posterior lobe. They concluded that FSH-RH is localized to the stalk–median eminence region in the rat (Watanabe and McCann, 1968).

B. Fluctuations in Hypothalamic Content of FSH-RH

Physiological studies suggest that in several species FSH-RH release may be affected by light, temperature, levels of circulating gonadal hormones, age, and other factors. Thus, light was reported to increase the FSH-RH content in rats (Negro-Vilar *et al.*, 1968c). The FSH-RH content of the hypothalamus falls at puberty in the female rat, concomitantly with a decrease in pituitary FSH (Corbin and Daniels, 1967). Corbin and Daniels (1969) also have shown that treatment with estradiol, which advanced the onset of puberty, significantly reduced FSH-RH concentration in the median eminence of immature female rats.

In rats of either sex, gonadectomy raises, and treatment with gonadal hormones lowers, the hypothalamic content of FSH-RH (David *et al.*, 1965b; Mittler and Meites, 1966). There are also changes in hypothalamic

FSH-RH content during the estrous cycle of the rat. A significant decline in hypothalamic FSH-RH content was observed between 11:00 AM and 4:30 PM on the day of proestrus (Negro-Vilar et al., 1970).

C. FSH-RH IN BLOOD

Saito et al. (1967b) examined peripheral blood from normal and hypophysectomized rats for FSH-RH activity. Assays for FSH-RH activity consisted of measurement of the depletion of FSH in the pituitaries of normal male rats or castrated rats pretreated with testosterone propionate. FSH-RH activity was found in the plasma of male rats hypophysectomized for 1 or 2 months. It was diminished after decapitation. No FSH-RH activity was detected in the peripheral blood of normal rats of either sex hypophysectomized 10 days previously or female rats hypophysectomized 10–90 days earlier.

Negro-Vilar et al. (1968a) used the more specific in vitro method for comparison of plasma from male rats hypophysectomized for 1 and 2 months with plasma from intact rats for FSH-RH activity. Only the plasma from the hypophysectomized rats induced release of FSH upon incubation with rat pituitaries. Exposure of hypophysectomized rats to constant light for 3 weeks increased FSH-RH activity in the plasma to levels greater than those found after hypophysectomy alone. Since the FSH-RH content in the hypothalamus remained unchanged, these results suggest that hypophysectomy and constant light stimulate release of FSH-RH from the hypothalamus into the blood (Negro-Vilar et al., 1968a). Treatment with reserpine or testosterone propionate inhibited FSH-RH release into plasma and also depressed hypothalamic FSH-RH content in the hypophysectomized rats (Negro-Vilar et al., 1968b). Similarly, destruction of the median eminence area in hypophysectomized rats will result in a disappearance of FSH-RH activity from blood (Corbin et al., 1970).

D. LOCALIZATION OF LH-RH

Early work suggested that LH-RH could be extracted from a medial, basal hypothalamic zone that extended as far rostrally as the optic chiasma (McCann, 1962). Schneider et al. (1969) and Crighton et al. (1969) confirmed this localization by sectioning frozen rat hypothalami and assaying the extracts prepared from discrete areas by means of the in vitro assay for LH-RH. They also concluded that LH-RH secreting neurons may be located in the suprachiasmatic area and may be responsible for the discharge of ovulatory amounts of LH.

E. FLUCTUATIONS IN HYPOTHALAMIC CONTENT OF LH-RH

In mature female rats, the hypothalamic content of LH-RH undergoes changes during the estrous cycle. Chowers and McCann (1965) and Ramirez and Sawyer (1965a) reported that hypothalamic LH-RH is highest late in diestrus and declines late at proestrus. At first it was reported that hypothalamic tissue of immature or mature rats of both sexes contains similar amounts of LH-RH (Ramirez and McCann, 1963a). Ramirez and Sawyer (1966) then showed increased LH-RH activity in the hypothalamus of female rats from the neonatal age up to a period between 25 and 35 days of age, coinciding with vaginal opening, when a sudden drop was seen. This fall in hypothalamic LH-RH was interpreted as a massive release into the portal vessels of this neurohormone, which therefore may play a key role in the onset of puberty. Recently, it was demonstrated that hypothalami of very old male rats contain about twice as much LH-RH activity as young mature rats (Debeljuk et al., 1972d). The pituitary of the old rat showed a decreased sensitivity to stimulation with LH-RH (Debeljuk et al., 1972d). These findings suggest that the aging process may impair hypothalamopituitary relationships. Ramirez and Sawyer (1965b) also showed that onset of puberty in the female rat is accompanied by a sharp drop in pituitary LH and increase in plasma LH levels. An effect of light on hypothalamic content of LH-RH has been reported in sheep (J. Pelletier and Ortavant, 1968).

The effects of gonadal hormones on hypothalamic LH-RH content are controversial. Chowers and McCann (1965) reported that castration and treatment with sex hormones were ineffective in altering the hypothalamic LH-RH content in the rat. Only implants of testosterone and estradiol into the median eminence lowered the LH-RH content. At variance with these results, Piacsek and Meites (1966) found in male rats that castration increased LH-RH content in the hypothalamus 2- to 3-fold. This increase could be prevented by administration of testosterone. In the female rat 3 weeks after ovariectomy, there was a fall in the LH-RH content. Similar results were reported by Moszkowska and Kordon (1965). Treatment of ovariectomized rats with estrogen further depressed the LH-RH content. Progesterone had no effect on LH-RH content when given alone, but together with estrogen prevented the latter from lowering LH-RH content. These results suggest that ovariectomy stimulates the release of LH-RH and estrogen inhibits the release and synthesis of LH-RH. Minaguchi and Meites (1967) demonstrated that administration of Enovid decreased pituitary FSH and LH as well as hypothalamic LH-RH and FSH-RH content. This suggests that the inhibitory effect of some antifertility steroids on LH and FSH release may be mediated through suppression of synthesis and release of hypothalamic LH-RH and

FSH-RH. The effects of castration and sex steroids on hypothalamic content of LH-RH and FSH-RH were discussed by Meites et al. (1967).

F. LH-RH in Blood

Plasma from normal rats or rats hypophysectomized for 1 week contains no detectable LH-RH activity. However, plasma from rats hypophysectomized for 2 or 3 months contains LH-RH activity (Nallar and McCann, 1965). This LH-RH activity disappears after a lesion in the hypothalamus. Fink et al. (1965, 1967) reported that blood collected from the cut pituitary stalk (termed hypophyseal portal blood) from rats in proestrus, or from hypophysectomized rats, had much higher LH-RH activity than peripheral plasma from the same animals. After repurification of portal blood, an "LH-free" fraction raised plasma LH in ovariectomized, estrogen- and progesterone-treated rats and caused ovulation in rabbits when infused directly into the anterior pituitary gland of these animals. The results of these experiments suggested the presence of LH-RH in the "LH-free" fraction of hypophyseal portal plasma (Fink and Harris, 1970). Harris and Ruf (1970) found that electrical stimulation of the hypothalamus increased the LH-RH activity of hypophyseal portal blood in proestrus and metestrus, but not in estrus. LH-RH activity has also been reported in the plasma of hypophysectomized cockerels (Frankel et al., 1965).

VII. Methods of Determination of LH-RH and FSH-RH Activity

A. LH-RH

Methods for measuring LH-RH activity have been reviewed in recent years (Schally and Kastin, 1970; Schally et al., 1967c, 1968a). Below are listed only some of the more specific methods currently used.

1. In Vivo

a. Elevation of Plasma LH Levels in Chronically Ovariectomized Pretreated Rats. Pretreatment was with (i) estrogen and progesterone (Ramirez and McCann, 1963b) and (ii) oral contraceptives (Schally et al., 1968b, 1970e).

The rats are ovariectomized 30–90 days previously and treated with 50 μg estradiol and 25 mg progesterone (or with oral contraceptive steroids; for dosages of these, see Schally et al., 1970e). LH-RH is given intravenously, into the carotid, or subcutaneously. This appears to be the most sensitive and the most convenient existing assay for LH-RH. Amounts as small as 0.0002 μg of pure natural or synthetic LH-RH administered intravenously have a significant effect on plasma LH (Schally *et al.*, 1971b, 1971i). The rise in plasma LH occurs soon after giving purified LH-RH (Schally *et al.*, 1970b) or crude hypothalamic extracts (Gay *et al.*, 1969), and the peak of response is reached 15–20 minutes after the injection.

b. *Elevation of Plasma LH Levels in Male Castrated, Treated Rats.* Rats were castrated 30 days, and treated with 1–2 mg of testosterone 4 and 2 days, before the experiment (Schally *et al.*, 1967b, 1970b). LH-RH can be given by vein or by the carotid artery.

c. *Elevation of Plasma LH in Immature Male Rats.* Rats 22–25 days old were tested by intravenous administration (Arimura *et al.*, 1972a). These rats are less sensitive to LH-RH than castrated rats treated with steroids, but this test can be used for the simultaneous determination of FSH-RH activity.

d. *Elevation of Plasma LH in Rats after Pituitary Portal Vessel Infusion.* In a very elegant study, Kamberi *et al.* (1971) showed that hypothalamic extracts infused into a stalk portal vessel of an anesthetized rat caused an increase in arterial levels of LH (and FSH).

In early work on LH-RH by McCann *et al.* (1965, 1968), Schally and Bowers (1964b), and Schally *et al.* (1967a, 1968a), plasma LH levels in rats were measured by the ovarian ascorbic acid depletion assay (Parlow, 1961). During the past few years specific radioimmunoassays for rat LH have been developed by Niswender *et al.* (1968) and Monroe *et al.* (1968). Results obtained by bioassay for LH were confirmed (Gay *et al.*, 1969, 1970a; Schally *et al.*, 1970a,b,e; Kerdelhue *et al.*, 1970) by the use of these specific radioimmunoassays for serum LH. Thus, criticism (Guillemin, 1967b) of the results on LH-RH based on measurement of LH by ascorbic acid depletion methods is no longer relevant (McCann *et al.*, 1968; Schally *et al.*, 1970b). However, the radioimmunoassay for LH is more accurate and precise and permits the convenient determination of a much larger number of samples than does the ovarian ascorbic acid depletion method.

e. *Induction of Ovulation in Proestrus Rabbits after Intrapituitary Infusion of Crude or Purified Hypothalamic Extracts.* LH-RH materials of high purity (Campbell *et al.*, 1961, 1964; Hilliard *et al.*, 1966, 1971; Spies *et al.*, 1969) were used. Ovulation offers a very desirable end point to measure the effect of LH-RH, but this technique may be more cumbersome to use than the methods based on elevation of plasma LH in rats. Recent development of a radioimmunoassay for rabbit LH (Bogdanove *et al.*, 1971) will make this method more convenient.

f. *Elevation of Plasma LH in Sheep.* The method (Amoss and Guillemin, 1969; Gay *et al.*, 1970a; Reeves *et al.*, 1970a,b, 1971a,b, 1972) was followed by radioimmunoassay for sheep LH (Niswender *et al.*, 1969). LH-RH can be given by intracarotid, intramuscular, and intravenous route. When LH-RH is given by intracarotid injection, the sheep are surgically prepared with a carotid loop. Blood is collected from a catheter placed in jugular vein (Reeves *et al.*, 1970b). Castrated sheep (wethers) give much larger responses to LH-RH than rams or ewes. The response in ewes increases during the onset of estrus.

g. *Elevation of Plasma LH in Humans.* The method (Kastin *et al.*, 1969, 1970a,b, 1971a,b) was followed by specific radioimmunoassay for human LH and FSH (Midgley, 1966, 1967). Men and women usually give excellent responses to LH-RH after intravenous or subcutaneous administration of LH-RH.

2. *In Vitro*

a. *Short-Term Incubation of Rat Pituitaries.* LH-RH stimulates LH release from rat anterior pituitaries incubated *in vitro* under various conditions. Schally and Bowers (1964a) modified the method of Saffran and Schally (1955) by using pituitaries from rats ovariectomized 30–45 days previously and treated with estrogen and progesterone. The method is highly specific and very sensitive to LH-RH, but it is less convenient than that utilizing pituitaries of normal male rats (Piacsek and Meites, 1966; Mittler and Meites, 1966; Schally *et al.*, 1970d, 1972c).

b. *Tissue Cultures of Rat Pituitaries.* Various methods were used.

(i) Cohen *et al.* (1966) cultured monolayers of rat pituitaries.

(ii) Mittler *et al.* (1970) used standard techniques of tissue culture. Each anterior pituitary was removed and cut into 4–6 explants. The cultures were performed for 3 days in sterile disposable plastic petri dishes in medium 199 (Difco, Detroit) with one part in 10 of newborn calf serum. The explants were supported in a gas–medium interface at 36°C.

(iii) Recently these methods were modified by Redding *et al.* (1971, 1972), who carried out pituitary tissue cultures in Erlenmeyer flasks with constant shaking in a gyrorotator incubator. The advantage of tissue culture methods is that they permit one to study the synthesis of LH in addition to the stimulation of its release.

B. FSH-RH

Only the specific methods currently used are listed below.

1. *In Vivo*

a. *Elevation of Plasma FSH in Castrated, Pretreated Male Rats.* The rats were pretreated with testosterone propionate by the intracarotid route (Saito *et al.*, 1967a). The conditions are the same as for LH-RH described in Section VII, A, 1, b).

b. *Elevation of Plasma FSH in Immature Male Rats* (Arimura *et al.*, 1972a). (For conditions, see Section VII, A, 1, c.) Male rats 22–25 days old are used. Elevation of plasma FSH can be observed 15 minutes after intravenous injection of FSH-RH. Plasma levels of FSH can be measured by the Steelman–Pohley (1953) bioassay, if enough plasma is available. However, routinely, the radioimmunoassay for rat FSH (Daane and Parlow, 1971) is used. The release of LH can be studied simultaneously.

c. *Elevation of Plasma FSH in the Human Being* (Kastin *et al.*, 1969, 1970a,b). This is detected conveniently by radioimmunoassay for human FSH (Midgley, 1967).

2. *In Vitro*

a. *Short-Term Incubation System.* Stimulation of FSH release *in vitro* from rat pituitaries can be studied in Krebs–Ringer bicarbonate glucose (KRBG) medium or T. C. Medium 199 and a gas phase of 95% oxygen, 5% carbon dioxide under the following conditions:

(i) Pituitaries from normal male rats. Mittler and Meites (1966) used T. C. medium 199. Schally *et al.* (1970d) used KRBG medium as originally recommended by Saffran and Schally (1955) for this type of pituitary incubation. Usually 10 pituitary halves with a total weight of 30–50 mg are incubated in 10 ml KRBG medium for 6 hours at 37°C. The pituitary halves are distributed randomly and not matched. Doses of LH-RH/FSH-RH as small as 0.2 ng/ml medium cause a significant stimulation of release of FSH.

(ii) Pituitaries from castrated male rats pretreated with testosterone propionate. The rats which had been castrated for 30–60 days are given subcutaneous injections of 1.5 mg of testosterone propionate 4 days and 2 days before the experiment. Pituitary halves are usually incubated in 10 ml KRBG for 4–6 hours (Schally *et al.*, 1970d).

(iii) Pituitaries from female rats ovariectomized 30–45 days previously and given 20 mg of progesterone and 50 μg of estradiol benzoate 3 days before the experiment. When 20 pituitaries are used, the incubation time can be reduced to 1 hour (Schally and Bowers, 1964a; Schally *et al.*, 1970d).

The FSH released into the incubation medium is routinely measured by the assay of Steelman and Pohley (1953). Five to 8 rats are used per group. The results can be given in terms of ovarian weight, since the response is linear with respect to dosage over a certain range. The control amount of FSH released in this system is close to the lower threshold of the Steelman–Pohley assay (1953). FSH in the medium can also be measured by radioimmunoassay for rat FSH (Daane and Parlow, 1971). In all these three systems, the release of LH can also be studied.

b. *Tissue Cultures of Rat Pituitaries.* These are conducted as described for LH-RH in Section VII, A, 2, b (Mittler *et al.*, 1970; Redding *et al.*, 1971, 1972). Both the release and the synthesis of FSH can be studied. The secreted FSH is measured by bioassay or radioimmunoassay methods (see above).

VIII. Effects of Natural and Synthetic Preparations of LH-RH/FSH-RH

This topic was also the subject of recent extensive reviews (Schally *et al.*, 1968a, 1970b, 1971g). Only the most recent results, nearly all obtained with "pure" homogeneous porcine LH-RH or synthetic preparations of LH-RH will be mentioned. These effects will be discussed together, since it is most important to understand that in most cases the release of LH and FSH is probably simultaneous. However, the different half-lives of LH and FSH (Gay and Bogdanove, 1968; Gay *et al.*, 1970b) and the different sensitivities of some animal preparations to the FSH-RH activity of LH-RH (in turn probably due to endogenous steroid levels or various pretreatment with exogenous gonadal steroids) may contribute to the great variations between LH and FSH release which are occasionally seen.

A. Effect of LH-RH/FSH-RH in Rats

1. *Elevation of Plasma LH in Ovariectomized Rats Pretreated with Estrogen and Progesterone*

Doses as small as 0.25 ng of pure porcine LH-RH will raise plasma LH levels in this animal preparation, as shown in Table III. Greater

TABLE III
Effect of Porcine LH-RH/FSH-RH on Plasma LH Levels of
Ovariectomized Rats Pretreated with Estrogen and Progesterone[a]

Preparation	Dose (dry weight) ng/rat	RIA for rat LH plasma LH level[a] (ng/ml ± SE)	P value
Saline	—	4.9 ± 0.6	—
LH-RH/FSH-RH	0.25	8.1 ± 0.8	0.01
LH-RH/FSH-RH	0.625	14.8 ± 0.8	0.001
LH-RH/FSH-RH	1.56	28.1 ± 2.3	0.001
LH-RH/FSH-RH	3.9	43.7 ± 2.9	0.001
LH-RH/FSH-RH	9.75	91.1 ± 11.2	0.001

[a] From Schally *et al.* (1971i), by permission of The American Society of Biological Chemists, Inc., Bethesda, Maryland.
[b] In terms of NIH-LH-S-14. RIA = radioimmunoassay.

doses cause greater elevations of plasma LH, close to 20-fold or occasionally even higher. These effects were obtained with two different preparations of homogeneous porcine LH-RH (Schally et al., 1971b, 1971i). Plasma LH was conveniently measured by radioimmunoassay (RIA) (Niswender et al., 1968). This rise in plasma LH occurred as early as 3 minutes after intravenous administration of LH-RH (Schally et al., 1970b).

Synthetic (pyro)Glu-His-Trp-Ser-Tyr-Gly-Leu-Arg-Pro-Gly-NH$_2$ is also active in nanogram doses (Table IV) and possesses identical activity with natural LH-RH. The dose-response regression lines for natural and synthetic LH-RH are parallel (Arimura et al., 1972e). In fact, since the natural preparation of LH-RH used contained only 70% peptide material, the potency of some synthetic preparation of LH-RH was about 10–30% higher, in agreement with theoretical values.

In this animal preparation, a significant effect of natural and synthetic LH-RH on the release of FSH can be obtained only occasionally. The suppressive effect of estrogen and progesterone on FSH release may play some part in this. If the duration of stimulation with LH-RH/FSH-RH is prolonged (e.g., 2 hour infusion), a 2- to 3-fold elevation of plasma FSH can be obtained (Arimura et al., 1972c).

TABLE IV

LH-RH ASSAY in Vivo ON NATURAL AND SYNTHETIC MATERIAL
USING OVARIECTOMIZED, ESTROGEN-PROGESTERONE
PRETREATED RATS[a]

Group No.	Sample	Dose (ng/rat)	Plasma LH levels RIA for rat LH (mean LH ng/ml[b] ± SE)
1	Saline	—	5.6 ± 1.1
2	Natural LH-RH AVS 77-33, No. 215–269	0.5	17.5 ± 4.5
3	Natural LH-RH AVS 77-33, No. 215–269	2.5	74.0 ± 6.9
4	Synthetic LH-RH AVS 77-49 No. 215–269	0.5	19.4 ± 6.3
5	Synthetic LH-RH AVS 77-49 No. 215–269	2.5	81.6 ± 10.7

[a] Potency of synthetic LH-RH made by Matsuo et al. (1971a) = 114% (95% confidence limits = 70%–180%) as compared with potency of natural LH-RH, AVS 77-33, No. 215–269. λ = 0.152; nonparallelism = not significant.
[b] As NIH-LH-S-14.

TABLE V

Effect of Natural LH-RH/FSH-RH on Plasma LH and FSH Levels in Castrated Male Rats Treated with Testosterone[a]

Sample	Dose (ng/rat)	Plasma FSH activity Steelman–Pohley assay Ovarian weight (mg)	Plasma FSH activity FSH[b] (μg/ml)	Radioimmunoassay FSH (μg/ml)[c] Before	Radioimmunoassay FSH (μg/ml)[c] After	Radioimmunoassay FSH (μg/ml)[c] P	Plasma LH activity RIA LH ng/ml[d]
Saline	—	89.4 ± 6	10 (6.5–15.3)	2.2 ± 0.1	2.2 ± 0.2	NS	0
LH-RH	1	—	—	2.9 ± 0.6	3.6 ± 0.9	NS	12 ± 4.5
LH-RH	5	—	—	2.6 ± 0.2	3.0 ± 0.2	NS	42 ± 4.0
LH-RH	25	134.2[e] ± 10.9	19 (12.1–28.9)	2.3 ± 0.2	3.2 ± 0.2	0.02	66 ± 5.9

[a] Modified from Schally et al. (1971b). Courtesy of Biochem. Biophys. Res. Commun. and Academic Press, New York.
[b] As NIH-FSH-S-8, 45 minutes after injection with 95% limits.
[c] As NIAMD-RAT-FSH-RP-1 45 minutes after the injection.
[d] As NIH-LH-S-14, 10 minutes after injection. RIA = radioimmunoassay.
[e] P = 0.05 vs. saline.

2. Elevation of Plasma LH and FSH in Castrated Male Rats Pretreated with Testosterone

A rise in both LH and FSH in plasma is readily detected 10 and 45 minutes after intravenous or intracarotid administration of natural or synthetic LH-RH/FSH-RH (Tables V and VI and Fig. 2). LH was measured by RIA and FSH both by bioassay and radioimmunoassay. The rise in plasma FSH is immediate, as seen in Fig. 2. The rise in LH in this animal preparation also occurs within 3–10 minutes after administration of LH-RH/FSH-RH as reported previously (Schally et al., 1970b). A 24-fold elevation can be seen in Table VI.

3. Elevation of Plasma LH and FSH in Immature Male Rats

The rise of plasma LH which occurs in this animal preparation after intravenous administration of either natural and synthetic LH-RH is very large (Table VII). The rise in plasma FSH is smaller than that of LH, but highly significant. It is interesting that rat hypothalamic extracts cannot induce a bigger rise in FSH than the pure natural or synthetic LH-RH/FSH-RH. This supports the concept that no other substance

TABLE VI

In Vivo Effect of Synthetic LH-RH/FSH-RH in Castrated Testosterone Propionate-Treated Rats[a]

		Plasma LH (ng/ml) as NIH-LH-S-17			
Sample	Dose	10 Min	P^d	45 Min	P^d
Saline	—	4.5 ± 0.6	—	5.5 ± 1.7	—
Natural LH-RH[b]	20	71.3 ± 6.4	0.01		
Natural LH-RH[b]	80	105.4 ± 9.4	0.01	39.5 ± 5.4	0.01
Synthetic LH-RH[c]	80	66.3 ± 10.9	0.01		
Synthetic LH-RH[c]	320	106.7 ± 3.6	0.01	35.6 ± 5.8	0.01

		Plasma FSH (μg/ml) as NIAMD-Rat FSH-RP-1			
Saline	—	2.24 ± 0.094	—	2.15 ± 0.09	—
Natural LH-RH[b]	20	2.49 ± 0.095	0.05		
Natural LH-RH[b]	80	2.70 ± 0.054	0.01	2.59 ± 0.09	0.01
Synthetic LH-RH[c]	80	2.61 ± 0.048	0.01		
Synthetic LH-RH[c]	320	2.78 ± 0.019	0.01	2.53 ± 0.26	NS

[a] From Arimura et al. (1972a). Courtesy of *Endocrinology* and J. B. Lippincott Co., Philadelphia, Pennsylvania.

[b] Natural LH-RH AVS 77-33 No. 215–269.

[c] Synthetic LH-RH AVS 77-45 No. 282–343 with potency of 24.7% of maximal potency of natural or synthetic LH-RH preparation.

[d] Duncan's new multiple range test.

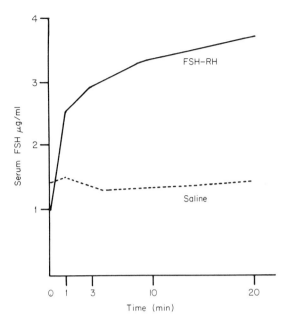

FIG. 2. Effect of administration of 0.1 μg of highly purified FSH-RH/LH-RH on plasma levels of FSH in castrated male rats pretreated with testosterone propionate. FSH was measured by radioimmunoassays for rat FSH and is expressed in terms of NIAMD RAT FSH-RP-1. From Schally *et al.* (1972c). Courtesy of *Fert. Steril.* and the Williams and Wilkins Co., Baltimore, Maryland.

with major FSH-RH activity exists in hypothalamic extracts (Schally *et al.*, 1971i; Arimura *et al.*, 1972a).

4. Stimulation of the Release of LH and FSH in Vitro

Table VIII illustrates that doses as small as 0.5 ng of natural LH-RH/per milliliter stimulated the release of both LH and FSH *in vitro* from pituitaries of male rats as measured by bioassay and radioimmunoassay of the media (Schally *et al.*, 1971b, 1972c). The stimulation of FSH and LH release is related to the log dose of natural LH-RH/FSH-RH over the range 1.5–13.5 ng/ml. The highest dose resulted in a 3- to 4-fold increase in both FSH and LH activity in the incubation medium.

Synthetic LH-RH/FSH-RH has an identical effect (Table IX) when assayed in this specific and accurate system. The FSH-RH activity of several preparations of synthetic pyro(Glu)-His-Trp-Ser-Tyr-Gly-Leu-Arg-Pro-Gly-NH₂ (our own, Hoechst and Abbott Laboratories) was the same as that of natural LH-RH/FSH-RH (Schally *et al.*, 1972c).

Stimulation of LH release during superfusion of rat pituitary glands

TABLE VII

In Vivo EFFECTS OF NATURAL AND SYNTHETIC LH-RH/FSH-RH ON PLASMA
LH AND FSH LEVELS IN NORMAL IMMATURE MALE RATS[a]

Sample	Dose	Plasma LH[b] (ng/ml ± SE)	P[c]	Plasma FSH[d] (μg/ml ± SE)	P[c]
Saline	—	0.2 ± 0.1	—	1.55 ± 0.09	—
Natural LH-RH[e]	25 ng	4.4 ± 0.9	0.01	1.94 ± 0.14	NS
Natural LH-RH[e]	100 ng	8.2 ± 0.8	0.01	2.16 ± 0.13	0.01
Synthetic LH-RH[f]	50 ng	5.4 ± 0.5	0.01	2.45 ± 0.17	0.01
Synthetic LH-RH[f]	200 ng	7.8 ± 0.8	0.01	2.49 ± 0.18	0.01
Rat SME[g]	0.5 SME	1.5 ± 0.3		2.09 ± 0.06	
Rat SME	1 SME	2.6 ± 0.3		2.02 ± 0.06	
Rat SME	2 SME	3.9 ± 0.1		2.31 ± 0.22	

[a] From Arimura et al. (1972a). Courtesy of Endocrinology and J. B. Lippincott Co., Philadelphia, Pennsylvania.
[b] As NIH-LH-S-17.
[c] Duncan's NMR Test.
[d] As NIAMD-RAT-FSH-RP-1.
[e] Pure material.
[f] = Hoechst.
[g] SME = stalk–median eminence.

TABLE VIII

STIMULATION BY NATURAL LH-RH/FSH-RH OF FSH AND LH RELEASE
in Vitro FROM PITUITARIES OF MALE RATS[a]

Sample	Dose	FSH content of medium[b] Steelman-Pohley assay Ovarian weight (mg ± SE)	P value	FSH[c] (μg/ml)	FSH content RIA (μg[d]/ml)	LH content RIA LH ng[e]/ml
Control	—	71.4 + 4.2	—	21	8.0	238
LH-RH	0.5	94.9 ± 4.9	0.01	28	9.6	362
LH-RH	1.5	101.6 ± 6.4	0.005	32	12.4	460
LH-RH	4.5	143.2 ± 20.0	0.01	53	16.2	628
LH-RH	13.5	169.6 ± 10.0	0.001	77	24	978

[a] Modified from Schally et al. (1971b). Courtesy of Biochem. Biophys. Res. Commun. and Academic Press, New York.
[b] Total volume 10 ml.
[c] Expressed as NIH-FSH-S-4.
[d] As NIAMD rat FSH-RP-1.
[e] As NIH-LH-S-14.

TABLE IX

EFFECT OF NATURAL AND SYNTHETIC LH- AND FSH-RELEASING HORMONE
(LH-RH/FSH-RH) ON THE STIMULATION OF RELEASE OF
FSH FROM RAT PITUITARIES[a,b]

			FSH content of medium		
Group	Addition LH-RH	Dose (ng/ml)	Ovarian weight (mg ± SE)	P value 1 vs. all	FSH (μg/ml)[c]
1	Control	—	38.7 ± 3.6	—	20
2	Control	—	42.1 ± 5.6	—	18
3	Natural[d]	1.0	63.4 ± 3.9	0.005	48
4	Natural	1.0	69.3 ± 2.7	0.001	61
5	Natural	4.0	89.1 ± 3.3	0.001	138.8
6	Natural	4.0	89.2 ± 1.9	0.001	138.8
7	Synthetic[e]	1.0	56.2 ± 5.7	0.05	38.9
8	Synthetic	1.0	61.7 ± 3.3	0.005	44.4
9	Synthetic	4.0	89.4 ± 8.6	0.001	138.9
10	Synthetic	4.0	99.1 ± 9.1	0.001	205.6

[a] From Schally et al. (1972c). Courtesy of Endocrinology and J. B. Lippincott Co., Philadelphia, Pennsylvania.
[b] Potency of synthetic vs. natural = 0.95 (0.65–1.38); λ = 0.24; deviation NS.
[c] As NIH-FSH-S8.
[d] Natural LH-RH/FSH-RH = AVS-77-33, No. 215–269.
[e] AVS synthetic LH-RH/FSH-RH/(Dr. H. Matsuo) AVS-77-49 No. 215–269.

has also been reported by Serra and Midgley (1970). Unfortunately, crude hypothalamic extracts were used, not the pure preparation.

5. Stimulation of Synthesis of LH and FSH in Tissue Cultures

It was postulated that the main effect of LH-RH may be on the release of LH rather than its synthesis (Samli and Geschwind, 1967). Evidence that the LH-RH/FSH-RH can induce both the release and synthesis of LH and FSH was obtained by the use of techniques for tissue cultures of rat anterior pituitaries (Mittler et al., 1970; Redding et al., 1971). Addition of minute amounts of highly purified porcine LH-RH/FSH-RH significantly increased the quantities of LH and FSH released. The total LH and FSH content of stimulated tissue and medium exceeded those of controls as measured by radioimmunoassays for LH and FSH and by bioassay for FSH (Mittler et al., 1970). These findings were confirmed and extended by modified organ cultures of rat anterior pituitaries using pure or synthetic preparations of LH-RH/FSH-RH (Redding et al., 1971, 1972). Measurement of medium and pituitary tissue for LH showed that addition of nanogram amounts of natural porcine or synthetic LH-RH to the medium stimulated LH release and synthesis as compared with the controls (Table X). A significant multiplier effect was obtained. LH-RH also significantly increased [³H]glucosamine incorporation into LH found in the medium, confirming de novo synthesis of LH. FSH synthesis was also stimulated (Table XI). Thus, natural porcine LH-RH/FSH-RH or synthetic LH-RH/FSH-RH is capable of stimulating both the release and synthesis of LH and FSH in vitro.

6. Other Studies with LH-RH/FSH-RH in the Rat

For induction of ovulation in rats, Arimura et al. (1967b) used partially purified LH-RH. Adult female rats in proestrus were given pentobarbital (Nembutal) in order to block spontaneous ovulation. Highly purified LH-RH was injected into their carotid arteries. Ten micrograms

TABLE X

EFFECT OF PURE NATURAL AND PURE SYNTHETIC LH-RH/FSH-RH ON MEDIUM AND TISSUE LH CONTENT IN RAT ANTERIOR PITUITARY CULTURES[a]

Group	Treatment LH-RH/ FSH-RH	Dose (total of 5 doses, μg/pituitary)	LH content (ng LH/pituitary)[b] by radioimmunoassay			
			Medium	Tissue	Total	Increase
1	Control	—	880 ± 23	989 ± 64	1869	
2	Natural[c]	0.02	2100 ± 33	229 ± 34	2329	460
			$P^e = 0.001$	$P^e = 0.001$		
3	Synthetic[d]	0.02	2450 ± 33	267 ± 37	2717	848
			$P^e = 0.001$	$P^e = 0.001$		
4	Control	—	1076 ± 32	1184 ± 19	2260	
5	Natural[c]	0.10	2900 ± 87	72 ± 5	2972	712
			$P^e = 0.001$	$P^e = 0.001$		
6	Synthetic[d]	0.10	2700 ± 115	180 ± 82	2880	620
			$P^e = 0.001$	$P^e = 0.001$		
7	Control	—	906 ± 14	1171 ± 37	2077	
8	Natural[c]	0.50	3400 ± 75	205 ± 5	3605	1528
			$P^e = 0.001$	$P^e = 0.001$		
9	Synthetic[d]	0.50	3750 ± 188	130 ± 17	3880	1803
			$P^e = 0.001$	$P^e = 0.001$		

[a] From Redding et al. (1972). Courtesy of Endocrinology and J. B. Lippincott Co., Philadelphia, Pennsylvania.
[b] Expressed in terms of NIH-LH-S-14, ± standard error of mean.
[c] Natural LH-RH/FSH-RH = AVS-77-33 No. 216–269.
[d] Synthetic LH-RH/FSH-RH = Hoechst.
[e] Student's t test, stimulated vs. control.

TABLE XI
EFFECT OF PURE NATURAL AND PURE SYNTHETIC LH-RH/FSH ON MEDIUM
AND TISSUE FSH CONTENT IN RAT ANTERIOR PITUITARY CULTURES[a]

Group	Treatment LH-RH/ FSH-RH	Dose (total of 5 doses, μg/ pituitary)	FSH content (ng FSH/pituitary)[b] by radioimmunoassay			
			Medium	Tissue	Total	Increase
1	Control	—	25,366 ± 1,433	5237 ± 278	30,603	
2	Natural[c]	0.02	33,267 ± 1,277 $P^e = 0.005$	1562 ± 502 $P^e = 0.001$	34,829	4,226
3	Synthetic[d]	0.02	36,433 ± 745 $P^e = 0.005$	620 ± 155 $P^e = 0.001$	37,053	6,450
4	Control	—	23,133 ± 566	7686 ± 642	30,819	
5	Natural[c]	0.10	43,400 ± 3,360 $P^e = 0.005$	288 ± 51 $P^e = 0.001$	43,688	12,869
6	Synthetic[d]	0.10	40,000 ± 845 $P^e = 0.001$	1488 ± 930 $P^e = 0.001$	41,209	10,390
7	Control	—	24,200 ± 330	5760 ± 437	29,960	
8	Natural[c]	0.50	38,393 ± 237 $P^e = 0.001$	738 ± 160 $P^e = 0.001$	39,131	9,171
9	Synthetic[d]	0.50	34,367 ± 2,283 $P^e = 0.01$	783 ± 83 $P^e = 0.001$	35,150	5,190

[a] From Redding et al. (1972). Courtesy of *Endocrinology* and J. B. Lippincott Co., Philadelphia, Pennsylvania.
[b] Expressed in terms of NIAMD-Rat-FSH-RP-1, ± standard error of mean.
[c] Natural LH-RH/FSH-RH = AVS-77-33 No. 216-269.
[d] Synthetic LH-RH/FSH-RH = Hoechst.
[e] Student's t test, stimulated vs. control.

of LH-RH, when injected over 30 minutes, induced full ovulation in all rats tested; 1 or 2 μg occasionally caused ovulation. Previously, Schiavi et al. (1963) induced ovulation with partially purified sheep LH-RH in rats rendered anovulatory by hypothalamic lesions.

Very few chronic studies have been done so far in view of the scarcity of natural LH-RH/FSH-RH. However, Beddow et al. (1970) reported that chronic administration of crude sheep hypothalamic extracts in hypophysectomized male rats with pituitary transplants caused significant increases in the weights of the testes and ventral prostate and corresponding increases in uterine and ovarian weight of similarly prepared female rats. Recently, Arimura et al. (1971b) treated with synthetic LH-RH/FSH-RH hypophysectomized female rats bearing a pituitary autograft under the kidney capsule and found a significant increase in ovarian weight as well as morphological evidence of an effect on the LH cells of the pituitary graft.

7. Morphological Changes in the Pituitary after LH-RH/FSH-RH

Von Lawzewitsch *et al.* (1970) examined the effects of hypothalamic extracts on the pituitary by histological means. They reported that intra-carotid administration of crude and semipurified beef hypothalamic extracts to normal male rats caused a degranulation of acidophile, thyro-tropic, and gonadotropic cells of the adenohypophysis. At 90 minutes, the gonadotrophs were still partially degranulated and vacuolized. How-ever, Rennels *et al.* (1971) could not detect any morphological signs of accelerated LH release by electron microscopy after administration of highly active preparations of porcine LH-RH to rats. In these rats, ovariectomized and steroid pretreated, serum levels of LH were elevated approximately 13-fold over control levels, 5 minutes after the injection of 100 ng of LH-RH while serum levels of FSH were elevated less than 2-fold. In spite of this evidence of intensive release of LH from the pituitary, no significant depletion of pituitary LH stores was seen, nor as mentioned above, were there any detectable changes in pituitary gonadotropic cells. Using crude rat hypothalamic extracts, G. Pelletier *et al.* (1971) could not find any extrusion from the gonadotrophs, al-though corticotrophs, somatotrophs, and thyrotrophs showed extrusion of granules by exocytosis after both intravenous injection *in vivo* and after short-term incubation *in vitro*. However, Shiino *et al.* (1972) re-cently observed extrusions of secretory granules from the LH-gonado-trophs, 15 minutes after administration of pure porcine LH-RH to androgen-lesioned persistent-estrus rats. Tixier-Vidal *et al.* (1971) also observed granule extrusion from LH cells of the lamb anterior pituitary gland after LH-RH.

B. Effects of LH-RH in the Golden Hamster

Synthetic LH-RH was tested for the induction of ovulation in golden hamsters pretreated with phenobarbital to prevent spontaneous ovulation. Subcutaneous injections of small amounts of synthetic LH-RH prepara-tion induced ovulation in these animals by stimulating the release of pituitary LH (Arimura *et al.*, 1971a).

C. Effects of LH-RH in Rabbits

Campbell *et al.* (1964) and Fawcett *et al.* (1965, 1968) reported that partially purified LH-RH obtained from beef or sheep hypothalami in-duced ovulation when infused into the pituitaries of estrous rabbits. Hilliard, Sawyer, and associates induced ovulation in estrous rabbits when crude rabbit median eminence extracts were infused directly into the adenohypophysis through stereotaxically implanted cannulae (Hilliard *et al.*, 1966; Spies *et al.*, 1969; Stevens *et al.*, 1970). Recently 0.2 μg of a highly purified preparation of porcine LH-RH was also shown to induce ovulation (Hilliard *et al.*, 1971).

D. Effects of LH-RH in Sheep

Several groups of workers have recently used crude or partially puri-fied preparations of LH-RH to induce a significant release of LH in sheep (Domanski and Kochman, 1968; Amoss and Guillemin, 1969; Reeves *et al.*, 1970b, 1971a,b). Reeves *et al.* (1970b) used three ewes, three wethers and one ram to study responses to LH-RH purified from porcine hypothalami. Serum LH was measured by a double antibody radioimmunoassay. The response to LH-RH in the ewes were first com-pared during diestrus. The animals received intracarotid doses of 1–27 μg LH-RH. At these dosages of LH-RH, each animal showed a sig-nificant increase in serum LH 2.5 minutes after LH-RH administration. The maximal responses in the ewes and ram appeared to be obtained with 3 μg of LH-RH. Greater doses (9–27 μg) of LH-RH could not further increase plasma LH in the ewes or the ram. The wethers showed much better responses to LH-RH than the ewes or the ram. Reeves *et al.* (1971a) showed that after administration of purified porcine LH-RH into ewes, an elevation of serum LH occurred at all stages of the estrous cycle. However, the same dose of LH-RH induced a greater change in serum LH during a 4–12 hour period on day 1 of the estrous cycle than at any other stage. This indicates that pituitary responsiveness to LH-RH at estrus is considerably greater than at other stages of the estrous cycle, and may be an important factor in the preovulatory surge of LH.

Recent studies indicate that administered synthetic LH-RH caused a great elevation in plasma LH in ewes and that it could also induce ovulation (Reeves *et al.*, 1972; Arimura *et al.*, 1972b). Thus, after injec-tion of very large doses (250 μg) of synthetic LH-RH, a rise of serum LH occurred within 5–10 minutes. These LH levels remained steady or rose very gradually for 25 minutes or longer and then increased sharply again. The peak levels of LH were observed at 1.5 hours after intra-carotid injection. Following this a gradual decrease was observed. The pattern and the magnitude of LH response after intramuscular injection of LH-RH was similar to that induced by the intracarotid injection of the same dose of LH-RH (Arimura *et al.*, 1972b).

E. Effects of LH-RH in Monkeys

Intravenous infusion of purified porcine LH-RH into an immature male chimpanzee resulted in marked rises in serum levels of both LH and FSH (Schally *et al.*, 1970b). The peaks of LH and FSH occurred within 10 minutes of the infusion. In rhesus monkeys natural and synthetic LH-RH injected intravenously or infused into the pituitary, increased serum LH significantly, as measured by radioimmunoassay (Arimura et al., 1972f).

F. EFFECT OF LH-RH IN HUMANS

Even though the quantity of natural LH-RH/FSH-RH available for testing in man was extremely limited, a reasonable amount of clinical information has been obtained. Using what the authors termed "partially purified beef hypothalamic FSH-releasing factor," Igarashi et al. (1968) found an increase in serum FSH levels 30 minutes after initiation of treatment. Unfortunately, the FSH values were determined by the bioassay method of Igarashi and McCann, the specificity of which has been questioned (deReviers and Mauleon, 1965; Lamond and Bindon, 1966). The actual weight of the administered hypothalamic extracts was not mentioned in the publication. This same preparation was given to 10 other women in a way similar to that in which human menopausal gonadotropin (HMG) or Pergonal is sometimes used in infertility cases. Thus, after an estrogenic effect was induced, human chorionic gonadotropin (HCG), a preparation high in LH activity, was administered. Ovulation occurred in one woman after FSH-RF treatment only and in 2 others after the subsequent HCG treatment.

Root et al. (1969) administered "crude ovine hypothalamic extract" to 3 abnormal children. A 7-month-old boy and a 5-week-old girl had chromosomal abnormalities while a 6-year-old boy had CNS damage with dwarfism. The weight of only one subject, the 6-year-old, was reported; from this it can be seen that, at the highest dose, this subject received 113 mg of material in a single injection. All 3 children seemed to respond to the hypothalamic extract with an increase in plasma LH levels, as determined by radioimmunoassay.

The first report of stimulation of LH release by highly purified porcine LH-RH was published in 1969 (Kastin et al., 1969). In an attempt to determine what type of subject would be most sensitive to LH-RH, 8 individuals were given a single injection of 1.5 mg of porcine LH-RH as well as 1 unit of lysine vasopressin as a control. The design was that of a 4-factor partially nested factorial experiment in which each subject served as his own control. Two men and 2 women were untreated, and 2 other men were pretreated with large doses of ethynylestradiol and 2 women received an oral contraceptive. Although there was a tendency for the men pretreated with the estrogen to show a greater release of LH and FSH, than the other groups, the differences between groups were not statistically significant. The significant release of both LH and FSH generally occurred between 16 and 32 minutes after the intravenous injection in all groups. The rise in both LH and FSH after LH-RH is interesting, since it is well known that in women, plasma LH levels and to a variable extent FSH levels rise sharply at mid-cycle (Cargile et al., 1969; Midgley and Jaffe, 1968).

The next study, using similar material at a dose of 0.7 to 1.4 mg, demonstrated that highly purified porcine LH-RH was effective in releasing LH and FSH in a number of clinical conditions (Kastin et al., 1970a). Lysine vasopressin, at a dose (0.1 unit) equivalent to that contained in the administered LH-RH, was without effect. Even though postmenopausal women already had elevated levels of LH and FSH, they released LH and FSH after injection of LH-RH, regardless of whether or not their serum LH levels had been suppressed by pretreatment with an oral contraceptive. Subcutaneous injection was found to be at least as effective as intravenous injection, and it is reasonable to expect that the intramuscular route of administration will also be effective. The question of putrescine representing FSH-RH (White et al., 1968) was again laid to rest on the basis of its lack of effect by itself or together with LH-RH in 2 subjects. Attempts to induce ovulation by a single intravenous injection of LH-RH in 2 women with secondary amenorrhea or 2 normal women on day 9 of the menstrual cycle, were unsuccessful, in spite of significant elevation of serum LH and FSH levels.

The efficacy of highly purified LH-RH in postmenopausal women prompted us to test the effects of this hypothalamic hormone in 6 men pretreated with clomiphene, a compound known to elevate plasma LH and FSH levels. The oral administration of 200 mg/day of clomiphene for 8 days caused a statistically significant increase in both LH and FSH levels which did not increase further when the treatment continued for an additional 8 days. When 0.7 mg of porcine LH-RH was injected on either day 8 or day 16, a significant increase in serum LH and FSH levels occurred, peaking between 16 and 32 minutes. The response to the LH-RH did not differ between the group taking clomiphene for 8 days and that taking it for 16 days (Kastin et al., 1970b).

The doses of highly purified porcine LH-RH used in these first 3 studies ranged between 0.7 and 1.4 mg. This dose was calculated on the basis of animal experiments so as to be reasonably sure of obtaining an adequate response (Kastin et al., 1971b). A study was then initiated to determine the minimum effective dose as well as the dose-response relationship. Accordingly, 3 normal men received 7 different doses of purified LH-RH ranging from 1.1 to 810 µg. Using analysis of variance followed by Duncan's New Multiple Range Test, it was found that as little as

10 μg of LH-RH caused a significant release of LH while 30 μg was required for a significant release of FSH. A linear trend ($p < 0.01$) was observed in the log dose-response curve. These doses were calculated to correspond to 1 and 3 μg of "pure" LH-RH, respectively.

Since our initial attempts to induce ovulation with a single injection of LH-RH were unsuccessful, a 24-hour continuous intravenous infusion was administered to a 34-year-old woman with secondary amenorrhea (Kastin et al., 1971c). The resulting elevations of LH were much higher than we ever observed with a single injection and more closely paralleled the increased mid-cycle elevations of LH observed to accompany ovulation naturally. The intravenous infusion of 600 μg of LH-RH was supplemented with acute injections of 300 μg LH-RH at 8 and 24 hours. The marked rise in urinary pregnanediol levels and basal body temperature indicated ovulation, and this was confirmed by pregnancy. In spite of the fact that a control cycle in which only HMG was administered did not result in ovulation, a cause and effect relationship between the LH-RH and ovulation was not proved. Additional cases are now being studied with various schedules of administration, including the omission of HMG (Pergonal). This result, though in a single patient, supports the possibility that LH-RH may be useful in the treatment of infertility in women.

Another potential use of LH-RH is in the diagnosis of pituitary dysfunction. TRH is now finding wide use in this area. We injected both LH-RH and TRH to 3 subjects, each of whom was an acromegalic with enlargement of the sella turcica. Three different patterns of response were found (Kastin et al., 1972b). One patient released LH in response to LH-RH, but no TSH in response to TRH. A second acromegalic showed the opposite type of response, namely, release of TSH but not LH. The third patient released both LH and TSH in response to LH-RH and TRH.

The responses of pituitary hormones other than LH and FSH to administration of LH-RH were also tested (Kastin et al., 1972d). No significant changes in plasma levels of TSH, GH, or cortisol were found. The amount of gonadotropin released by the LH-RH, however, was sufficient to elevate plasma estradiol levels in the males. In this same study, it was also demonstrated that the prepubertal pituitary is as responsive to LH-RH as the adult pituitary. Since the gonads are known to respond to gonadotropins in children, that leaves the hypothalamus as the likely center responsible for the onset of puberty.

Porcine LH-RH has also been tested in subjects with Turner's and Klinefelter's syndromes, both conditions usually characterized by elevation of gonadotropin levels. LH-RH induced release of both LH and FSH in each condition (Gual et al., 1970, 1971).

Hypothalamic tissue from humans obtained at autopsy has been purified and tested in 2 men (Kastin *et al.*, 1971a). A significant increase in LH values was found, although the FSH release was relatively insignificant. Arginine vasopressin (0.2 unit) was essentially without effect. The older subject was much less responsive to the human LH-RH than the younger volunteer. This 50-year-old man was the oldest yet tested, and further tests will be required to determine whether there is a changing sensitivity of the pituitary to LH-RH with increasing age.

A small, but significant increase in gonadotropin release has also been observed in patients with hypogonadotropic hypogonadism with varying degrees of hyposmia after administration of LH-RH (Naftolin *et al.*, 1971; Zarate *et al.*, 1972; Kastin *et al.*, 1972a).

The first clinical trials involving synthetic LH-RH FSH-RH have just been completed (Kastin *et al.*, 1972c). The synthetic decapeptide was tested in 12 subjects, divided into groups of untreated men, untreated women, men pretreated with ethynylestradiol, and women pretreated with an oral contraceptive. A marked increase in plasma LH levels and a smaller, but significant increase in plasma FSH levels was found (Figs. 3 and 4). As was the case in our first study (Kastin *et al.*, 1969), the increased gonadotropin levels did not differ among the groups. It must be pointed out, however, that relatively few subjects were tested and that individual variation was large. Since synthetic LH-RH/FSH-RH is effective in releasing gonadotropins in man, and since this decapeptide can be made in large quantities, a wide variety of clinical studies of the diagnostic and therapeutic effects of LH-RH should be possible.

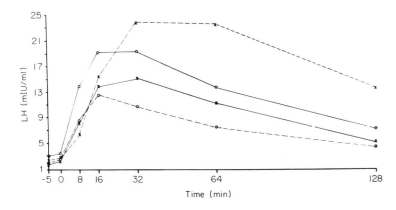

Fig. 3. Elevation of plasma LH levels in humans after administration of synthetic LH-RH/FSH-RH. From Kastin *et al.* (1972c). Courtesy of *J. Clin. Endocrinol. Metab.* and J. B. Lippincott Co., Philadelphia, Pennsylvania. X——X, Untreated men; O——O, untreated women; X- - -X, treated men; O- - -O, treated women.

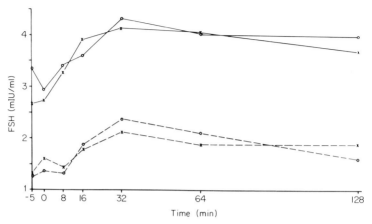

FIG. 4. Elevation of plasma FSH level in humans after administration of synthetic LH-RH/FSH-RH. See Fig. 3 for explanation of symbols. From Kastin *et al.* (1972c). Courtesy of *J. Clin. Endocrinol. Metab.* and J. B. Lippincott Co., Philadelphia, Pennsylvania.

G. APPLICATION OF LH-RH

The potential application of LH-RH as a drug for the enhancement of fertility as well as possible uses of LH-RH and its derivatives for fertility control were recently discussed in detail by Schally and Kastin (1971).

IX. EFFECT OF SEX STEROIDS AND CLOMIPHENE ON THE RESPONSE TO LH-RH/FSH-RH

A. SEX STEROIDS

The action of sex steroids on LH and FSH secretion has been discussed in Section V. The effects of steroids on the response to LH-RH/FSH-RH will be described here in some detail in order to formulate a hypothesis of how the interaction of sex steroids with a single hypothalamic gonadotropic releasing hormone (LH-RH/FSH-RH) regulates the secretion of both LH and FSH for the pituitary.

The interaction between LH-RH/FSH-RH and contraceptive steroids was studied in an attempt to find the site(s) of action of these compounds. Very large doses of 12 commonly used estrogen–progestogen oral contraceptive preparations did not block the stimulatory effect of a minute dose of LH-RH/FSH-RH on LH and FSH release in ovariectomized rats (Schally *et al.*, 1968b, 1970e). These contraceptive steroidal preparations lowered plasma LH to about one-fourth of its basal level, but administration of LH-RH/FSH-RH invariably resulted in a 6- to 13-fold elevation in plasma LH. A moderate suppression of basal FSH levels and a small rise in plasma FSH levels also occurred in ovariectomized rats treated with some of the contraceptive preparations. Some progestogens by themselves were not effective in suppressing plasma FSH levels in these ovariectomized rats. Addition of estrogen suppressed plasma FSH and also may have inhibited the rise in FSH after LH-RH.

Since these steroids did not block the release of LH (and in some cases, FSH) after administration of LH-RH, we suggested that they acted principally on the hypothalamus or another brain center rather than on the pituitary (Schally et al., 1968b, 1970e). This view is probably correct.

Recent observations, however, indicate some probable direct inhibitory effect of progesterone on the pituitary (Arimura and Schally, 1970; Hilliard et al., 1971). Arimura and Schally (1970) studied the effects of progesterone on LH release in cycling rats. Doses of 25 mg of progesterone were injected subcutaneous into intact adult female rats (proestrus rats were excluded). Forty-eight hours after the injection, a preparation of highly purified porcine LH-RH was injected into the carotid artery or infused into the pituitary. Intracarotid injection of 10 and 50 ng of LH-RH into the untreated rats raised serum LH concentrations. The same doses in the progesterone-treated animals caused a much smaller increase in serum LH. Intrapituitary infusion of LH-RH also caused a smaller rise in LH in progesterone-pretreated rats than in untreated rats. Statistical analyses indicated that progesterone significantly suppressed the LH release induced by intracarotid or intrapituitary administration of LH-RH. Thus, although large doses of progesterone do not abolish LH-RH-induced LH release in rats, they significantly suppress it. This probably indicates a direct inhibitory effect of progesterone on the pituitary (Arimura and Schally, 1970).

The studies of Hilliard et al. (1971) in rabbits also suggest some direct effect of progesterone on the pituitary. They first showed that ovulation was readily induced in estrous rabbits in response to 0.2 μg of a highly purified preparation of porcine LH-RH when it was infused directly into the adenohypophysis through stereotaxically implanted cannulae. Pretreatment with a single injection of 2 mg of progesterone 16–19 hours before infusion blocked ovulation in response to the 0.2 μg dose of LH-RH in 14/20 cases (70% block). Four of the 6 rabbits which had ovulated in spite of progesterone subsequently ovulated to a smaller dose (0.1 μg) of LH-RH in the absence of progesterone. On the other hand, when the dose of LH-RH was increased to 1.0 μg, 4 of 6 animals in which progesterone had blocked ovulation to the 0.2 μg dose now ovulated in spite of progesterone. Endogenous progesterone released during pregnancy or pseudopregnancy was effective in blocking ovulation in response to

LH-RH. Pretreatment with estradiol benzoate counteracted the blocking action of progesterone in 5/6 rabbits. These data indicate that the ability of LH-RH to overcome progesterone blockade is directly related to the dose of LH-RH administered. They also support the hypothesis that progestogens exert part of their suppressive effect on LH release directly on the pituitary.

In summary, the results in the rat and rabbit are in agreement with the concept that progesterone is involved in the inhibition of LH secretion. This may take place under physiological conditions after ovulation has occurred.

In contrast to the partial blockade by progesterone of the responses to small doses of LH-RH in rabbits, studies in rats (Arimura and Schally, 1971), sheep (Reeves et al., 1971b), and man (Kastin et al., 1969, 1970a) indicate that small doses of estrogen may increase the response to LH-RH. The effect of pretreatment with estrogen on the LH-RH induced release of LH was first investigated in diestrus rats. Small doses of estradiol were injected into 5-day cycling female rats on day 1 (diestrus). On day 2 (diestrus), 0.1 μg of LH-RH was injected into the carotid artery. Serum LH levels before and 20 minutes after the injection of LH-RH were determined by radioimmunoassay. In control rats, LH-RH injection induced only a small rise in serum LH. In the estrogen-pretreated rats, the same dose of LH-RH caused a much greater rise in serum LH levels. Estrogen by itself did not affect the level of serum LH. The results suggested that in female rats, pretreatment with estrogen results in an increased responsiveness of the pituitary to LH-RH (Arimura and Schally, 1971). In the male rat, however, pretreatment with estradiol benzoate not only failed to augment the FSH and LH release induced by LH-RH, but even slightly suppressed that response (Debeljuk et al., 1972c). On the other hand, pretreatment of male rats with testosterone propionate clearly suppressed the FSH and LH release after LH-RH. The combination of testosterone propionate with estradiol benzoate suppressed the response to LH-RH more than testosterone alone (Debeljuk et al., 1972c). Treatment of men with ethynylestradiol lowered plasma LH and FSH levels, but testosterone administration lowered only serum LH (Peterson et al., 1968).

The effects of estrogen on the response to LH-RH were also studied in sheep. Pretreatment of anestrous ewes with 250 and 500 μg estradiol benzoate increased baseline levels of LH. Doses of 250 and 500 μg estradiol benzoate augmented the LH release after LH-RH as compared to control ewes (Reeves et al., 1971b). These data add further support to the hypothesis that part of the stimulatory effects of estrogens on LH-release may be due to an increase in pituitary responsiveness to LH-RH.

It is interesting that the peak of plasma estradiol precedes the ovulatory surge of LH in rats (Brown-Grant et al., 1970). Similarly, a peak of plasma or urinary estrogen also precedes the surge of FSH and LH in women at mid-cycle and may be responsible for it (Goebelsmann et al., 1969; Corker et al., 1969; Burger et al., 1968).

On the other hand, there is fairly good evidence that increased estrogen secretion may suppress FSH release (Flerko, 1971; Davidson, 1969; Speroff and Van de Wiele, 1971). Indirect evidence from studies on contraceptive steroids (Schally et al., 1970e), which were reviewed above, (Section IX, A) supports this view. Moreover, the positive feedback of estrogen may stimulate mostly LH but not FSH secretion (Speroff and Van de Wiele, 1971). Treatment of castrated rats with estrogen and progesterone may impair the release and synthesis of FSH (Gay and Bogdanove, 1969). Recent results of Schally et al. (1972c) clearly demonstrate that addition of small amounts of ethynylestradiol to rat pituitaries incubated in vitro significantly inhibits the stimulatory effect of LH-RH/FSH-RH on the release of FSH. LH release is also inhibited, but apparently to a lesser extent than that of FSH. This proves that estrogen can inhibit the release of FSH and LH and that one of the sites of this negative feedback is the pituitary gland. In conclusion, FSH secretion, particularly after LH-RH/FSH-RH, appears to be more readily suppressed by estrogen (or a combination of estrogen and progesterone, see also below) than either LH secretion or the effects of LH-RH/FSH-RH on LH release (Speroff and Van de Wiele, 1971; Schally et al., 1970b, 1972c).

The effects of the estrogen–progesterone combination on the response to LH-RH/FSH-RH were also investigated. Debeljuk et al. (1972b) investigated the effect of pretreatment with estradiol, progesterone, or a combination of both steroids on the response of LH and FSH to LH-RH in female rats and ewes. In intact diestrous rats, estradiol augmented the LH release induced by LH-RH. Progesterone did not block the LH release induced by 1 μg of LH-RH, but suppressed that caused by 0.05 μg LH-RH. In these rats, as well as in anestrous ewes, the combination of estradiol and progesterone unmistakably suppressed the release of LH in response to moderate doses of LH-RH (Debeljuk et al., 1972b).

The blocking effect of the combination of estrogen plus progesterone on LH release may have a physiological meaning, since large amounts of these steroids, especially progesterone, are secreted after ovulation in rats (Lisk, 1969), monkeys (Monroe et al., 1970), and women (Neill et al., 1967; Cargille et al., 1969; Saxena et al., 1968; Midgley and Jaffe, 1968; Odell et al., 1968; Johansson and Wide, 1969). It is well known that concentrations of serum LH and FSH increase dramatically during mid-cycle in women (Midgley and Jaffe, 1968; Cargille et al., 1969; Taymor *et al.*, 1968) and in the afternoon of proestrus in rats (Gay *et al.*, 1970b; Parlow *et al.*, 1969; Schwartz and Calderelli, 1965; McCann and Ramirez, 1964; McClintock and Schwartz, 1968) and then decline. The peak of plasma LH is also associated with estrus and ovulation in cows, sheep, and pigs (Gay *et al.*, 1970b). Estrogens combined with high levels of progesterone secreted after ovulation, may lower serum LH and FSH concentrations, perhaps by decreasing the pituitary responsiveness to LH-RH/FSH-RH. They may also suppress the further release of endogenous LH-RH/FSH-RH by an inhibitory feedback exerted at the hypothalamus.

At the time this review is being written (September–October, 1971) no other results are available on the effects of steroids on the response to LH-RH, and it is not possible to construct a detailed and complete model of the interactions of sex steroids with LH-RH/FSH-RH. Nevertheless, the interactions of sex steroids with a single hypothalamic LH- and FSH-releasing hormone are likely to be responsible for the entire regulation of LH and FSH secretion. The responsiveness of the pituitary to LH-RH/FSH-RH, the synthesis of pituitary LH and FSH, and the consequent levels of LH and FSH may be due to interactions with sex steroids as originally suggested by Bogdanove (1964).

B. CLOMIPHENE

Clomiphene citrate is a synthetic nonsteroidal substance having a triarylhaloethylenic chemical structure and is comprised of the two geometric isomers, cisclomiphene and transclomiphene. It has been extensively evaluated in animals and in man and reported to affect the hypophyseal–gonadal system (S. Roy *et al.*, 1964; Greenblatt and Mahesh, 1965; Kistner, 1966; Bardin *et al.*, 1967). A study was undertaken to try to elucidate the effect of clomiphene and its isomers on the release of LH and FSH as well as their effect on the responses to LH-RH (Schally *et al.*, 1970c).

The effects of subcutaneous administration of clomiphene citrate and its isomers were evaluated in ovariectomized adult rats. At doses of 2500 and 10,000 μg per day for 3 days, the three compounds lowered plasma LH levels. Transclomiphene was more effective in suppressing LH levels than cisclomiphene. However, administration of LH-RH to rats treated with these high doses of clomiphene and its isomers raised plasma LH levels. Lower doses of the compounds (15–135 μg per rat per day for 3 days) appeared to further increase the high plasma LH found in ovariectomized rats; cisclomiphene gave the greatest and most consistent elevation. The low doses of clomiphene and cisclomiphene also seemed to enhance slightly the response to LH-RH. Serum FSH was raised by low doses of clomiphene and its isomers and decreased by the high doses of transclomiphene. Thus, clomiphene and its isomers exert a dual dose-dependent effect. At high doses they inhibit LH release, but at low doses stimulate either LH release or facilitate the effect of LH-RH on the pituitary. The stimulatory effect of clomiphene on LH and FSH secretion may be mediated by the release of hypothalamic LH-RH/FSH-RH (Schneider et al., 1968; Baier and Taubert, 1968). The response to LH-RH/FSH-RH was not blocked by the high doses of clomiphene. This provides evidence that the blocking action of clomiphene is exerted not on the pituitary, but on a CNS center, possibly the hypothalamus (Schally et al., 1970c). Similar results were obtained by Igarashi et al. (1967), Boyar (1970), and Koch et al. (1971). However, in sheep, cis-clomiphene inhibited LH release induced by LH-RH (Debeljuk et al., 1972a). This finding is in agreement with that recently reported by Lindsay and Robinson (1970), who observed that the injection of clomiphene in sheep evoked ovarian and uterine inhibition.

X. Mechanism of Action of LH-RH/FSH-RH

Several groups of investigators attempted to study the mechanism of action of LH-RH and FSH-RH. This subject has been recently expertly reviewed by Geschwind (1970).

Samli and Geschwind (1968) showed that the stimulatory effect of the hypothalamic extract on the release of LH from the rat pituitary incubated *in vitro* was dependent upon the presence of Ca^{2+} in the medium. Jutisz and De La Llosa (1970) showed the same effect for FSH. The many possible explanations for this effect were discussed by Geschwind (1970). Samli and Geschwind also showed that when the K^+ concentration of the medium was increased 10 times, the release of LH was stimulated as compared to controls in isotonic (normal) K^+. Jutisz and De La Llosa (1970) observed the same effect for FSH.

The effects of "optimal" high (K^+) concentration are enhanced by LH-RH (Samli and Geschwind, 1968). This may mean that high (K^+) facilitates the release of LH in a different way than does LH-RH. The release of neural hormones by a high (K^+) was attributed by Douglas (1963) to the depolarization of the specific cell membranes. Therefore, LH-RH may not act by the same mechanism.

Since energy transfer inhibitors such as dinitrophenol and oligomycin, which block or uncouple oxidative phosphorylations, inhibited incorporation of [^{14}C]leucine into LH but did not affect the release of LH, the synthesis and release of LH were said to be separate phenomena (Samli and Geschwind, 1968). Nevertheless, some energy may be required for the process of LH release (Geschwind, 1970).

The dependence of the release of LH and FSH on the protein on RNA synthesis has also been studied. Crighton *et al.* (1968) reported that neither puromycin nor actinomycin D interfered with the stimulatory effect of LH-RH on the release of LH *in vitro*. Jutisz *et al.* (1966) showed that the stimulatory effect of LH-RH on the release of LH *in vitro* by pituitary tissue is partially but significantly inhibited by puromycin, which is an inhibitor of protein synthesis. Actinomycin D (an inhibitor of RNA synthesis) seems to have no significant effect. As puromycin does not inhibit the LH-releasing activity of LH-RH to the same extent as it inhibits the total synthesis of proteins (95%), Jutisz *et al.* (1966) suggested that LH-RH may act not by stimulation of the synthesis of the LH polypeptide chain, but at a different stage of the completion of the LH molecule.

Watanabe *et al.* (1968) reported that puromycin and actinomycin D almost completely inhibited the release of FSH from adult male anterior pituitaries incubated *in vitro* in the presence of hypothalamic extracts. Puromycin and actinomycin D interfered with the incorporation of labeled substrates into the protein and RNA fractions of the incubated pituitaries. Neither antibiotic affected the release of FSH which occurred in the absence ' of hypothalamic extract. They suggested that protein synthesis may be required for the action of FSH-RH in inducing release of FSH from the anterior pituitary (Watanabe *et al.*, 1968). On the other hand, Jutisz and De La Llosa (1969) showed that puromycin and actinomycin D partially inhibited the stimulatory action of FSH-RH on FSH release *in vitro*. As inhibition of FSH-release after FSH-RH by puromycin and actinomycin D was not equivalent to that of the total synthesis of proteins and RNA, they suggested that FSH-RH does not act directly on stimulation of either biosynthesis of the FSH-polypeptide chain or synthesis of the messenger RNA specific for FSH. It was said that FSH-RH acted only on the stimulation of the release of FSH. They suggested that the synthesis of FSH during the incubation of pituitary tissue with FSH-RH may be explained by resynthesis after the process of the release of FSH. However, a dual action of FSH-RH on release and synthesis of FSH was not excluded.

The stimulatory effects of cyclic AMP on LH and FSH release were also studied by Jutisz and De La Llosa (1970). The stimulatory effect of cyclic AMP was found to be Ca^{2+} dependent. Jutisz *et al.* (1970) showed that the amounts of LH and FSH released in the presence of cyclic AMP were much lower than those released by the stimulatory effect of LH-RH/FSH-RH preparations. This may be because of rapid destruction by phosphodiesterase (Robison *et al.*, 1968). Although the action of cyclic AMP on the release of LH was slower than the action of

LH-RH, Jutisz *et al.* (1970) concluded that potentiation of the action of LH-RH by theophylline is good presumptive evidence of the participation of cyclic AMP in the processes of release of LH and FSH. How cyclic AMP promotes LH and FSH release is uncertain (Geschwind, 1970).

In conclusion the mechanism of action of LH-RH/FSH-RH is still obscure. Moreover, although there is much evidence that the synthesis of LH and FSH is stimulated by LH-RH/FSH-RH, the experiments on the mechanism of action do not yield clear evidence how this effect is exerted.

XI. CONTROL OF RELEASE OF LH-RH AND FSH-RH

EFFECT OF MONOAMINES ON FSH-RH AND LH-RH SECRETION

Recent evidence implicates dopamine in the control of release of LH-RH and FSH-RH. Hypothalamic neurons are known to contain dopamine, norepinephrine, and serotonin. These amines by themselves do not alter LH release from rat pituitaries. If hypothalamic and pituitary tissue together were incubated with dopamine, the LH release was stimulated. These results were explained by an enhanced LH-RH release by incubated hypothalamic tissue in the presence of dopamine (Schneider and McCann, 1969). The authors also suggested that hypothalamic dopaminergic neurons "synapse" with the neurosecretory neurons which secrete the LH-RH and stimulate its release (Schneider and McCann, 1969).

The action of dopamine in inducing release of FSH-RH from hypothalamic tissue *in vitro* was also studied (Kamberi *et al.*, 1970b). If the combined hypothalamic and anterior pituitary tissue were incubated together with 1–5 μg/ml of serotonin, epinephrine, or norepinephrine, basal release of FSH was unaltered. When dopamine was added to the incubation medium in doses of 2.5–5 μg/ml, FSH release was significantly increased and a dose-response relationship was observed. The response to dopamine was completely inhibited by the α-adrenergic blocker, phentolamine (Kamberi *et al.*, 1970b).

Schneider and McCann (1970) studied the effect of intraventricular injection of dopamine on LH release in rats. Dopamine raised LH to levels as high as 8- or 10-fold above controls in rats on day 2 of diestrus or in proestrus. In normal males, it raised plasma LH in most animals. Kamberi *et al.* (1970a) compared the effect of anterior pituitary perfusion and intraventricular injection of dopamine on LH release. Within 10 minutes after injection of dopamine hydrochloride into the third ventricle, the serum LH concentration had increased 9-fold. When dopamine was perfused into the anterior pituitary for 30 minutes via a microcannula inserted into a hypophyseal portal vein, LH release was not affected. Furthermore, when dopamine was infused into the stalk–median eminence complex via the basilar artery, no significant effect on serum LH concentration was observed. These findings indicate that dopamine does not affect LH release by a direct action on the anterior pituitary but indirectly through the hypothalamus (Kamberi et al., 1970a). Perhaps the most conclusive proof that dopamine affects the release of LH-RH was provided by the demonstration in rats of increased levels of LH-RH in blood from hypophyseal stalk after administration of dopamine (Kamberi et al., 1969). However, it should be noted that Ahren et al. (1971) used the histochemical fluorescence analysis of dopamine to find opposite results. That is, they describe decreased dopamine turnover in the median eminence during proestrus and early estrus. They therefore propose an inhibitory dopaminergic input to the hypothalamus.

XII. A CHANGE IN NOMENCLATURE?

In 1967 we proposed (Schally et al., 1968a) a new nomenclature for hypothalamic neurohumors involved in the control of anterior pituitary gland, which was based on the term releasing hormone, rather than factor. Since then, more evidence has accumulated suggesting strongly that the hypothalamic releasing hormones regulate the synthesis of anterior pituitary hormones as well as their release. We are suggesting now further revision of our nomenclature by recommending the use of the name "regulating hormone." The abbreviation would remain the same. Thus, LH-RH/FSH-RH would stand for LH- and FSH-regulating hormone. The abbreviation Gn-RH for gonadotropin-releasing hormone is inconvenient and confusing, since it is too similar to GH-RH (growth hormone-releasing hormone).

XIII. SUMMARY AND CONCLUSIONS

Early physiological and anatomical studies in the 1930s, 1940s, and early 1950s suggested the existence of agent(s), formed in the hypothalamus and secreted into the hypophyseal portal blood, which acted as key regulators of secretion of gonadotropin from the anterior pituitary gland. This hypothesis proved to be correct, and during the 1960s we have seen the preparation of highly potent concentrates of hypothalamic tissue which stimulated the release of follicle-stimulating hormone and luteinizing hormone in vivo and in vitro. Recently, we isolated from pig hypothalami a decapeptide which has both FSH-releasing hormone (FSH-RH) activity and LH-releasing hormone (LH-RH) activity. Its amino acid sequence was determined to be (pyro)Glu-His-Trp-Ser-Tyr-

Gly-Leu-Arg-Pro-Gly-NH₂. The decapeptide corresponding to this structure was synthesized and shown to release LH and FSH in animals and man. Natural and synthetic FSH-RH/LH-RH also stimulated the synthesis of both gonadotropins in tissue cultures of rat pituitaries *in vitro*. This polypeptide appears to represent the single hypothalamic hormone which controls the secretion of both LH and FSH from the anterior pituitary gland. The overall control of release and synthesis of FSH and LH is most likely mediated by the interactions of this hypothalamic FSH- and LH-releasing hormone with sex steroids. Clinical studies carried out with natural and synthetic LH-RH/FSH-RH indicate that this substance should find practical application in the treatment of sterility. The availability of synthetic LH-RH/FSH-RH should now make possible large-scale clinical evaluation of this hormone.

ACKNOWLEDGMENTS

We are grateful to Dr. Luciano Debeljuk, Professors C. H. Sawyer, and E. M. Bogdanove for editorial suggestions, and Mrs. Linda Lawler for expert editing and typing.

REFERENCES

Ahren, K., Fuxe, K., Hamberger, L., and Hokfelt, T. (1971). *Endocrinology* **88**, 1415.
Amoss, M. S., and Guillemin, R. (1969). *Endocrinology* **84**, 1517.
Amoss, M., Burgus, R., Ward, D. N., Fellows, R. E., and Guillemin, R. (1970). *Proc. 52nd Meet. Endocrine Soc.* Abstract, p. 61, No. 50.
Amoss, M. S., Burgus, R., Blackwell, R., Vale, W., Fellows, R., and Guillemin, R. (1971). *Biochem. Biophys. Res. Commun.* **44**, 205.
Antunez-Rodrigues, J., and McCann, S. M. (1967). *Endocrinology* **81**, 666.
Arai, Y., and Gorski, R. A. (1968). *Endocrinology* **82**, 871.
Arimura, A., and Schally, A. V. (1970). *Endocrinology* **87**, 653.
Arimura, A., and Schally, A. V. (1971). *Proc. Soc. Exp. Biol. Med.* **136**, 290.
Arimura, A., Saito, T., Muller, E., Bowers, C. Y., Sawano, S., and Schally, A. V. (1967a). *Endocrinology* **80**, 972.
Arimura, A., Schally, A. V., Saito, T., Muller, E. E., and Bowers, C. Y. (1967b). *Endocrinology* **80**, 515.
Arimura, A., Matsuo, H., Baba, Y., and Schally, A. V. (1971a). *Science* **174**, 511.
Arimura, A., Rennels, E. G., Shiino, M., and Schally, A. V. (1971b). *Congr. Physiol. Sci.* [*Proc.*], *25th, 1971* Vol. IX, No. 57, p. 23.
Arimura, A., Debeljuk, L., Matsuo, H., and Schally, A. V. (1972a). *Endocrinology* (submitted for publication).
Arimura, A., Debeljuk, L., Matsuo, H., and Schally, A. V. (1972b). *Proc. Soc. Exp. Biol. Med.* **139**, 851.
Arimura, A., Debeljuk, L., and Schally, A. V. (1972c). *Endocrinology* **91** (in press).
Arimura, A., Kastin, A. J., and Schally, A. V. (1972d). *In* "Gonadotropins" (B. Saxena, C. G. Beling, and H. M. Gandy, eds.), p. 32. Wiley (Interscience), New York.
Arimura, A., Matsuo, H., Baba, Y., Debeljuk, L., Sandow, J., and Schally, A. V. (1972e). *Endocrinology* **90**, 163.
Arimura, A., Spies, H. G., Debeljuk, L., and Schally, A. V. (1972f). In preparation.

Baba, Y., Matsuo, H., and Schally, A. V. (1971a). *Biochem. Biophys. Res. Commun.* **44,** 459.

Baba, Y., Arimura, A., and Schally, A. V. (1971b). *Biochem. Biophys. Res. Commun.* **45,** 483.

Baba, Y., Arimura, A., and Schally, A. V. (1971c). *J. Biol. Chem.* **264,** 7581.

Baier, H., and Taubert, H.-D. (1968). *Experientia* **24,** 1165.

Baker, J. R., and Ranson, R. M. (1932). *Proc. Roy. Soc., Ser. B* **110,** 313.

Bardin, C. W., Ross, G. T., and Lipsett, M. B. (1967). *J. Clin. Endocrinol. Metab.* **27,** 558.

Bargman, W. (1949). *Z. Zellforsch. Mikrosk. Anat.* **34,** 610.

Barraclough, C. A. (1963). *Advan. Neuroendocrinol., Proc. Symp., 1961* p. 224.

Barraclough, C. A., and Haller, E. W. (1970). *Endocrinology* **86,** 542.

Barraclough, C. A., and Sawyer, C. H. (1957). *Endocrinology* **61,** 341.

Barry, J., Moschetto, Y., and Leonardelli, J. (1967). *C. R. Acad. Sci.* **265,** 1141.

Beddow, D. G., and McCann, S. M. (1969). *Endocrinology* **84,** 595.

Beddow, D., Dhariwal, A. P. S., and McCann, S. M. (1970). *Proc. Soc. Exp. Biol. Med.* **135,** 671.

Benoit, J. (1935). *C. R. Soc. Biol.* **120,** 1326.

Benoit, J., and Assenmacher, I. (1951). *Arch. Anat. Microsc. Morphol. Exp.* **40,** 27.

Benoit, J., and Assenmacher, I. (1953). *Arch. Anat. Microsc. Morphol. Exp.* **42,** 334.

Bissonnette, T. H. (1932). *Proc. Roy. Soc., Ser. B* **110,** 332.

Bogdanove, E. M. (1957). *Endocrinology* **60,** 689.

Bogdanove, E. M. (1963). *Endocrinology* **73,** 696.

Bogdanove, E. M. (1964). *Vitam. Horm. (New York)* **22,** 205.

Bogdanove, E. M. (1967). *Anat. Rec.* **157,** 117.

Bogdanove, E. M., and Gay, V. L. (1967). *Endocrinology* **81,** 930.

Bogdanove, E. M., Spirtos, B. N., and Halmi, N. S. (1955). *Endocrinology* **57,** 302.

Bogdanove, E. M., Hilliard, J., and Sawyer, C. H. (1971). *Endocrinology* **88,** A-76.

Bogentoft, C., Currie, B. L., Sievertsson, H., Chang, J-K., Folkers, K., and Bowers, C. Y. (1971). *Biochem. Biophys. Res. Commun.* **44,** 403.

Bowers, C. Y., Redding, T. W., and Schally, A. V. (1964). *Endocrinology* **74,** 559.

Bowers, C. Y., Chang, J-K., Sievertsson, H., Bogentoft, C., Currie, B. L., and Folkers, K. (1971). *Biochem. Biophys. Res. Commun.* **44,** 414.

Boyar, R. M. (1970). *Endocrinology* **86,** 629.

Brown-Grant, K. (1969). *J. Endocrinol.* **43,** 553.

Brown-Grant, K., Exley, D., and Naftolin, F. (1970). *J. Endocrinol.* **48,** 295.

Burger, H. G., Catt, K. J., and Brown, J. B. (1968). *J. Clin. Endocrinol. Metab.* **28,** 1508.

Byrnes, W. W., and Meyer, R. K. (1951). *Endocrinology* **49,** 449.

Caligaris, L., Astrada, J. J., and Taleisnik, S. (1968). *Acta Endocrinol. (Copenhagen)* **59,** 177.

Callantine, M. R., Humphrey, R. R., and Nesset, B. L. (1966). *Endocrinology* **79,** 455.

Campbell, H. J., Feuer, G., Garcia, J., and Harris, G. W. (1961). *J. Physiol. (London)* **157,** 30P.

Campbell, H. J., Feuer, G., and Harris, G. W. (1964). *J. Physiol. (London)* **170,** 474.

Cargille, C. M., Ross, G. T., and Yoshimi, T. (1969). *J. Clin. Endocrinol. Metab.* **29,** 12.

Chang, J-K., Sievertsson, H., Bogentoft, C., Currie, B. L., Folkers, K., and Bowers, C. Y. (1971). *Biochem. Biophys. Res. Commun.* 44, 409.
Chowers, I., and McCann, S. M. (1965). *Endocrinology* 76, 700.
Cohen, A. I., Nicol, E., and White, W. F. (1966). *Fed. Proc., Fed. Amer. Soc. Exp. Biol.* 25, 315.
Corbin, A., and Cohen, A. I. (1966). *Endocrinology* 78, 41.
Corbin, A., and Daniels, E. L. (1967). *Neuroendocrinology* 2, 304.
Corbin, A., and Daniels, E. L. (1969). *Neuroendocrinology* 4, 65.
Corbin, A., and Story, J. C. (1966). *Experientia* 22, 694.
Corbin, A., and Story, J. C. (1967). *Endocrinology* 80, 1006.
Corbin, A., Daniels, E. L., and Milmore, J. E. (1970). *Endocrinology* 86, 735.
Corker, C. S., Naftolin, F., and Exley, D. (1969). *Nature (London)* 222, 1063.
Courrier, R., Guillemin, R., Jutisz, M., Sakiz, E., and Aschheim, P. (1961). *C. R. Acad. Sci.* 253, 922.
Courrier, R., Jutisz, M., and Colonge, A. (1963). *C. R. Acad. Sci.* 257, 3774.
Crighton, D. B., Watanabe, S., Dhariwal, A. P. S., and McCann, S. M. (1968). *Proc. Soc. Exp. Biol. Med.* 128, 537.
Crighton, D. B., Schneider, H. P. G., and McCann, S. M. (1969). *J. Endocrinol.* 44, 405.
Critchlow, V. (1958). *Amer. J. Physiol.* 195, 171.
Critchlow, V. (1963). *Advan. Neuroendocrinol., Proc. Symp., 1961* p. 377.
Daane, T. A., and Parlow, A. F. (1971). *Endocrinology* 88, 653.
David, M. A., Fraschini, F., and Martini, L. (1965a). *Experientia* 21, 483.
David, M. A., Fraschini, F., and Martini, L. (1965b). *C. R. Acad. Sci.* 261, 2249.
David, M., Fraschini, F., and Martini, L. (1966). *Endocrinology* 78, 55.
Davidson, J. M. (1966). In "Neuroendocrinology" (L. Martini and W. F. Ganong, eds.), Vol. 1, p. 565. Academic Press, New York.
Davidson, J. M. (1969). In "Frontiers in Neuroendocrinology" (W. F. Ganong and L. Martini, eds.), pp. 343–388. Oxford Univ. Press, London and New York.
Davidson, J. M., and Sawyer, C. H. (1961a). *Proc. Soc. Exp. Biol. Med.* 107, 4.
Davidson, J. M., and Sawyer, C. H. (1961b). *Acta Endocrinol. (Copenhagen)* 37, 385.
Davidson, J. M., Contopoulos, A. N., and Ganong, W. F. (1960). *Endocrinology* 66, 735.
Debeljuk, L., Arimura, A., Sandow, J. K., and Schally, A. V. (1972a). *J. Anim. Sci.* 34, 294.
Debeljuk, L., Arimura, A., and Schally, A. V. (1972b). *Proc. Soc. Exp. Biol. Med.* 139, 774.
Debeljuk, L., Arimura, A., and Schally, A. V. (1972c). *Endocrinology* 90, 1578.
Debeljuk, L., Arimura, A., and Schally, A. V. (1972d). *Endocrinology* 90, 585.
deReviers, M. M., and Mauleon, P. (1965). *C. R. Acad. Sci.* 261, 540.
Deuben, R. R., and Meites, J. (1964). *Endocrinology* 74, 408.
Dey, F. L. (1941). *Amer. J. Anat.* 69, 61.
Dey, F. L. (1943). *Endocrinology* 33, 75.
Dey, F. L., Fisher, C., Berry, C. M., and Ranson, S. W. (1940). *Amer. J. Physiol.* 129, 39.
Dhariwal, A. P. S., Antunes-Rodriguez, J., and McCann, S. M. (1965a). *Proc. Soc. Exp. Biol. Med.* 118, 999.
Dhariwal, A. P. S., Nallar, R., Batt, M., and McCann, S. M. (1965b). *Endocrinology* 76, 290.

154   A. V. SCHALLY, A. J. KASTIN, AND A. ARIMURA

Docke, F., and Dorner, G. (1965). *J. Endocrinol.* 33, 491.
Docke, F., and Dorner, G. (1969). *Neuroendocrinology* 4, 139.
Docke, F., Dorner, G., and Voigt, K. H. (1968). *J. Endocrinol.* 41, 353.
Domanski, E., and Kochman, K. (1968). *J. Endocrinol.* 42, 383.
Donovan, B. T. (1971). *Acta Endocrinol. (Copenhagen)* 66, 1.
Donovan, B. T., and Harris, G. W. (1954). *Nature (London)* 174, 503.
Donovan, B. T., and Harris, G. W. (1956). *J. Physiol. (London)* 131, 102.
Doolittle, R. F., and Armentrout, R. W. (1968). *Biochemistry* 7, 463.
Douglas, W. W. (1963). *Nature (London)* 197, 81.
Ectors, F., and Pasteels, J. L. (1967). *C. R. Acad. Sci.* 265, 758.
Eisenfeld, A. J., and Axelrod, J. (1965). *J. Pharmacol. Exp. Ther.* 150, 469.
Endroczi, E., and Hilliard, J. (1965). *Endocrinology* 77, 667.
Eshkol, A., and Lunenfeld, B. (1967). *Acta Endocrinol. (Copenhagen)* 54, 91.
Everett, J. W. (1948). *Endocrinology* 43, 389.
Everett, J. W. (1951). *Anat. Rec.* 109, 291.
Everett, J. W. (1956a). *Endocrinology* 58, 786.
Everett, J. W. (1956b). *Endocrinology* 59, 580.
Everett, J. W. (1961). In "Sex and Internal Secretions" (W. C. Young, ed.), 3rd ed.,
    Volume 1, p. 497. Williams & Wilkins, Baltimore, Maryland.
Everett, J. W. (1964). *Physiol. Rev.* 44, 373.
Everett, J. W. (1969). *Annu. Rev. Physiol.* 31, 383.
Everett, J. W. (1970). In "La photoregulation de la reproduction chez les oiseaux
    et les mammifères" (J. Benoit and I. Assenmacher, eds.), p. 387. CNRS, Paris.
Everett, J. W., and Quinn, D. L. (1966). *Endocrinology* 78, 141.
Everett, J. W., and Sawyer, C. H. (1949). *Endocrinology* 45, 581.
Everett, J. W., and Sawyer, C. H. (1950). *Endocrinology* 47, 198.
Everett, J. W., and Sawyer, C. H. (1953). *Endocrinology* 52, 83.
Everett, J. W., Sawyer, C. H., and Markee, J. E. (1949). *Endocrinology* 44, 234.
Everett, J. W., Holsinger, J. W., Zeilmaker, G. H., Redmond, W. C., and Quinn,
    D. L. (1970). *Neuroendocrinology* 6, 98.
Exley, D., Gellert, R. J., Harris, G. W., and Nadler, R. D. (1968). *J. Physiol.
    (London)* 195, 697.
Farner, D. S. (1965). In "Circadian Clocks" (J. Aschoff, ed.), p. 357. North-Holland
    Publ., Amsterdam.
Farner, D. S., and Follett, B. K. (1966). *J. Anim. Sci.* 25, 90.
Faure, J., Vincent, D., and Bensch, C. (1966). *C. R. Soc. Biol.* 160, 1557.
Fawcett, C. P. (1970). In "Hypophysiotropic Hormones of the Hypothalamus: Assay
    and Chemistry" (J. Meites, ed.), p. 242. Williams & Wilkins, Baltimore,
    Maryland.
Fawcett, C. P., and McCann, S. M. (1972). Private communication.
Fawcett, C. P., and McCann, S. M. (1971). *Int. Congr. Physiol. Sci. [Proc.], 25th,
    1971* No. 503, p. 172.
Fawcett, C. P., Harris, G. W., and Reed, M. (1965). *Int. Congr. Physiol. Sci. Lect.
    Symp., 23rd, 1965 Int. Congr. Ser. No. 87,* p. 300.
Fawcett, C. P., Reed, M., Charlton, H. M., and Harris, G. W. (1968). *Biochem. J.*
    106, 229.
Fevold, H. L. (1943). *Ann. N. Y. Acad. Sci.* 43, 321.
Fevold, H. L., Hisaw, F. L., and Leonard, S. L. (1931). *Amer. J. Physiol.* 104, 291.
Fevold, H. L., Hisaw, F. L., Hellbaum, A., and Hertz, R. (1933). *Amer. J. Physiol.*
    104, 710.
Fevold, H. L., Hisaw, F. L., and Greep, R. O. (1937). *Endocrinology* 21, 343.

Fevold, H. L., Lee, M., Hisaw, F. L., and Cohn, E. J. (1940). *Endocrinology* **26**, 999.

Fink, G., and Harris, G. W. (1970). *J. Physiol. (London)* **208**, 221.

Fink, G., Nallar, R., and Worthington, W. C., Jr. (1965). *J. Physiol. (London)* **183**, 20p.

Fink, G., Nallar, R., and Worthington, W. C., Jr. (1967). *J. Physiol. (London)* **191**, 407.

Fiske, V. M. (1941). *Endocrinology* **29**, 187.

Flerko, B. (1963). *Advan. Neuroendocrinol., Proc. Symp., 1961* p. 211.

Flerko, B. (1971). *In* "The Hypothalamus" (L. Martini, M. Motta, and F. Fraschini, eds.), p. 351. Academic Press, New York.

Flerko, B., and Szentágothai, J. (1957). *Acta Endocrinol. (Copenhagen)* **26**, 121.

Flouret, G., Arnold, W., Cole, J. W., Morgan, R., Nedland, M., and White, W. F. (1972). *J. Med. Chem.* (in press).

Follett, B. K. (1970). *Gen. Comp. Endocrinol.* **15**, 165.

Follett, B. K., and Farner, D. S. (1966). *Gen. Comp. Endocrinol.* **7**, 111.

Follett, B. K., and Sharp, P. J. (1969). *Nature (London)* **223**, 968.

Frankel, A. I., Gibson, W. R., Graber, J. W., Nelson, D. M., Reichert, L. E., Jr., and Nalbandov, A. V. (1965). *Endocrinology* **77**, 651.

Fuerstner, P. G. (1944). *J. Nerv. Ment. Dis.* **99**, 588.

Gans, E. (1959). *Acta Endocrinol. (Copenhagen)* **32**, 362.

Gay, V. L., and Bogdanove, E. M. (1968). *Endocrinology* **82**, 359.

Gay, V. L., and Bogdanove, E. M. (1969). *Endocrinology* **84**, 1132.

Gay, V. L., Rebar, R. W., and Midgley, A. R., Jr. (1969). *Proc. Soc. Exp. Biol. Med.* **130**, 1344.

Gay, V. L., Niswender, G. D., and Midgley, A. R., Jr. (1970a). *Endocrinology* **86**, 1305.

Gay, V. L., Midgley, A. R., Jr., and Niswender, G. D. (1970b). *Fed. Proc., Fed. Amer. Soc. Exp. Biol.* **29**, 1880.

Geiger, R., Konig, W., Wissman, H., Geisin, K., and Enzmann, F. (1971). *Biochem. Biophys. Res. Commun.* **45**, 767.

Gellert, R. J., Bass, E., Jacobs, C., Smith, R., and Ganong, W. F. (1964). *Endocrinology* **75**, 861.

Geschwind, I. I. (1970). *In* "Hypophysiotropic Hormones of the Hypothalamus: Assay and Chemistry" (J. Meites, ed.), p. 298. Williams & Wilkins, Baltimore, Maryland.

Gittes, R. F., and Kastin, A. J. (1966). *Endocrinology* **78**, 1023.

Goebelsmann, U., Midgley, A. R., Jr., and Jaffe, R. B. (1969). *J. Clin. Endocrinol. Metab.* **29**, 1222.

Gorski, R. A., and Barraclough, C. A. (1962). *Proc. Soc. Exp. Biol. Med.* **110**, 298.

Gray, W. F. (1967). *In* "Methods in Enzymology" (C. H. W. Hirs, ed.), Vol. 11, p. 139. Academic Press, New York.

Green, J., and Harris, G. W. (1947). *J. Endocrinol.* **5**, 136.

Greenblatt, R. B., and Mahesh, V. B. (1965). *In* "Yearbook of Endocrinology 1964–1965" (T. B. Schwartz, ed.), p. 248. Yearbook Publ., Chicago, Illinois.

Greep, R. O. (1936). *Proc. Soc. Exp. Biol. Med.* **34**, 754.

Greep, R. O. (1961). *In* "Sex and Internal Secretions" (W. C. Young, ed.), 3rd ed., Vol. 1, p. 242. Williams & Wilkins, Baltimore, Maryland.

Greep, R. O., and Barrnett, R. J. (1951). *Endocrinology* **49**, 172.

Greep, R. O., and Chester-Jones, I. (1950). *Recent Progr. Horm. Res.* **5**, 197.

Gual, C., Flores, F., Kastin, A. J., Schally, A. V., and Midgley, A. R., Jr. (1970). *Reunion Anual Soc. Mex. Nutr. Endocrinol., 10th* p. 331.

Gual, C., Kastin, A. J., Midgley, A. R., Jr., and Flores, F. (1971). *Endocrinology* Suppl. 88, A-128.

Guillemin, R. (1967a). *Int. J. Fert.* 12, 359.

Guillemin, R. (1967b). *Annu. Rev. Physiol.* 29, 313.

Guillemin, R., Jutisz, M., and Sakiz, E. (1963a). *C. R. Acad. Sci.* 256, 504.

Guillemin, R., Yamazaki, E., Gard, G., Jutisz, M., and Sakiz, E. (1963b). *Endocrinology* 73, 564.

Guillemin, R., Burgus, R., Sakiz, E., and Ward, D. (1966). *C. R. Acad. Sci.* 262, 2278.

Halasz, B. (1962). *In* "Hypothalamic Control of the Anterior Pituitary" (J. Szentágothai, ed.), p. 106. Akadémiai Kiadó, Budapest.

Halasz, B., and Gorski, R. A. (1967). *Endocrinology* 80, 608.

Hamburger, C. (1957). *Acta Endocrinol. (Copenhagen)* 31, Suppl., 59.

Harris, G. W. (1937). *Proc. Roy. Soc., Ser. B* 122, 374.

Harris, G. W. (1948a). *J. Physiol. (London)* 107, 418.

Harris, G. W. (1948b). *Physiol. Rev.* 28, 139.

Harris, G. W. (1955). *In* "Neural Control of the Pituitary Gland." Arnold, London.

Harris, G. W. (1961). *In* "Control of Ovulation" (C. A. Villee, ed.), p. 56. Pergamon, Oxford.

Harris, G. W., and Jacobsohn, D. (1952). *Proc. Roy. Soc., Ser. B* 139, 263.

Harris, G. W., and Naftolin, F. (1970). *Brit. Med. Bull.* 26, 3.

Harris, G. W., and Ruf, K. B. (1970). *J. Physiol. (London)* 208, 243.

Harris, G. W., and Sherratt, R. M. (1969). *J. Physiol. (London)* 203, 59.

Hartley, B. S. (1970). *Biochem. J.* 119, 805.

Haterius, H. O., and Derbyshire, A. J., Jr. (1937). *Amer. J. Physiol.* 119, 329.

Haun, C. K., and Sawyer, C. H. (1960). *Endocrinology* 67, 270.

Hertz, R. (1960). *Endocrinology* 66, 842.

Hertz, R., and Meyer, R. K. (1937). *Endocrinology* 21, 756.

Hill, N. M., and Parkes, A. S. (1933). *Proc. Roy. Soc., Ser. B* 113, 537.

Hillarp, N. A. (1949). *Acta Endocrinol. (Copenhagen)* 2, 11.

Hilliard, J., Croxatto, H. B., Hayward, J. W., and Sawyer, C. H. (1966). *Endocrinology* 79, 411.

Hilliard, J., Schally, A. V., and Sawyer, C. H. (1971). *Endocrinology* 88, 730.

Hinsey, J. C., and Markee, J. E. (1963). *Proc. Soc. Exp. Biol. Med.* 31, 270.

Holsinger, J. W., and Everett, J. W. (1970). *Endocrinology* 86, 251.

Holweg, W., and Junkmann, K. (1932). *Klin. Wochenschr.* 11, 32.

Hooper, K. C. (1968). *Biochem. J.* 110, 151.

Hotchkiss, J., Atkinson, L. E., and Knobil, E. (1971). *Endocrinology* 89, 177.

Igarashi, M. (1971). *Proc. World Congr. Fert. Steril. 7th, 1971* p. 31.

Igarashi, M., and McCann, S. M. (1964a). *Endocrinology* 74, 440.

Igarashi, M., and McCann, S. M. (1964b). *Endocrinology* 74, 446.

Igarashi, M., Ibuki, Y., Kubo, H., Kamioka, J., Yokota, N., Ebara, Y., and Matsumoto, S. (1967). *Amer. J. Obstet. Gynecol.* 97, 120.

Igarashi, M., Yokota, N., Ehara, Y., Mayuzumi, R., Hirano, T., Matsumoto, S., and Yamasaki, M. (1968). *Amer. J. Obstet. Gynecol.* 100, 867.

Johansson, E. D. B., and Wide, L. (1969). *Acta Endocrinol. (Copenhagen)* 62, 82.

Jorgensen, C. B. (1965). *Arch. Anat. Microsc. Morphol. Exp.* 54, 261.

Jutisz, M., and De La Llosa, M. P. (1967). *Endocrinology* 81, 1193.

Jutisz, M., and De La Llosa, M. P. (1969). *C. R. Acad. Sci., Ser. D* 268, 1636.

Jutisz, M., and De La Llosa, M. P. (1970). *Endocrinology* **86,** 761.
Jutisz, M., Berault, A., Novella, M-A., and Chaperville, F. (1966). *C. R. Acad. Sci.* **263,** 664.
Jutisz, M., Berault, A., Novella, M-A., and Ribot, G. (1967). *Acta Endocrinol. (Copenhagen)* **55,** 481.
Jutisz, M., Kerdelhue, B., and Berault, A. (1970). "The Human Testis," p. 221. Plenum, New York.
Kalra, S. P., Ajika, K., Krulich, L., Fawcett, C. P., Quijada, M., and McCann, S. M. (1971). *Endocrinology* **88,** 1150.
Kamberi, I. A., and McCann, S. M. (1969). *Endocrinology* **85,** 815.
Kamberi, I. A., Mical, R. S., and Porter, J. C. (1969). *Science* **166,** 388.
Kamberi, I. A., Mical, R. S., and Porter, J. C. (1970a). *Endocrinology* **87,** 1.
Kamberi, I. A., Schneider, H. P. G., and McCann, S. M. (1970b). *Endocrinology* **86,** 278.
Kamberi, I. A., Mical, R. S., and Porter, J. C. (1971). *Endocrinology* **88,** 1294.
Kanematsu, S., and Sawyer, C. H. (1963a). *Endocrinology* **72,** 243.
Kanematsu, S., and Sawyer, C. H. (1963b). *Endocrinology* **73,** 687.
Kastin, A. J., and Schally, A. V. (1966). *Gen. Comp. Endocrinol.* **7,** 452.
Kastin, A. J., Schally, A. V., Gual, C., Midgley, A. R., Jr., Bowers, C. Y., and Diaz-Infante, A., Jr. (1969). *J. Clin. Endocrinol. Metab.* **29,** 1046.
Kastin, A. J., Schally, A. V., Gual, C., Midgley, A. R., Jr., Bowers, C. Y., and Gomez-Perez, E. (1970a). *Amer. J. Obstet. Gynecol.* **108,** 177.
Kastin, A. J., Schally, A. V., Gual, C., Midgley, A. R., Jr., Miller, M. C., III, and Flores, F. (1970b). *J. Clin. Endocrinol. Metab.* **31,** 689.
Kastin, A. J., Schally, A. V., Gual, C., Midgley, A. R., Jr., Arimura, A., Miller, M. C., III, and Cabeza, A. (1971a). *J. Clin. Endocrinol. Metab.* **32,** 287.
Kastin, A. J., Schally, A. V., Gual, C., Midgley, A. R., Jr., Miller, M. C., III, and Cabeza, A. (1971b). *J. Clin. Invest.* **50,** 1551.
Kastin, A. J., Zarate, A., Midgley, A. R., Canales, E. S., and Schally, A. V. (1971c). *J. Clin. Endocrinol. Metab.* **33,** 980.
Kastin, A. J., Gual, C., and Schally, A. V. (1972a). *Recent Progr. Horm. Res.* **28,** 201.
Kastin, A. J., Schally, A. V., Gonzales-Barcena, D., Schalch, D. S., and Lee, L. (1972b). *Arch. Intern. Med.* (in press).
Kastin, A. J., Schally, A. V., Gual, C., and Arimura, A. (1972c). *J. Clin. Endocrinol. Metab.* **34,** 753.
Kastin, A. J., Schally, A. V., Schalch, D. S., Korenman, S. G., Gual, C., and Perez-Pasten, E. (1972d). *Pediat. Res.* **6,** 481.
Kato, J. (1970). *Acta Endocrinol. (Copenhagen)* **64,** 687.
Kato, J., and Villee, C. A. (1967). *Endocrinology* **80,** 1133.
Kawakami, M., and Sawyer, C. H. (1959). *Endocrinology* **65,** 631.
Kerdelhue, M., Berault, A., Ribot, G., and Jutisz, M. (1970). *C. R. Acad. Sci.* **270,** 1010.
Keyes, P. L. (1969). *Science* **164,** 846.
Kimura, K., Kishida, Y., Hiuma, T., and Sakakibara, S. (1971). *Program 9th Symp. Peptide Chem., 1971* Abstract No. 19, p. 15.
Kingsley, T. R., and Bogdanove, E. M. (1971). *Fed. Proc., Fed. Amer. Soc. Exp. Biol.* **30,** 253.
Kistner, R. W. (1966). *Fert. Steril.* **17,** 569.
Knigge, K. (1962). *Amer. J. Physiol.* **208,** 387.

Koch, Y., Dikstein, S., Superstine, E., and Sulman, F. G. (1971). *J. Endocrinol.* **49**, 13.

Korenman, S., Perrin, L., and Rao, B. R. (1969). *Abstr., 51st Meet. Endocrine Soc.* p. 116.

Kuroshima, A., Ishida, Y., Bowers, C. Y., and Schally, A. V. (1964). *Abstr. Program, 46th Meet. Endocrine Soc.* p. 110.

Kuroshima, A., Ishida, Y., Bowers, C. Y., and Schally, A. V. (1965). *Endocrinology* **76**, 614.

Kuroshima, A., Arimura, A., Saito, T., Ishida, Y., Bowers, C. Y., and Schally, A. V. (1966). *Endocrinology* **78**, 1105.

Lamond, D. R., and Bindon, B. M. (1966). *J. Endocrinol.* **34**, 365.

Laumas, K. R., and Faroog, A. (1966). *J. Endocrinol.* **36**, 95.

Leavitt, W. W., Friend, J. P., and Robinson, J. A. (1969). *Science* **165**, 496.

Li, C. H. (1949). *Fed. Proc., Fed. Amer. Soc. Exp. Biol.* **8**, 219.

Li, C. H., and Yamashiro, D. (1970). *J. Amer. Chem. Soc.* **92**, 7608.

Li, C. H., Simpson, M. E., and Evans, H. M. (1940). *Science* **92**, 355.

Li, C. H., Simpson, M. E., and Evans, H. M. (1949). *Science* **109**, 445.

Libertun, C., Moguilevsky, J. A., Schiaffini, O., and Christot, J. (1969). *J. Endocrinol.* **43**, 317.

Lindsay, D. R., and Robinson, T. J. (1970). *J. Reprod. Fert.* **23**, 277.

Lisk, R. D. (1960). *J. Exp. Zool.* **145**, 147.

Lisk, R. D. (1962a). *Amer. J. Physiol.* **203**, 493.

Lisk, R. D. (1962b). *Acta Endocrinol. (Copenhagen)* **41**, 195.

Lisk, R. D. (1967). *Endocrinology* **80**, 754.

Lisk, R. D. (1969). *Trans. N. Y. Acad. Sci.* [2] **31**, 593.

Lisk, R. D., and Newlon, M. (1963). *Science* **139**, 222.

Lostroh, A. J. (1969). *Endocrinology* **85**, 438.

McCann, S. M. (1962). *Amer. J. Physiol.* **202**, 395.

McCann, S. M. (1963). *Amer. J. Med.* **34**, 379.

McCann, S. M., and Ramirez, V. D. (1964). *Recent Progr. Horm. Res.* **20**, 131.

McCann, S. M., and Taleisnik, S. (1961). *Endocrinology* **69**, 909.

McCann, S. M., and Taleisnik, S. (1962). *Amer. J. Physiol.* **202**, 395.

McCann, S. M., Taleisnik, S., and Friedman, H. M. (1960). *Proc. Soc. Exp. Biol. Med.* **104**, 432.

McCann, S. M., Taleisnik, S., and Friedman, H. M. (1961). *Endocrinology* **68**, 1071.

McCann, S. M., Antunes-Rodrigues, J., and Dhariwal, A. P. S. (1965). *Int. Congr. Physiol. Sci., Lect. Symp., 23rd, 1965* Int. Congr. Ser. No. 87, p. 292.

McCann, S. M., Dhariwal, A. P. S., and Porter, J. C. (1968). *Annu. Rev. Physiol.* **30**, 589.

McClintock, J. A., and Schwartz, N. B. (1968). *Endocrinology* **83**, 433.

McEwen, B. S., Pfaff, D. W., and Zigmond, R. E. (1970). *Brain Res.* **21**, 17.

McGuire, J. L., and Lisk, R. D. (1969). *Neuroendocrinology* **4**, 289.

Mancini, R. E., Seigner, A. C., and Perez-Lloret, A. (1969). *J. Clin. Endocrinol. Metab.* **29**, 467.

Manning, M. (1968). *J. Amer. Chem. Soc.* **90**, 1348.

Markee, J. E., Sawyer, C. H., and Hollinshead, W. H. (1946). *Endocrinology* **38**, 345.

Markee, J. E., Sawyer, C. H., and Hollinshead, W H. (1948). *Recent Progr. Horm. Res.* **2**, 117.

Markee, J. E., Everett, J. W., and Sawyer, C. H. (1952). *Recent Progr. Horm. Res.* **7**, 139.

Marshall, F. H. A. (1936). *Phil. Trans. Roy. Soc. London, Ser. B* **226**, 423.

Marshall, F. H. A. (1942). *Biol. Rev.* **17**, 68.

Marshall, F. H. A. (1956). "Physiology of Reproduction," 3rd ed. Longmans, Green, New York.

Marshall, F. H. A., and Verney, E. B. (1936). *J. Physiol. (London)* **86**, 327.

Marshall, G. R. (1968). *In* "Pharmacology of Hormonal Polypeptides and Proteins" (N. Back, R. Paoletti, and L. Martini, eds.). Plenum, New York.

Martini, L., Fraschini, F., and Motta, M. (1968). *Recent Progr. Horm. Res.* **24**, 439.

Mather, F. B., and Wilson, W. O. (1964). *Poultry Sci.* **43**, 860.

Matsubara, H., and Sasaki, R. (1969). *Biochem. Biophys. Res. Commun.* **35**, 175.

Matsuo, H., Fujimoto, Y., and Tatsuno, T. (1966). *Biochem. Biophys. Res. Commun.* **22**, 69.

Matsuo, H., Arimura, A., Nair, R. M. G., and Schally, A. V. (1971a). *Biochem. Biophys. Res. Commun.* **45**, 822.

Matsuo, H., Baba, Y., Nair, R. M. G., Arimura, A., and Schally, A. V. (1971b). *Biochem. Biophys. Res. Commun.* **43**, 1334.

Meites, J., and Nicoll, C. S. (1966). *Annu. Rev. Physiol.* **28**, 57.

Meites, J., Piacsek, B. E., and Mittler, J. C. (1967). *Proc. Int. Congr. Horm. Steroids, 2nd, 1966* Int. Congr. Ser. No. 132, p. 958.

Merrifield, R. B. (1967). *Recent Progr. Horm. Res.* **23**, 451.

Meyer, R. K., Leonard, S. L., Hisaw, F. L., and Martin, S. J. (1932). *Endocrinology* **16**, 655.

Midgley, A. R., Jr. (1966). *Endocrinology* **79**, 10.

Midgley, A. R., Jr. (1967). *J. Clin. Endocrinol. Metab.* **27**, 295.

Midgley, A. R., and Jaffe, R. B. (1968). *J. Clin. Endocrinol. Metab.* **28**, 1699.

Minaguchi, H., and Meites, J. (1967). *Endocrinology* **81**, 826.

Mittler, J. C., and Meites, J. (1964). *Proc. Soc. Exp. Biol. Med.* **117**, 309.

Mittler, J. C., and Meites, J. (1966). *Endocrinology* **78**, 500.

Mittler, J. C., Arimura, A., and Schally, A. V. (1970). *Proc. Soc. Exp. Biol. Med.* **133**, 1321.

Moguilevsky, J. A., Kolbermann, L. E., Libertun, C., and Gomez, C. J. (1971). *Proc. Soc. Exp. Biol. Med.* **136**, 1115.

Monahan, M., Riviers, J., Burgus, R., Amoss, M., Blackwell, R., Vale, W., and Guillemin, R. (1971). *C. R. Acad. Sci.* **273**, 508.

Monroe, S. E., Parlow, A. F., and Midgley, A. R., Jr. (1968). *Endocrinology* **83**, 1004.

Monroe, S. E., Atkinson, L. E., and Knobil, E. (1970). *Endocrinology* **87**, 453.

Moore, C. R., and Price, D. (1932). *Amer. J. Anat.* **50**, 13.

Moszkowska, A., and Kordon, C. (1965). *Gen. Comp. Endocrinol.* **5**, 596.

Motta, M., Frachini, F., Giuliani, G., and Martini, L. (1968). *Endocrinology* **83**, 1101.

Naftolin, F., Harris, G. W., and Bobrow, M. (1971). *Nature (London)* **232**, 496.

Nair, R. M. G., and Schally, A. V. (1972). *Int. J. Pept. Res.* (in press).

Nallar, R., and McCann, S. M. (1965). *Endocrinology* **76**, 272.

Nallar, R., Antunes-Rodrigues, J., and McCann, S. M. (1966). *Endocrinology* **79**, 907.

Negro-Vilar, A., Dickerman, E., and Meites, J. (1968a). *Endocrinology* **82**, 939.

Negro-Vilar, A., Dickerman, E., and Meites, J. (1968b). *Endocrinology* **83**, 1349.

Negro-Vilar, A., Dickerman, E., and Meites, J. (1968c). *Proc. Soc. Exp. Biol. Med.* **127**, 751.

Negro-Vilar, A., Sar, M., and Meites, J. (1970). *Endocrinology* **87**, 1091.
Neill, J. D., Johansson, E. D. B., Dotta, J. K., and Knobil, E. (1967). *J. Clin. Endocrinol. Metab.* **27**, 1167.
Nikitovitch-Winer, M. B. (1960). *Mem. Soc. Endocrinol.* **9**, 70.
Nikitovitch-Winer, M. B. (1962). *Endocrinology* **70**, 350.
Nikitovitch-Winer, M. B., and Everett, J. W. (1957). *Nature (London)* **180**, 1434.
Nikitovitch-Winer, M. B., and Everett, J. W. (1958). *Endocrinology* **63**, 916.
Nikitovitch-Winer, M. B., and Everett, J. W. (1959). *Endocrinology* **65**, 357.
Niswender, G. D., Midgley, A. R., Jr., Monroe, S. E., and Reichert, L. E., Jr. (1968). *Proc. Soc. Exp. Biol. Med.* **128**, 807.
Niswender, G. D., Reichert, L. E., Jr., Midgley, A. R., Jr., and Nalbandov, A. V. (1969). *Endocrinology* **84**, 1166.
Odell, W. D., Ross, G. T., and Rayford, P. L. (1968). *J. Clin. Invest.* **46**, 248.
Ojeda, S. R., and Ramirez, V. D. (1969). *Endocrinology* **84**, 786.
Palka, Y. S., Ramirez, V. D., and Sawyer, C. H. (1966). *Endocrinology* **78**, 487.
Papkoff, H., and Ekblad, M. (1970). *Biochem. Biophys. Res. Commun.* **40**, 614, 1970.
Papkoff, H., Sairam, M. R., and Li, C. H. (1971). *J. Amer. Chem. Soc.* **93**, 1531.
Parlow, A. F. (1961). *In* "Human Pituitary Gonadotropins" (A. Albert, ed.), pp. 300–310. Thomas, Springfield, Illinois.
Parlow, A. F., Daane, T. A., and Schally, A. V. (1969). *Abstr., 51st Meet. Endocrine Soc.* p. 83.
Pasteels, J. L. (1962). *C. R. Acad. Sci.* **254**, 2664.
Peake, G. T., and Daughaday, W. (1968). *Med. Clin. N. Amer.* **52**, 357.
Pelletier, G., Peillon, F., and Vila-Porcile, E. (1971). *Z. Zellforsch. Mikrosk. Anat.* **115**, 501.
Pelletier, J. (1970). *Acta Endocrinol. (Copenhagen)* **63**, 290.
Pelletier, J., and Ortavant, R. (1968). *C. R. Acad. Sci.* **266**, 1604.
Peterson, N. T., Jr., Midgley, A. R., Jr., and Jaffe, R. B. (1968). *J. Clin. Endocrinol. Metab.* **28**, 1473.
Pfaff, D. W. (1968a). *Science* **161**, 1355.
Pfaff, D. W. (1968b). *Endocrinology* **82**, 1149.
Piacsek, B. E., and Meites, J. (1966). *Endocrinology* **79**, 432.
Piacsek, B. E., Armstrong, D. T., and Greep, R. O. (1969). *Endocrinology* **84**, 1184.
Popa, G., and Fielding, V. (1930). *J. Anat.* **65**, 88.
Popa, G., and Fielding, V. (1935). *J. Anat.* **67**, 227.
Porath, J. (1957). *Ark. Kemi* **11**, 259.
Purves, H. D. (1961). *In* "Sex and Internal Secretions" (W. C. Young, ed.), 3rd ed., Vol. 1, p. 161. Williams & Wilkins, Baltimore, Maryland.
Quinn, D. L. (1961). *Nature (London)* **209**, 891.
Quinn, D. L. (1969). *Neuroendocrinology* **4**, 254.
Ramirez, V. D., and McCann, S. M. (1963a). *Endocrinology* **72**, 452.
Ramirez, V. D., and McCann, S. M. (1963b). *Endocrinology* **73**, 193.
Ramirez, V. D., and McCann, S. M. (1964). *Endocrinology* **74**, 814.
Ramirez, V. D., and Sawyer, C. H. (1965a). *Endocrinology* **76**, 282.
Ramirez, V. D., and Sawyer, C. H. (1965b). *Endocrinology* **76**, 1158.
Ramirez, V. D., and Sawyer, C. H. (1966). *Endocrinology* **78**, 958.
Ramirez, V. D., Abrams, R. M., and McCann, S. M. (1964). *Endocrinology* **75**, 243.
Redding, T. W., Schally, A. V., and Locke, W. (1971). *Endocrinology* **88**, A-75.
Redding, T. W., Schally, A. V., Arimura, A., and Matsuo, H. (1972). *Endocrinology* **90**, 764.

Reeves, J. J., Arimura, A., and Schally, A. V. (1970a). *Proc. Soc. Exp. Biol. Med.* **134**, 938.

Reeves, J. J., Arimura, A., and Schally, A. V. (1970b). *J. Anim. Sci.* **31**, 933.

Reeves, J. J., Arimura, A., and Schally, A. V. (1971a). *J. Anim. Sci.* **32**, 123.

Reeves, J. J., Arimura, A., and Schally, A. V. (1971b). *Biol. Reprod.* **4**, 88.

Reeves, J. J., Arimura, A., Schally, A. V., Kragt, C., Beck, T. W., and Casey, J. M. (1972). *J. Anim. Sci.* **35**, 84.

Reichert, L. E., Jr., Rasco, M. A., Ward, D. N., Niswender, G. D., and Midgley, A. R., Jr. (1969). *J. Biol. Chem.* **244**, 5110

Reichlin, S. (1963). *N. Engl. J. Med.* **269**, 1182.

Reichlin, S. (1968). *In* "Textbook of Endocrinology" (R. H. Williams, ed.), p. 967. Saunders, Philadelphia, Pennsylvania.

Rennels, E. G., Bogdanove, E. M., Arimura, A., Saito, M., and Schally, A. V. (1971). *Endocrinology* **88**, 1318.

Robison, G. A., Butcher, R. W., and Sutherland, E. W. (1968). *Annu. Rev. Biochem.* **37**, 149.

Root, A. W., Smith, G. P. Dhariwal, A. P. S., and McCann, S. M. (1969). *Nature* (*London*) **221**, 570.

Rothchild, I. (1960). *Endocrinology* **67**, 9.

Rothchild, I. (1965). *Vitam. Horm.* (*New York*) **23**, 209.

Rowan, W. (1925). *Nature* (*London*) **115**, 494.

Rowan, W. (1928). *Nature* (*London*) **122**, 11.

Roy, S., Greenblatt, R. B., and Mahesh, V. B. (1964). *Acta Endocrinol* (*Copenhagen*) **47**, 657.

Roy, S. K., Jr., and Laumas, K. R. (1969). *Acta Endocrinol.* (*Copenhagen*) **61**, 629.

Saffran, M., and Schally, A. V. (1955). *Can. J. Biochem. Physiol.* **33**, 408.

Saffran, M., Schally, A. V., and Benfey, B. G. (1955). *Endocrinology* **57**, 439.

Saito, T., Arimura, A., Muller, E. E., Bowers, C. Y., and Schally, A. V. (1967a). *Endocrinology* **80**, 313.

Saito, T., Sawano, S., Arimura, A., and Schally, A. V. (1967b). *Endocrinology* **81**, 1226.

Sakakibara, S., Shimonishi, Y., Kishida, Y., Okada, M., and Sugihara, H. (1967). *Bull. Chem. Soc. Jap.* **40**, 2164.

Samli, M. H., and Geschwind, I. I. (1967). *Endocrinology* **81**, 835.

Samli, M. H., and Geschwind, I. I. (1968). *Endocrinology* **82**, 225.

Sawyer, C. H. (1959). *J. Exp. Zool.* **142**, 227.

Sawyer, C. H. (1963). *Advan. Neuroendocrinol. Proc. Symp., 1961* p. 451.

Sawyer, C. H. (1965). *Proc. Congr. Endocrinol. 2nd, 1964* Int. Congr. Ser. No. 83, p. 629.

Sawyer, C. H. (1969a). *In* "The Hypothalamus" (W. Haymaker, E. Anderson, and W. J. H. Nauta, eds.), p. 389. Thomas, Springfield, Illinois.

Sawyer, C. H. (1969b). *In* "Perspectives in Reproduction and Sexual Behavior" (M. Diamond, ed.), pp. 13–23. Indiana Univ. Press, Bloomington.

Sawyer, C. H. (1970). *Fed. Proc., Fed. Amer. Soc. Exp. Biol.* **29**, 1895.

Sawyer, C. H. (1971). *In* "The Hypothalamus" (L. Martini, M. Motta, and F. Fraschini, eds.), p. 83. Academic Press, New York.

Sawyer, C. H., and Everett, J. W. (1959). *Endocrinology* **65**, 644.

Sawyer, C. H., and Kawakami, M. (1959). *Endocrinology* **65**, 622.

Sawyer, C. H., and Kawakami, M. (1961). *In* "Control of Ovulation" (C. A. Villee, ed.), p. 79. Pergamon, Oxford.

Sawyer, C. H., Markee, J. E., and Townsend, B. F. (1949). *Endocrinology* **44**, 18.

Sawyer, C. H., Markee, J. E., and Everett, J. W. (1950). *J. Exp. Zool.* **113**, 659.

Sawyer, C. H., Markee, J. E., and Everett, J. W. (1951). *Amer. J. Physiol.* **166**, 223.

Saxena, B. B., Demura, H., Gandy, H. M., and Peterson, R. E. (1968). *J. Clin. Endocrinol. Metab.* **28**, 519.

Scacchi, P., Moguilevsky, J. A., and Szwarcfarb, B. (1971). *Proc. Soc. Exp. Biol. Med.* **136**, 1068.

Schally, A. V., and Bowers, C. Y. (1964a). *Endocrinology* **75**, 312.

Schally, A. V., and Bowers, C. Y. (1964b). *Endocrinology* **75**, 608.

Schally, A. V., and Kastin, A. J. (1970). In "Advances in Steroid Biochemistry and Pharmacology" (M. H. Briggs, ed.), Vol. 2, p. 41. Academic Press, New York.

Schally, A. V., and Kastin, A. J. (1971). *Drug Ther.* **1**, 39.

Schally, A. V., Saffran, M., and Zimmermann, N. (1958). *Biochem. J.* **70**, 97.

Schally, A. V., Meites, J., Bowers, C. Y., and Ratner, A. (1964). *Proc. Soc. Exp. Biol. Med.* **117**, 252.

Schally, A. V., Bowers, C. Y., Kuroshima, A., Ishida, Y., Redding, T. W., and Kastin, A. J. (1965a). *Int. Congr. Physiol. Sci., Lect. Symp., 23rd, 1965* Int. Congr. Ser. No. 87, p. 275.

Schally, A. V., Kuroshima, A., Ishida, Y., Redding, T. W., and Bowers, C. Y. (1965b). *Proc. Soc. Erp. Biol. Med.* **118**, 350.

Schally, A. V., Steelman, S. L., and Bowers, C. Y. (1965c). *Proc. Soc. Exp. Biol. Med.* **119**, 208.

Schally, A. V., Bowers, C. Y., Redding, T. W., and Barrett, J. F. (1966a). *Biochem. Biophys. Res. Commun.* **25**, 165.

Schally, A. V., Saito, T., Arimura, A., Muller, E. E., Bowers, C. Y., and White, W. F. (1966b). *Endocrinology* **79**, 1087.

Schally, A. V., Bowers, C. Y., White, W. F., and Cohen, A. I. (1967a). *Endocrinology* **81**, 77.

Schally, A. V., Carter, W. H., Arimura, A., and Bowers, C. Y. (1967b). *Endocrinology* **81**, 1173.

Schally, A. V., Kastin, A. J., Locke, W., and Bowers, C. Y. (1967c). In "Hormones in Blood" (C. H. Gray and A. L. Bacharach, eds.), 2nd rev. ed. Vol. 1, p. 491. Academic Press, New York.

Schally, A. V., Saito, T., Arimura, A., Sawano, S., Bowers, C. Y., White, W. F., and Cohen, A. I. (1967d). *Endocrinology* **81**, 882.

Schally, A. V., Muller, E. E., Arimura, A., Bowers, C. Y., Saito, T., Redding, T. W., Sawano, S., and Pizzolato, P. (1967e). *J. Clin. Endocrinol. Metab.* **27**, 755.

Schally A. V., Arimura, A., Bowers, C. Y., Kastin, A. J., Sawano, S., and Redding, T. W. (1968a). *Recent Progr. Horm. Res.* **24**, 497.

Schally, A. V., Carter, W. H., Saito, M., Arimura, A., and Bowers, C. Y. (1968b). *J. Clin. Endocrinol. Metab.* **28**, 1747.

Schally, A. V., Bowers, C. Y., Carter, W. H., Arimura, A., Redding, T. W., and Saito, M. (1969). *Endocrinology* **85**, 290.

Schally, A. V., Arimura, A., Bowers, C. Y., Wakabayashi, I., Kastin, A. J., Redding, T. W., Mittler, J. C., Nair, R. M. G., Pizzolato, P., and Segal, A. J. (1970a). *J. Clin. Endocrinol. Metab.* **31**, 291.

Schally, A. V., Arimura, A., Kastin, A. J., Reeves, J. J., Bowers, C. Y., and Baba, Y. (1970b). In "Mammalian Reproduction" (H. Gibian and E. J. Plotz, eds.), p. 45. Springer-Verlag, Berlin and New York.

Schally, A. V., Carter, W. H., Parlow, A. F., Saito, M., Arimura, A., Bowers, C. Y., and Holtkamp, D. E. (1970c). *Amer. J. Obstet. Gynecol.* **107**, 1156.

Schally, A. V., Mittler, J. C., and White, W. F. (1970d). *Endocrinology* **86**, 903.

Schally, A. V., Parlow, A. F., Carter, W. H., Saito, M., Bowers, C. Y., and Arimura, A. (1970e). *Endocrinology* **86**, 530.

Schally, A. V., Arimura, A., Kastin, A. J., Matsuo, H., Baba, Y., Redding, T. W., Nair, R. M. G., Debeljuk, L., and White, W. F. (1971a). *Science* **173**, 1036.

Schally, A. V., Arimura, A., Baba, Y., Nair, R. M. G., Matsuo, H., Redding, T. W., and Debeljuk L. (1971b). *Biochem Biophys. Res. Commun.* **43**, 393.

Schally A. V., Arimura, A., Baba, Y., Nair, R. M. G., Matsuo, H., Redding, T. W., Debeljuk, L., and White, W. F. (1971c). *Endocrinology* **88**, A-70.

Schally A. V., Baba, Y., Arimura, A., Redding, T. W., and White, W. F. (1971d). *Biochem. Biophys. Res. Commun.* **42**, 50.

Schally, A. V., Baba, Y., Matsuo, H., Arimura, A., and Redding, T. W. (1971e). *Neuroendocrinology* **8**, 347.

Schally, A. V., Baba, Y., and Redding, T. W. (1971f). *Neuroendocrinology* **8**, 70.

Schally, A. V., Kastin, A. J., and Arimura, A. (1971g). *Fert. Steril.* **27**, 703.

Schally, A. V., Nair, R. M. G., and Carter, W. H. (1971h). *Anal. Chem.* **43**, 1527.

Schally, A. V., Nair, R. M. G., Redding T. W., and Arimura, A. (1971i). *J. Biol. Chem.* **246**, 7230.

Schally, A. V., Arimura, A., Carter, W. H., Redding, T. W., Geiger, R., Koenig, W., Wissman, H., Jaeger, G., Sandow, J., Yanaihara, N., Yanaihara, C., Hashimoto, T., and Sakagami, N. (1972a). *Biochem. Biophys. Res. Commun.* **48**, 366.

Schally, A. V., Kastin, A. J., and Arimura, A. (1972b). *Am. J. Obstet. Gynecol.* (in press).

Schally, A. V., Redding, T. W., Matsuo, H., and Arimura, A. (1972c). *Endocrinology* **90**, 1561.

Scharrer, E., and Scharrer, B. (1954). *Recent Progr. Horm. Res.* **10**, 183.

Scharrer, E., and Scharrer, B. (1963). *In* "Neuroendocrinology," p. 289. Columbia Univ. Press, New York.

Schiavi, R., Jutisz, M., Sakiz, E., and Guillemin, R. (1963). *Proc. Soc. Exp. Biol. Med.* **114**, 426.

Schneider, H. P. G., and McCann, S. M. (1969). *Endocrinology* **85**, 121.

Schneider, H. P. G., and McCann, S. M. (1970). *Endocrinology* **86**, 1127.

Schneider, H. P. G., Staemmler, H.-J., Straehler-Pohl, K., and Sachs, L. (1968). *Acta Endocrinol.* (Copenhagen) **58**, 347.

Schneider, H. P. G., Crighton, D. B., and McCann, S. M. (1969). *Neuroendocrinology* **5**, 271.

Schreiber, V., Rybak, M., Eckertova, A., Jirgl, A., Koci, V., Franc, Z., and Kementova, V. (1962). *Experientia* **18**, 338.

Schwartz N. B., and Calderelli, D. (1965). *Proc. Soc. Exp. Biol. Med.* **119**, 16.

Seiki, K., Higashida, M., Imanaski, Y., Myamoto, M., Kitagawa, T., and Kotani, M. (1968). *J. Endocrinol.* **41**, 109.

Serra, G. B., and Midgley, A. R., Jr. (1970). *Proc. Soc. Exp. Biol. Med.* **133**, 1370.

Sharp, P. J., and Follett, B. K. (1969). *Neuroendocrinology* **5**, 205.

Sherwood, O. D., Grimek, H. J., and McShan, W. H. (1970). *J. Biol. Chem.* **245**, 2328.

Shiino, M., Arimura, A., Schally, A. V., and Rennels, E. G. (1972). *Zellforsch. Mikrosk. Anat.* **128**, 152.

Smith, E. R., and Davidson, J. M. (1967). *Endocrinology* **80**, 725.
Smith, P. E. (1926). *Proc. Soc. Exp. Biol. Med.* **24**, 131.
Smith, P. E., and Engle, E. T. (1927). *Amer. J. Anat.* **40**, 159.
Speroff, L., and Van de Wiele, R. L. (1971). *Amer. J. Obstet. Gynecol.* **109**, 234.
Spies, H. G., Stevens, K. R., Hilliard, J., and Sawyer, C. S. (1969). *Endocrinology* **84**, 277.
Steelman, S. L., and Pohley, F. M. (1953). *Endocrinology* **53**, 604.
Steinberger, E., and Duckett, G. (1968). *Acta Endocrinol. (Copenhagen)* **57**, 289.
Stevens, K. R., Jackson, G. L., and Nalbandov, A. V. (1968). *Endocrinology* **83**, 225.
Stevens, K. R., Spies, H. G., Hilliard, J., and Sawyer, C. H. (1970). *Endocrinology* **86**, 970.
Stewart, J. M., and Young, J. P. (1969). *In* "Solid State Peptide Synthesis." Freeman, San Francisco, California.
Stumpf, W. E. (1968). *Science* **162**, 1001.
Taleisnik, S., and McCann, S. M. (1961). *Endocrinology* **68**, 263.
Talwalker, P. K., Ratner, A., and Meites, J. (1963). *Amer. J. Physiol.* **205**, 213.
Taymor, M. L., Aono, T., and Pheteplace, C. (1968). *Acta Endocrinol. (Copenhagen)* **59**, 298.
Thomson, A. P. D., and Zuckerman, S. (1953). *Nature (London)* **171**, 970.
Tixier-Vidal, A., Kerdelhue, B., Berault, A., Picart, R., and Jutisz, M. (1971). *Gen. Comp. Endocrinol.* **17**, 33.
von Lawzewitsch, I., Debeljuk, L., and Puig, R. (1970). *Neuroendocrinology* **6**, 65.
Ward, D. N., Sweeney, C. M., Holcomb, G. N., Lamkin, W. M., and Fujino, M. (1968). *Proc. Int. Congr. Endocrinol., 3rd, 1968* p. 385.
Watanabe, S., and McCann, S. M. (1968). *Endocrinology* **82**, 664.
Watanabe, S., Dhariwal, A. P. S., and McCann, S. M. (1968). *Endocrinology* **82**, 674.
Weick, R. F., and Davidson, J. M. (1970). *Endocrinology* **87**, 693.
Weick, R. F., Smith, E. R., Dominguez, R., Dhariwal, A. P. S., and Davidson, J. M. (1971). *Endocrinology* **88**, 293.
Westman, A., and Jacobsohn, D. (1938). *Acta Pathol. Microbiol. Scand.* **15**, 301.
Westman, A., and Jacobsohn, D. (1940). *Acta Obstet. Gynecol. Scand.* **20**, 392.
White, W. F. (1970a). *In* "Mammalian Reproduction" (H. Gibian and E. J. Plotz, eds.), p. 84. Springer-Verlag, Berlin and New York.
White, W. F. (1970b). *In* "Hypophysiotropic Hormones of the Hypothalamus: Assay and Chemistry" (J. Meites, ed.), p. 249. Williams & Wilkins, Baltimore, Maryland.
White, W. F., Cohen, A. I., Rippel, R. H., Story, J. C., and Schally, A. V. (1968). *Endocrinology* **82**, 742.
Wieland, T., Determann, H., and Kahle, W. (1963). *Angew. Chem.* **75**, 209.
Wolfson, A. (1963). *Advan. Neuroendocrinol. Proc. Symp., 1961* p. 402.
Yamamoto, M., Diebel, N. D., and Bogdanove, E. M. (1970). *Endocrinology* **86**, 1102.
Yanaihara, N., Sakagami, M., Kaneko, T., Saito, S., Abe, K., Nagata, N., and Oka, H. (1971). *Program Symp. Peptide Chem., 9th, 1971* Abstract No. 20, p. 15.
Zarate, A., Kastin, A. J., Arimura, A., Canales, E., Miller, M. C., and Schally, A. V. (1972). *Clin. Res.* **20**, 446.
Zondek, B., and Aschheim, S. (1926). *Deut. Med. Wochenschr.* **52**, 343.
Zondek, B., and Aschheim, S. (1927). *Klin. Wochenschr.* **6**, 248.

Hypothalamic Control of Prolactin Secretion

JOSEPH MEITES AND JAMES A. CLEMENS

Department of Physiology, Michigan State University, East Lansing, Michigan, and Department of Physiological Research, Eli Lilly and Company, Indianapolis, Indiana

I. Introduction

Several reviews on the control of prolactin secretion have been published recently (Meites and Nicoll, 1966; Meites, 1966, 1970; Meites et al., 1972; Nicoll, 1971). The present chapter will not attempt to cover all aspects of prolactin control, and will emphasize newer observations and concepts. Regulation of prolactin secretion is exerted mainly via the hypothalamus, and this appears to involve the actions of a prolactin-inhibiting factor (PIF), a possible prolactin-releasing factor (PRF), catecholamines, serotonin, and perhaps other biogenic amines—all produced in the hypothalamus. Most other agents that stimulate or inhibit prolactin secretion, including estrogen, the suckling stimulus, stresses, many drugs, and prolactin itself, act through hypothalamic mechanisms. However, there are some hormones and drugs that can directly influence the anterior pituitary to increase or decrease prolactin secretion, although several of these also can act through the hypothalamus.

In mammals, prolactin is best known for its stimulatory effects on mammary growth and lactation, for its luteotropic action on the ovaries of several rodent species, and more recently, for its luteolytic effects on old corpora lutea in rats, and for its important role in development and growth of mammary tumors in rats and mice. Many metabolic actions have been attributed to prolactin, but these have not been definitely established as specific activities of prolactin in mammals. In submammalian species, more functions have been reported for prolactin than for any other single hormone (Bern and Nicoll, 1968).

The relation of prolactin to secretion of other anterior pituitary hormones also is of interest. A reciprocal relationship exists between the secretion of prolactin and the two gonadotropins, LH and FSH, in many physiological states. When prolactin secretion is high, as a result of estrogen action, the suckling stimulus or after administration of such drugs as reserpine or chlorpromazine, LH and FSH secretion are low. On the other hand, when prolactin secretion is inhibited, as a result of an implant of a small amount of prolactin in the median eminence or administration of L-dopa, secretion of the gonadotropins is apt to be increased. Prolactin also is related to secretion of growth hormone. Both are produced by acidophiles in the anterior pituitary, both lack a negative feedback from any of the target tissues they stimulate, and both have a number of functions in common (both stimulate mammary growth, and in ruminant species, GH stimulates lactation; prolactin exerts a limited stimulatory effect on growth processes in some species; etc.). It also is of interest that prolactin secretion, like ACTH, can be stimulated by many physical and psychic stresses and that both hormones are released by many of the same stresses, as first observed by Nicoll, Talwalker, and Meites (1960) in rats and more recently confirmed by radioimmunoassay of prolactin in man and animals. Prolactin secretion in humans is controlled essentially by the same mechanisms as in animals, as will be indicated here. It is apparent, therefore, that knowledge of the control of prolactin secretion is important.

II. PROLACTIN SECRETION DURING DIFFERENT PHYSIOLOGICAL STATES

A. PROLACTIN IN SEXUALLY IMMATURE ANIMALS

Small amounts of prolactin have been detected in the pituitary of 18-day-old fetal mice (Komoto and Bern, 1971). Prolactin levels in the pituitary of prepubertal female rats (Minaguchi *et al.*, 1968; Voogt *et al.*, 1970) and sexually immature female guinea pigs and rabbits (Meites and Turner, 1950) were found to be very low as compared to levels in mature animals of the same species. A pronounced rise in pituitary and serum prolactin occurs in female rats with the onset of puberty (Fig. 1). This appears to be due to estrogen stimulation, since administration of small doses of estrogen to prepubertal female rats elevates pituitary and serum prolactin values (Voogt *et al.*, 1970). Relatively large amounts of prolactin have been detected in amniotic fluid and blood of newborn human infants of both sexes, but prolactin disappears rapidly from these fluids after birth (Frantz *et al.*, 1972). This is in agreement with an early report by Lyons (1937), who found prolactin in the urine of newborn human infants, and this probably accounts for the transitory appearance of "witches milk" in the breasts of infants.

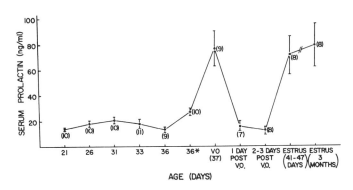

FIG. 1. Serum prolactin concentration before and after onset of puberty in Sprague-Dawley rats. V.O., vagina open; * = rats with ballooned uteri. Bars show standard errors. After Voogt *et al.* (1970).

B. Prolactin during Estrous and Menstrual Cycles

During each estrous cycle in the rat and other species, regular fluctuations in pituitary and blood prolactin levels are found. In the rat, pituitary content and concentration of prolactin are highest on the days of proestrus and estrus, and lowest on the days of diestrus (Reece and Turner, 1937; Sar and Meites, 1967). Serum levels of prolactin in the rat are low during diestrus; a peak rise is seen on the late afternoon of proestrus; and a decline occurs on the day of estrus, with values higher than in diestrus (Kwa and Verhofstad, 1967; Niswender et al., 1969; Wuttke and Meites, 1970b; Gay et al., 1970). Serum LH and FSH also show peak elevations on the late afternoon of proestrus in the rat (Gay et al., 1970; Wuttke and Meites, 1970b) (Fig. 2). Serum, but not pituitary GH, rises on the day of estrus (Dickerman and Meites, 1971) (Fig. 3), and this increase appears to be due to estrogen. Thus estrogen increases both prolactin and GH in the serum of rats.

Serum levels of prolactin also were reported to be elevated during proestrus or estrus in the sheep (Bryant and Greenwood, 1968) and cow (Raud et al., 1971), although Karg and Schams (1970) observed no

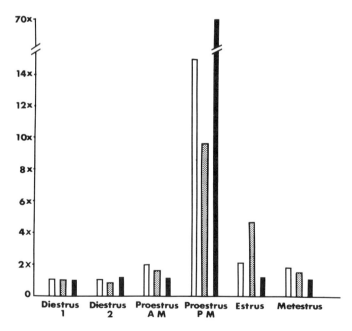

Fig. 2. Serum prolactin, □, LH, ■, and FSH, ▨, during the estrous cycle in the rat. X = multiple increase on PM of proestrus over diestrous values. After Wuttke and Meites (1970a).

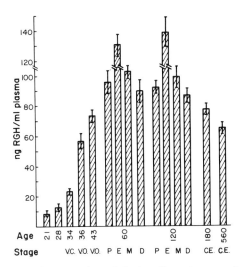

Fig. 3. Serum GH during growth and during the estrous cycle of the rat. Note marked rise in serum GH with onset of puberty (V.O.) on day 36; also on day 43. During the estrous cycle, GH rises on the day of estrus in rats 60 or 120 days old. P = proestrus; E = estrus; M = metestrus; D = diestrus; C.E. = constant estrus; V.C. = vagina closed; V.O. = vagina open. After Dickerman and Meites (1971).

change in blood prolactin values during the estrous cycle in cows. The failure of Karg and Schams (1970) to find any cyclic rise in prolactin may be due to the stress of chronic cannulation of the jugular vein, with a resultant elevation of blood prolactin that masked any rise during the cycle. Stressful stimuli of many types have been reported to elevate secretion of prolactin in animals and man (Nicoll et al., 1960; Raud et al., 1971; Frantz et al., 1972). During the menstrual cycle in women, no apparent changes in serum prolactin have been observed (Jaffe and Midgley, 1971; Frantz and Kleinberg, 1970). Estrogen is believed to be responsible for the rise in blood prolactin during the estrous cycle, and injections of estrogen have been demonstrated to increase pituitary prolactin levels in the rat, guinea pig, rabbit, goat, and cow (Reece and Turner, 1937; Meites, 1966; Chen and Meites, 1970a). Estrogen administration also increases blood prolactin levels in the rat (Chen and Meites, 1970a) (Fig. 4) and in the human (Frantz et al., 1972). Ovariectomy (Clark and Meites, 1971) or injection of an antiestrogen (Neill et al., 1971) on the day before proestrus in the rat prevents the normal rise in serum prolactin on the next day, whereas ovariectomy followed by an injection of estrogen produces a rise in prolactin (and LH) by the next day. Ovariectomy results in reduced pituitary and blood prolactin values (Chen and Meites, 1970a).

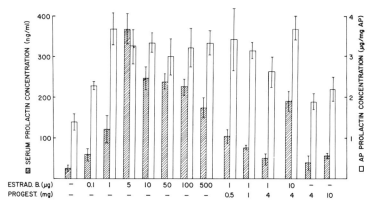

FIG. 4. Effects of daily subcutaneous injections for 5 days of estradiol benzoate on serum prolactin in mature ovariectomized rats. Note that even highest dose of estradiol benzoate (500 μg daily) did not reduce serum or pituitary prolactin values. Progesterone has little ability to increase serum prolactin, but can partially counteract the stimulatory action of estrogen. After Chen and Meites (1970a).

C. PROLACTIN DURING PSEUDOPREGNANCY AND PREGNANCY

During pseudopregnancy and pregnancy in the rat, serum prolactin values are elevated only for about the first 2 to 3 days (Kwa and Verhofstad, 1967; Amenomori et al., 1970; Wuttke and Meites, 1972). Thereafter serum prolactin in pseudopregnant rats is as low or lower than in diestrus. In pregnant rats prolactin remains low until about the last day of gestation. On the day of parturition there is a pronounced rise in serum prolactin in the rat (Amenomori et al., 1970), goat (Johke, 1970), and cow (Johke et al., 1971; Karg and Schams, 1970). Low blood levels of prolactin also have been found during most of pregnancy in the sheep and goat (Bryant and Greenwood, 1968) and cow (Karg and Schams, 1970) and in women (Frantz and Kleinberg, 1970). A rise in blood prolactin was observed in all these species at the end of pregnancy and on the day of parturition. Increases in pituitary content of prolactin also have been observed at the time of parturition in the mouse, rat, guinea pig, rabbit, goat, and cow (Meites and Turner, 1950; Meites, 1966).

The low levels of blood prolactin during most of pseudopregnancy and pregnancy in the rat may be associated with low estrogen secretion, since Yoshinaga et al. (1970) found that ovarian blood estrogen during most of pregnancy was depressed. Low prolactin values during most of pregnancy also may be associated with the ability of large amounts of progesterone to overcome the stimulatory action of small levels of estrogen on prolactin secretion (Meites, 1966; Chen and Meites, 1970a), and with the possible inhibitory action of placental lactogen on pituitary prolactin secretion. Human placental lactogen has been shown to rise in the blood during gestation in women (Friesen *et al.*, 1972). The rise in prolactin at the end of gestation and on the day of parturition may be associated with an increase in estrogen secretion and the stress of labor (Meites, 1966). There also is a pronounced rise in pituitary ACTH and blood corticosterone levels at the end of pregnancy and on the day of parturition in the rat (Voogt *et al.*, 1969), which together with the elevation in prolactin secretion, are believed to be responsible for initiation of lactation. Both adrenal cortical hormones and prolactin are essential for initiation of lactation in most species (Meites, 1966).

D. PROLACTIN DURING LACTATION

After parturition, the principal stimulus responsible for high prolactin secretion (and elevated ACTH-adrenal cortical hormones) is the suckling or milking act. Excitation of the numerous sensory nerves in the nipples and surrounding skin results in reflex release of prolactin and ACTH from the pituitary via the hypothalamus (Meites, 1966). Suckling evokes a significant reduction in pituitary prolactin and ACTH content in the rat (Reece and Turner, 1937; Grosvenor and Turner, 1958; Sar and Meites, 1967; Voogt *et al.*, 1969), and this is reflected in a marked rise in serum prolactin values (Fig. 5) (Amenomori *et al.*, 1970) and corticosterone values. Milking also elevates blood prolactin levels in the goat (Bryant and Greenwood, 1968), cow (Johke *et al.*, 1971; Karg and Schams, 1970),

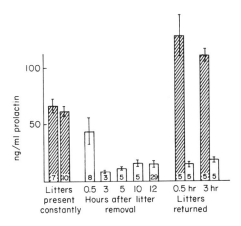

FIG. 5. Effects of suckling on serum prolactin values in postpartum lactating rats. Note marked decrease in serum prolactin 3, 5, 10, and 12 hours after litter removal, and rise in serum prolactin after 0.5 hour and 3.0 hours of suckling (Amenomori *et al.*, 1970).

and women (Frantz and Kleinberg, 1970). Exteroceptive stimuli (smell or sight of the young) and stresses also can induce prolactin release (Meites *et al.*, 1963; Grosvenor, 1965; Nicoll *et al.*, 1960; Wuttke and Meites, 1970b) and may have a role in maintenance of lactation. The suckling stimulus also induces release of ACTH and corticosterone (Voogt *et al.*, 1969), of oxytocin and vasopressin (Cross, 1961) and possibly GH (Grosvenor, 1967; Sar and Meites, 1967), but inhibits release of LH and FSH (Meites, 1966; Minaguchi and Meites, 1967). Inhibition of LH and FSH secretion by the suckling stimulus is believed to account for the temporary inhibition of cyclic ovarian function after parturition, and the degree of inhibition appears to depend on the *intensity* of the suckling stimulus. Prolongation of postpartum breast feeding constitutes one of the oldest methods of fertility control practiced by women, although it is not considered an efficient method for preventing conception.

Lactation can be initiated in virgin animals and nonpregnant women by prolonged stimulation of the nipples, and once initiated can be prolonged indefinitely by continuous application of the suckling stimulus (Meites, 1966). Even in the absence of milk removal, the suckling stimulus can maintain secretory activity in the mammary glands and inhibit involution of mammary lobuloalveolar tissue. In the absence of the milking stimulus and milk removal, limited secretory function can be maintained by administration of prolactin, adrenal cortical hormones and oxytocin, particularly when all three hormones are given together.

In women, spontaneous galactorrhea associated with absence of menstrual cycles (Chiari-Frommel and Forbes-Albright syndromes) has been shown to be associated with high blood prolactin values (Frantz and Kleinberg, 1970; Turkington, 1971). Administration of L-dopa was reported to inhibit lactation in such women and to result in resumption of menstrual cycles (Turkington, 1971).

E. PROLACTIN IN OLD RATS

Few studies have yet been reported on prolactin secretion in animals and man in the postreproductive phases of life. In female rats about 21 months of age showing constant vaginal estrus, pituitary levels of prolactin were found to be about twice as high as in 3-month-old rats on the day of estrus (Clemens and Meites, 1971). Pituitary LH levels were low whereas pituitary FSH was higher than in the young rats. Serum prolactin values in these old rats were at least as high as in the young rats on the day of estrus (Wuttke and Meites, 1970a). Continued elevation of prolactin secretion in these old rats may account at least in part for the rise in incidence of spontaneous mammary tumors and may be associated with increased size of the pituitary (and pituitary tumors). We have postulated that a fundamental change occurs in hypothalamic regulation of anterior pituitary function in old rats, which may be associated with changes in the sensitivity of the hypothalamus to hormonal and environmental stimuli (Clemens et al., 1970a; Clemens and Meites, 1971).

F. Prolactin in Male Animals

Male animals usually contain less prolactin in their pituitaries than female animals of the same species (Meites and Turner, 1948, 1950). Thus mature male rats and rabbits have less than half as much prolactin in their pituitaries as mature females. There is also less serum prolactin in male than in female rats, and no cyclic fluctuations are observed (Amenomori et al., 1970). Prolactin also is lower in the blood of men than of women (Frantz and Kleinberg, 1970). The pituitaries of male rats and rabbits also are less responsive to the stimulatory action of administered estrogen on prolactin secretion, probably reflecting the early influence of androgen on sexual differentiation of the hypothalamus in the newborn male animals. Castration of male rats results in reduced pituitary prolactin content, and injections of androgen evoke relatively small increases in pituitary prolactin levels. No definite functions have yet been established for prolactin in male animals, although it may stimulate growth of the reproductive tract.

G. Diurnal Rhythm in Prolactin Secretion

In both male and female rats, and in ovariectomized rats, a diurnal rhythm in serum prolactin has been observed, with values about twice as high in the late afternoon as in the morning (Koch et al., 1971) (Table I).

TABLE I
Morning and Afternoon Serum Prolactin Concentrations and Secretion Rates[a]

Experimental group	No. of rats	Serum prolactin (ng/ml) 9:45–10:15 AM	Serum prolactin (ng/ml) 5:45–6:15 PM	Secretion rate (ng/min) AM	Secretion rate (ng/min) PM
Diestrus	23	24.6 ± 2.4[b]	55.4 ± 4.9	32.4	73.1
Proestrus	23	26.0 ± 3.0	178.6 ± 14.3[c]	34.3	235.8
Estrus	19	48.8 ± 7.6	105.1 ± 11.1	64.4	138.7
Metestrus	24	26.8 ± 2.5	53.5 ± 3.7	35.4	70.6
Ovariectomized	10	20.0 ± 1.8	42.5 ± 5.9	26.4	56.2
Males	15	25.7 ± 2.5	46.2 ± 4.5	33.9	60.0

[a] After Koch et al. (1971).
[b] Mean ± SE.
[c] The proestrous rise is about 7-fold.

A similar diurnal rhythm in blood prolactin levels has been observed in lactating cows, with values between 4 and 7 PM about twice as high as values from 4 to 10 AM (Koprowski et al., 1972). Diurnal rhythms also have been reported in pituitary prolactin content in rats, again with higher levels in the afternoon than in the morning (Clark and Baker, 1964). The increase in secretion of prolactin during the late afternoon or evening may be associated with diurnal changes in some of the biogenic amines in the hypothalamus.

H. EFFECTS OF STRESS

The lability of prolactin release in response to many stresses is of considerable interest. Nicoll et al. (1960) reported that estrogen-primed female rats subjected to 5 days of continuous stresses responded by initiation of lactation, adrenal enlargement, and thymus involution. They concluded that these stresses promoted release of both prolactin and ACTH. Subsequently it was observed that stress induced by prolonged etherization or shortly after sodium pentobarbital injection, elevated serum prolactin in rats (Wuttke and Meites, 1970b; Neil et al., 1971). Stresses in cows (Raud et al., 1971; Johke et al., 1971) and both psychic and surgical stresses in human patients (Frantz et al., 1972) raised blood prolactin values in these species. The mechanism(s) by which stresses increase prolactin release, and the physiological purposes which this may serve, remain to be clarified. Obviously, it is an important consideration in collecting blood for assay of prolactin not to stress animals and humans.

III. EFFECTS OF THE HYPOTHALAMUS ON PROLACTIN SECRETION

A. EFFECTS OF REMOVAL OF HYPOTHALAMIC CONNECTIONS TO THE PITUITARY

Early studies by Desclin (1950) and Everett (1954) indicated that transplantation of the pituitary underneath the kidney capsule resulted in continuous prolactin secretion, as indicated by prolonged maintenance of luteal function in rats. Secretion of the other five anterior pituitary hormones (FSH, LH, TSH, ACTH, GH) was profoundly reduced, as judged by appearance of the target organs and decreased body growth. Subsequently many other investigations have confirmed these observations and also have shown that the pituitary is capable of autonomous secretion of prolactin after pituitary stalk section, after placement of lesions in the hypothalamus, and upon culture or incubation of the pituitary (Meites et al., 1963; Meites and Nicoll, 1966). With the recent availability of radioimmunoassays for measuring serum prolactin in a variety of species (rat, mouse, goat, sheep, cow, man), it has become possible to make even more precise observations of the role of the hypothalamus in regulation of prolactin secretion. These studies indicate that the predominant action of the mammalian hypothalamus on prolactin secretion is inhibitory in nature.

Transplantation of 1 to 4 heterologous anterior pituitaries underneath the kidney capsule of female hypophysectomized ovariectomized rats, resulted in continuous prolactin release during 10 weeks (Chen *et al.*, 1970) (Fig. 6). Rats with no pituitary grafts had barely detectable levels of serum prolactin, whereas rats with 1 pituitary graft had levels about as high as on the day of estrus. Rats with 2 pituitary grafts had about twice as much serum prolactin as rats with 1 pituitary, and rats with 4 pituitary grafts about 4 times as much serum prolactin during most of the 10-week period of observation as rats with 1 pituitary graft. Injections of small doses of estradiol benzoate (1 μg/day) for 5 days at the end of 10 weeks increased prolactin release by the grafted pituitaries, suggesting a direct action of the estrogen on the pituitary.

Placement of bilateral lesions in the median eminence, or anterior or posterior hypothalamus of ovariectomized rats, resulted in significant elevations of serum prolactin levels above control values (Fig. 7). This suggests that all these areas participate in regulation of prolactin secretion, and it is of interest that they all lie in the "hypophysiotropic area"

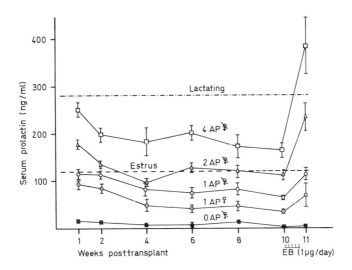

FIG. 6. Effects of transplantation of 1 to 4 rat anterior pituitaries on serum prolactin concentration in ovariectomized (⚥) or nonovariectomized (♀) hypophysectomized rats. The lactating values are those taken from rats immediately after suckling. Note that injection of 1 μg of estradiol benzoate daily for 5 days increased serum prolactin values. After Chen *et al.* (1970).

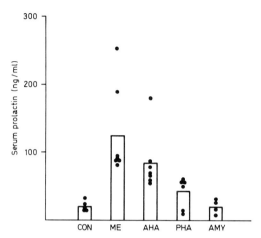

FIG. 7. Effects of placing bilateral lesions in the median eminence (ME), anterior hypothalamus (AHA), posterior hypothalamus (PHA), or amygdala (AMY) on serum prolactin. CON = control. After Chen *et al.* (1970).

of the hypothalamus as defined by Halasz (1962). The "hypophysiotropic area" is believed to control basal secretion of anterior pituitary hormones. Bilateral lesions placed in the amygdaloid nuclei had no effect on serum prolactin values. In a more recent experiment, Welsch *et al.* (1971b) demonstrated that placement of bilateral lesions in the median eminence in intact female rats resulted in about a 10-fold increase in serum prolactin by the end of 30 minutes and a subsequent fall to levels still above those of controls; this elevation in serum prolactin persisted during approximately 6 months of observation. Lesions placed in the medial basal hypothalamus were found to result in initiation of lactation in the rabbit (Haun and Sawyer, 1960), cat (Grosz and Rothballer, 1961), and rat (DeVoe *et al.*, 1966) and in early appearance of spontaneous mammary tumors in rats (Welsch *et al.*, 1970). It appears probable that placement of lesions in the median eminence or stalk section results in greater release of prolactin by the *in situ* pituitary than when the pituitary is transplanted to another site in the body. Apart from the possible damage to the pituitary during transplantation, the rat pituitary is known to shrink to one-half to one-third of its original size after transplantation to the kidney. Mouse anterior pituitaries grafted underneath the kidney capsule eventually become enlarged and tumorous (Boot, 1969), but grafted rat pituitaries remain shrunken in size. Prolonged administration of estrogen into intact female rats with a pituitary graft underneath the kidney capsule results in appearance of pituitary tumors both in the graft and *in situ* pituitary (Welsch *et al.*, 1971a).

B. Presence of a Prolactin-Inhibiting Factor (PIF) in the Hypothalamus

Since prolactin release is increased after removal of hypothalamic influence, it early became of interest to determine whether a factor was present in the hypothalamus that could inhibit prolactin release. A preliminary report indicated that injection of a crude rat hypothalamic extract for 5 days into estrogen-primed female rats initiated mammary secretion (Meites *et al.*, 1960), but prolactin levels were not measured either in the pituitary or blood—the latter because sufficiently sensitive bioassays or radioimmunoassays were not available at that time. In addition, lactation cannot be considered a specific response to prolactin alone, and many other agents can initiate mammary secretion in estrogen-primed rats (Meites *et al.*, 1963). Subsequently, it was shown that when crude hypothalamic extracts were added to incubations (Meites *et al.*, 1963; Talwalker *et al.*, 1963) or cultures (Pasteels, 1961) of rat pituitary, prolactin release was decreased. Hypothalamic extracts from the sheep,

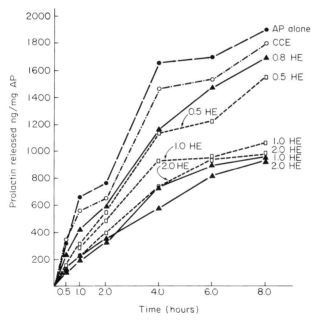

Fig. 8. Effects of an extract of rat hypothalamus on release of prolactin by male rat pituitary *in vitro*. CCE = cerebral cortical extract; HE = hypothalamic extract. Arrows at 4 hours indicate that additional amounts of HE were added at this time. An equivalent of 1 HE appeared to produce maximum inhibition of prolactin release. After Chen and Meites (1970b).

bovine, pig, and human also were demonstrated to inhibit release of prolactin (Schally et al., 1967). A negative dose-response relationship was reported between the amount of rat hypothalamic extract added to an incubation medium containing pituitary halves from the male rats and the amount of prolactin released into the medium (Kragt and Meites, 1965). The effect of adding a neutralized acid extract of rat hypothalamus on release of incubated male rat pituitary is shown in Fig. 8. It can be seen that when greater amounts of hypothalamic extract were added to the medium they produced larger decreases in prolactin release as measured by radioimmunoassay. Hypothalamic extracts also are effective in depressing prolactin release when injected into rats, as shown in Fig. 9. Other workers also have reported that hypothalamic extracts can inhibit prolactin release in vivo (Grosvenor et al., 1964; Schally et al., 1967; Watson et al., 1971).

The prolactin-inhibiting factor (PIF) (Talwalker et al., 1963) in the hypothalamus has not been characterized chemically, although it is probably a small polypeptide like the other hypothalamic hypophysiotropic hormones. Recent work by Nicoll (1971) indicates that 3',5' cyclic AMP can overcome the inhibitory action of hypothalamic extract on pituitary prolactin release in vitro, and that hypothalamic extract is as effective in inhibiting prolactin release in the absence as in the presence of theophylline. These results suggest that an action of PIF on the adenyl cyclase–phosphodiesterase system is unlikely. It is of interest that pro-

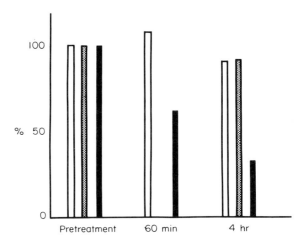

FIG. 9. Effects of an injection of the equivalent of 8 rat hypothalami (■, 8 HE) or similar amount of rat cerebral cortical tissue (▨, 8 CCE) on the morning of proestrus, on serum prolactin concentration. Note that the 8 HE reduced serum prolactin more at the end of 4 hours than at the end of 60 minutes, whereas the 8 CCE had no significant effect. □ = Saline. After Amenomori and Meites (1970).

lactin release in response to elevated potassium ion concentration is relatively small as compared to other pituitary hormones (Parsons, 1970). However, when hypothalamic extract was added in the presence of elevated potassium ions *in vitro*, the effects of each were reduced, suggesting that they each may influence release of prolactin through the same mechanism. One of the effects of elevated potassium ions is believed to be increased entry of Ca ions into the cells, and Ca ions have been shown to be essential for prolactin release by the pituitary *in vitro* (Parsons, 1970). Nicoll (1971) suggested that PIF acts on the prolactin secreting cell membrane to inhibit Ca influx. The cell is believed to depolarize spontaneously when it is freed from hypothalamic influence, with a resultant increase in Ca entry into the cell and consequent release of secretory granules (Parsons, 1970). Thus PIF may act by preventing spontaneous depolarization of the prolactin cells.

If prolactin secretion is controlled mainly by a PIF in the hypothalamus, the question may be asked: What controls PIF secretion? As discussed in Section IV, PIF secretion appears to be regulated mainly by biogenic amines in the hypothalamus. Stimuli that result in increased prolactin release usually have been found to be associated with a decrease in hypothalamic catecholamines and PIF content. These include the suckling stimulus, stresses, estrogen, testosterone, progesterone, Enovid, cortisol, reserpine, perphenazine, and haloperidol (Meites, 1970). An anesthetic dose of Na pentobarbital increases prolactin release for the first 30 minutes and this is associated with a fall in hypothalamic PIF; thereafter prolactin release is depressed but this appears to be due mainly to direct inhibition of the pituitary (Wuttke and Meites, 1970b; Wuttke *et al.*, 1971b).

Agents that depress prolactin secretion may produce increases in hypothalamic catecholamines and PIF activity. These include prolactin itself (Chen *et al.*, 1967; Voogt and Meites, 1971), ergot drugs (Wuttke *et al.*, 1971a), L-dopa, and monoamine oxidase inhibitors such as iproniazid and pargyline (Lu and Meites, 1971b). Kamberi *et al.* (1970) reported that an injection of dopamine into the third ventricle of rats increased PIF release in the hypothalamopituitary portal circulation and decreased serum prolactin values. We observed that a systemic injection of L-dopa into rats not only decreased serum prolactin values, but also released PIF into the systemic circulation of hypophysectomized and intact rats (Lu and Meites, 1971a).

C. Possible Presence of a Prolactin-Releasing Factor (PRF) in the Hypothalamus

Benson and Folley (1956) hypothesized that oxytocin may be the hypothalamic factor responsible for prolactin release, based on their observation that injections of oxytocin, like prolactin, could inhibit involution of the mammary glands in postpartum rats after litter removal. They believed that oxytocin induced prolactin release, although prolactin was not actually measured. Subsequently it was shown that oxytocin prevented mammary involution by a different action than prolactin, and that it did not alter pituitary prolactin levels (Meites *et al.,* 1963). More recently, Bryant and Greenwood (1972) reported that oxytocin failed to elevate blood prolactin values significantly in sheep. Thus oxytocin does not appear to be an important factor in prolactin release.

Our laboratory reported that injections of crude hypothalamic extracts could initiate mammary secretion in estrogen-primed female rats (Meites *et al.,* 1960). However, we could not definitely conclude that such extracts contained a prolactin-releasing factor (PRF), since many other substances were found to initiate mammary secretion in these rat preparations. Initiation of lactation is not a specific response to prolactin alone, but also requires the action of adrenal cortical steroids as well. In our early studies a crude CRF preparation was found to be more effective for inducing mammary secretion in estrogen-primed rats than crude hypothalamic extracts (Meites, 1962). Subsequently, Mishkinsky *et al.* (1968) confirmed our observations on the effects of crude hypothalamic extract on mammary secretion in estrogen-primed rats, and concluded that this constituted evidence for the existence of a PRF in the rat hypothalamus.

Other evidence for the possible existence of a PRF has come from more recent studies. Nicoll *et al.* (1970) reported that when they incubated rat pituitary tissue with crude hypothalamic extract, they observed inhibition of prolactin release for the first 4 hours and increased prolactin during the subsequent 4 hours. They concluded that their hypothalamic extract contained both PIF and PRF activities. Using a somewhat different system of incubation, our laboratory observed only inhibition of prolactin release throughout an 8-hour period of incubation (Meites, 1970) (see Fig. 8). Krulich *et al.* (1971) sectioned freshly frozen rat hypothalamus and reported that PIF activity was predominant in the dorsolateral part of the preoptic area, and that PRF activity was predominant in the median eminence area. The latter appears difficult to reconcile with the many observations that placement of lesions in the median eminence area results in increased release of prolactin (see Meites, 1970). If PRF activity predominated in this area, then lesions placed in the median eminence might be expected to result in decreased release of prolactin. It also is of interest that the preoptic area, which Krulich *et al.* (1971) reported contains PIF activity, has been observed to be concerned with the release of LH but not of prolactin by Everett and Quinn (1966) and Kordon (1966). The latter workers showed that stimulation of the preoptic area produced ovulation but not pseudopregnancy in the rat.

Valverde and Chieffo (1971) reported that relatively large doses of an extract of porcine hypothalamus increased serum prolactin levels in male rats pretreated with estrogen and progesterone. However, although full details of this work have not yet been published, equivalent amounts of cerebral cortical extract were not given and injections of physiological saline alone produced a significant decrease in serum prolactin. Also, injections of porcine hypothalamic extract into untreated male rats had no effect on serum prolactin. These observations are not in agreement with the earlier work of Schally et al. (1967), who reported that porcine hypothalamic extracts depressed prolactin release in rats under both in vitro and in vivo conditions.

Several recent reports have suggested that synthetic TRF (TRH) may be capable of inducing release of prolactin in rats and human subjects. Tashjian et al. (1971) made the interesting observation that addition of synthetic TRH to an incubation medium containing two clonal strains of cells from rat pituitary tumors, stimulated release of prolactin and inhibited release of GH. We have added several doses of synthetic TRH to an incubation medium containing normal rat anterior pituitary halves instead of cells from pituitary tumors, and observed no effect on prolactin release (Lu et al., 1972). Single injections of TRH into normal intact rats also failed to alter serum prolactin values, but when TRH was injected daily for 6 days there was a small increase in pituitary and serum prolactin levels. Such increases were not observed when TRH was injected for 6 days into thyroidectomized rats, suggesting that its effects were mediated through the TSH-thyroid system. In women, a single injection of synthetic TRH was reported to induce a rapid elevation of serum prolactin values (Friesen, 1971). Although this shows that TRH can increase prolactin in human subjects, no direct effect on the anterior pituitary has been demonstrated and the possibility cannot be excluded that its action is mediated through the TSH-thyroid system or by another mechanism. It was reported that thyroid hormones are stimulatory to prolactin secretion in rats (Chen and Meites, 1969) and can act directly on the rat anterior pituitary to increase prolactin release (Nicoll and Meites, 1963).

In contrast to mammals, the avian hypothalamus has been reported to contain prolactin-releasing activity, and there is evidence that the avian pituitary requires hypothalamic stimulation to secrete prolactin (Meites and Nicoll, 1966). Pigeons, for example, do not respond to estrogen or reserpine with increased prolactin release, and when the pigeon pituitary is transplanted to the crop sac there is no apparent stimulation of the crop sac epithelium (Kragt and Meites, 1965). Hypothalamic extracts from the pigeon, chicken, Japanese quail, turkey, tricolored blackbird, and duck have been shown to stimulate prolactin release by the pituitaries of each of these species *in vitro* (Meites, 1967). It is not clear why these differences exist in hypothalamic control of prolactin secretion between mammals and birds, and it is possible that PIF and PRF activities are present in the hypothalamus of both classes of animals. However, the predominant hypothalamic regulation appears to be inhibitory in mammals and stimulatory in birds.

IV. The Role of Biogenic Amines

A. Catecholamines

Early work suggested that biogenic amines may influence the release of anterior pituitary hormones. Thus, Markee *et al.* (1948) and Sawyer *et al.* (1949) reported that adrenergic and cholinergic drugs induced ovulation in rats or rabbits, whereas antiadrenergic and anticholinergic drugs blocked ovulation. Injections of epinephrine evoked ACTH release (Munson, 1963). We observed that administration of epinephrine, norepinephrine, acetylcholine, and serotonin induced lactation in estrogen-primed rats and rabbits, but this could not be considered as definite evidence that these drugs stimulated prolactin release since antagonists of these drugs and other drugs (dibenamine, atropine, reserpine, chlorpromazine, morphine, amphetamine, etc.) also promoted lactation (Meites, 1962). In addition, lactation is not a specific response to prolactin stimulation alone but also requires the action of adrenal cortical hormones. A better indication that catecholamines are involved in release of prolactin came from the observation that iproniazid, a recognized monoamine oxidase inhibitor and therefore a depressor of catecholamine metabolism, inhibited postpartum lactation in rats (Mizuno *et al.*, 1964). Subsequently, iproniazid was shown to increase hypothalamic PIF and reduce serum prolactin values (Lu and Meites, 1971b).

Participation of biogenic amines in release of anterior pituitary hormones appeared more plausible when it was demonstrated that norepinephrine and serotonin were highly concentrated in the hypothalamus (Vogt, 1954; Brodie *et al.*, 1959), and when it was shown that the median eminence (the "final common pathway" to the pituitary) was rich in dopaminergic nerve terminals (Fuxe, 1964; Carlsson *et al.*, 1965). It subsequently was found that various drugs and different physiological states (the estrous cycle, pregnancy, lactation, etc.) could alter catecholamine concentration in the hypothalamus and median eminence, and secretion of prolactin, LH, and FSH (Mizuno *et al.*, 1964; Schneider and

McCann, 1970; Lu *et al.*, 1970). Corresponding changes were found in hypothalamic release of PIF (Ratner *et al.*, 1965) and LRF and FRF (Schneider and McCann, 1970; Kamberi *et al.*, 1970). From these and related investigations the present concept arose that the catecholamines in the hypothalamus, particularly those in the median eminence, act as neurotransmitters to control the release of the hypothalamic hypophysiotropic hormones and their entry into the hypothalamopituitary portal vessels, which in turn regulate the release of anterior pituitary hormones (Coppola, 1968; Fuxe and Hokfelt, 1969; Wurtman, 1970).

Dopamine, epinephrine, norepinephrine, and serotonin do not readily pass through the blood–brain barrier upon systemic administration (Innes and Nickerson, 1970), and hence were not observed to have any effect on serum prolactin values after systemic injection in rats (Lu *et al.*, 1970). However, use of precursors of catecholamines and serotonin, inhibitors of catecholamine metabolism, and drugs that inhibit catecholamine receptors in the hypothalamus, were found to alter serum prolactin values significantly. Thus a single intraperitoneal injection of L-dopa (the precursor of dopamine) or of iproniazid, pargyline, or Eli Lilly

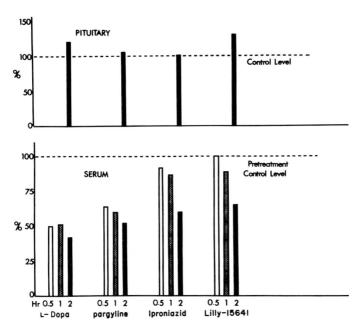

FIG. 10. Effects of L-dopa and 3 monoamine oxidase inhibitors (all increase hypothalamic catecholamines) on serum and pituitary prolactin values. All drugs decreased serum prolactin, but only L-dopa and Lilly 15641 increased pituitary prolactin content. After Lu and Meites (1971b).

compound 15641 (all monoamine oxidase inhibitors) and therefore inhibitors of catecholamine metabolism, resulted in significant elevations in hypothalamic PIF content and reductions in serum prolactin concentration (Fig. 10). These four drugs increase hypothalamic catecholamines. More recently, pyrogallol (an inhibitor of catechol-O-methyl transferase, another enzyme that metabolizes catecholamines), also was found to depress serum prolactin in rats (Quadri and Meites, 1971b).

A single injection of drugs that inhibit hypothalamic catecholamine activity, including reserpine, chlorpromazine, α-methyl-p-tyrosine, α-methyl-m-tyrosine, m-dopa, and d-amphetamine, all markedly increased serum prolactin values (Lu et al., 1970; Lu and Meites, 1971b) (Fig. 11). Several of these compounds, including reserpine, chlorpromazine, m-dopa, and d-amphetamine, were found to decrease hypothalamic PIF activity. Perphenazine, a compound related to chlorpromazine, and reserpine were demonstrated to act directly on rat hypothalamic tissue in vitro to reduce PIF release into the medium (Danon et al., 1963; Ratner et al.,

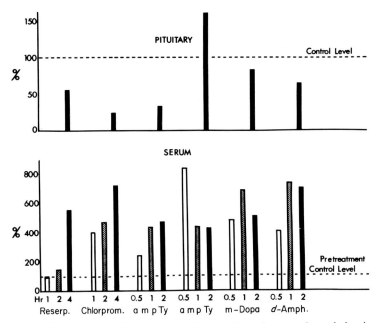

FIG. 11. Effects of a single injection of drugs that decrease hypothalamic catecholamine activity on serum and pituitary prolactin levels. All drugs greatly elevated serum prolactin, and all reduced pituitary prolactin content with the exception of α-methyl-m-tyrosine (a m m Ty). The latter may induce rapid synthesis as well as release of prolactin. Chlorprom. = chlorpromazine; d-Amph. = d-amphetamine; Reserp. = reserpine; a m p Ty = α-methyl-p-tyrosine. After Lu et al. (1970); and Lu and Meites (1971b).

1965). In related experiments, Kamberi *et al.* (1970) reported that an injection of dopamine into the third ventricle of male rats increased PIF release into the portal vessels and depressed serum prolactin values. These observations indicate that hypothalamic catecholamines act as neurotransmitters to increase PIF release, and this results in reduced release of prolactin. A decrease in hypothalamic catecholamines results in reduced PIF release and increased blood prolactin values.

Horn and Snyder (1971) carefully pointed to the conformational similarities of the chlorpromazine and dopamine molecules. Based on studies utilizing quantum mechanics, it was shown that a phenothiazine drug such as chlorpromazine could assume a conformation resembling dopamine. They suggested that the neuroleptic activity of chlorpromazine was due to inhibition of dopamine action at the receptor site. Although the similarity of the chlorpromazine conformation to that of dopamine would also apply to norepinephrine, whose X-ray structure is similar to dopamine, chlorpromazine seems to have a greater apparent blocking action at dopamine rather than at norepinephrine receptors (Carlsson and Lindquist, 1963; Nyback and Sedvall, 1968; Anden *et al.*, 1970). One of the most potent neuroleptic drugs is pimozide. A unique action of pimozide is its ability to block the action of dopamine at its receptor without inhibiting appreciably the interaction of norepinephrine with its receptor (Janssen *et al.*, 1968). As a norepinephrine antagonist, it is about 63 to 364 times less potent than chlorpromazine, while as a dopamine antagonist it is more potent than chlorpromazine. The following study was performed to test the effects of these drugs on prolactin secretion (Clemens *et al.*, 1971c): Adult female rats were ovariectomized and on day 10 after ovariectomy they were treated with chlorpromazine, 9.2

TABLE II

EFFECTS OF SEVERAL DRUGS ON PROLACTIN RELEASE IN OVARIECTOMIZED RATS[a]

Treatment	No. of rats	Prolactin[b] levels (ng/ml)
Controls, saline treated	10	13.1 ± 1.1
Chlorpromazine, 18.0 mg/kg	10	75.2 ± 2.2^c
Pimozide, 2.5 mg/kg	10	62.2 ± 3.9^c
Disulfiram, 200 mg/kg	10	7.0 ± 0.9^d
Lilly 78335, 30 mg/kg	8	10.5 ± 1.2

[a] Clemens *et al.* (1971c).
[b] Expressed as nanograms of NIAMD-prolactin-RP-1 per milliliter.
[c] $P < 0.0001$, treated vs. control using Student's t test.
[d] $P < 0.001$.

mg/kg; pimozide, 2.5 mg/kg; disulfiram (an inhibitor of norepinephrine synthesis), 200 mg/kg; and Lilly compound 78335 (an inhibitor of epinephrine synthesis), 30 mg/kg.

Table II shows the results of this study. Lilly compound 78335 did not influence prolactin levels. This is suggestive of little or no participation by epinephrine in the inhibition of prolactin secretion. Both agents that theoretically block the dopamine-receptor interaction (chlorpromazine and pimozide) significantly stimulated prolactin secretion. The potency of these compounds as norepinephrine antagonists had no relationship to their ability to stimulate prolactin. These results provide strong support for the view that dopaminergic neurons tonically stimulate PIF secretion, and that this tonic stimulation of PIF is not a nonspecific alpha-adrenergic phenomenon. In addition, it is possible that norepinephrine is stimulatory to prolactin secretion under normal conditions, since disulfiram caused a significant inhibition of prolactin release. This is in agreement with the results recently reported by Donoso et al. (1971).

Several investigators have reported that catecholamines can act directly on the rat pituitary to alter prolactin release, but it is doubtful that these observations are of physiological significance. Thus MacLeod (1969) and Birge et al. (1970) observed that when norepinephrine, epinephrine, and dopamine were incorporated into incubation media containing rat pituitary tissue, prolactin release was inhibited. Subsequently, it was demonstrated by us that smaller doses of norepinephrine and epinephrine than used by preceding workers could stimulate prolactin release by rat pituitary in vitro (Koch et al., 1970). There is no evidence that catecholamines are present in the hypothalamo-pituitary portal circulation (see Wurtman, 1970; Ruf et al., 1970) making it appear unlikely that hypothalamic catecholamines exert any direct effect on pituitary prolactin release.

B. OTHER BIOGENIC AMINES

The role of other biogenic amines is less clear. Recent work by Kamberi et al. (1971) showed that a single injection of serotonin or melatonin into the third ventricle of rats elevated serum prolactin levels. We have found that systemic injection of serotonin has no definite effect on serum prolactin concentration (Lu et al., 1970), but injection of tryptophan and particularly 5-hydroxytryptophan (precursors of serotonin) produced significant elevations in serum prolactin (Lu and Meites, 1971a). Thus hypothalamic serotonin may act in opposition to catecholamines on prolactin release. The observation that serum prolactin values in male and female rats show a diurnal rhythm, with greater values on the evening than on the morning (Koch et al., 1971), may be related to diurnal changes in hypothalamic serotonin levels. It is of interest that catecholamines and serotonin (also melatonin) have been reported to have opposite effects on release of LH and FSH, the former stimulating and the latter inhibiting release of the two gonadotropins (Kamberi et al., 1970, 1971). The influence of other biogenic amines in the hypothalamus such as acetylcholine on PIF and prolactin release remain to be investigated.

V. INHIBITORY FEEDBACK BY PROLACTIN ON PROLACTIN SECRETION

A. EFFECTS OF PROLACTIN-SECRETING PITUITARY TUMORS ON PROLACTIN SECRETION BY THE *in Situ* PITUITARY AND ON PIF

Prolactin secretion appears to be controlled, at least in part, by an autoregulatory mechanism. This was first hypothesized by Sgouris and Meites (1953), based on the view that prolactin had no target organ or tissue that could inhibit prolactin secretion, and that the circulating levels of prolactin might therefore help regulate prolactin secretion. Transplanted pituitary tumors that secrete large amounts of prolactin and growth hormone were able to reduce the prolactin content of the *in situ* pituitary (MacLeod et al., 1966, 1968; Chen et al., 1967). In addition to finding less prolactin in the pituitary, Chen et al. (1967) found more PIF in the hypothalamus of rats bearing pituitary tumor transplants (Table III). Although the pituitary tumor secreted GH as well as prolactin, the results were suggestive of an autoregulatory or

TABLE III

EFFECT OF "MAMMOSOMATOTROPIC" PITUITARY TUMOR TRANSPLANTS ($M_T TW_5$ AND $M_T TW_{15}$) ON PITUITARY PROLACTIN AND HYPOTHALAMIC PIF[a]

Expt. No.	Treatment	AP weight (mg)	AP Prolactin (IU/AP)	Hypothalamic PIF (prolactin released into medium, IU/100 mg AP)
1	Controls	8.71 ± 0.23	0.21 ± 0.14	1.34 ± 0.23^c
	$M_T TW_{15}$	6.24 ± 0.30	0.17 ± 0.07	0.80 ± 0.11^c
2	Controls	10.67 ± 0.29	0.42 ± 0.09^b	1.06 ± 0.21^c
	$M_T TW_{15}$	6.76 ± 0.96	0.11 ± 0.04^b	0.49 ± 0.11^c
3	Controls	8.38 ± 0.55	0.43 ± 0.03^c	4.01 ± 2.0^b
	$M_T TW_{15}$	6.22 ± 0.45	0.11 ± 0.01^c	1.27 ± 3.4^b

[a] After Chen et al. (1967).
[b] Significant difference ($P < 0.05$).
[c] Significant difference ($P < 0.001$).

"short loop" feedback mechanism for the control of prolactin secretion. An action on the brain by prolactin was indicated by the increase in PIF.

B. EFFECTS OF INJECTIONS OF PROLACTIN AND PITUITARY GRAFTS ON PROLACTIN SECRETION BY THE *in Situ* PITUITARY

Daily injection of 1 or 10 mg of NIH-P-S₇ prolactin markedly reduced pituitary weight and prolactin concentration in mature female rats (Sinha and Tucker, 1968). Multiple pituitary grafts under the kidney capsule for 2 weeks lowered pituitary weight and prolactin concentration of the *in situ* pituitary in intact and ovariectomized rats (Sinha and Tucker, 1968). In contrast, long-term pituitary grafts (2 months) decreased pituitary prolactin content and concentration but did not change hypothalamic PIF content in ovariectomized rats (Welsch *et al.*, 1968a).

A pituitary graft placed in the hypothalamus also was able to inhibit prolactin secretion by the *in situ* pituitary (Averill, 1969). Many of these grafts were situated distant from the medial basal hypothalamus and portal circulation, and the grafts themselves did not produce luteotropic effects similar to grafts placed beneath the kidney capsule. This is strongly indicative of a local feedback between the graft and neural tissue that produces PIF. In view of these results and those of Chen *et al.* (1970) showing that pituitaries transplanted to the kidney capsule secrete abundant amounts of prolactin and do not inhibit their own secretion, it appears that the feedback between the brain and pituitary prolactin is much more sensitive than the direct feedback of prolactin on the pituitary postulated by Spies and Clegg (1971). Fuxe and Hokfelt (1971) have shown that prolactin injections into rats activates tuberoinfundibular *dopaminergic* neurons. It is therefore probable that prolactin normally acts via the hypothalamus to increase dopamine activity, resulting in increased release of PIF into the portal vessels and consequent inhibition of prolactin release.

C. EFFECTS OF IMPLANTS OF PROLACTIN IN THE MEDIAN EMINENCE ON SECRETION OF PROLACTIN

1. *Implants in Cycling and Ovariectomized Rats*

The first study utilizing prolactin implants in the hypothalamus was reported by Clemens and Meites (1968). Implantation of small amounts of prolactin into the median eminence of mature intact and ovariectomized rats resulted in increased hypothalamic PIF content and reduced pituitary weight and prolactin concentration (Table IV). The ovaries of intact rats with prolactin implants were characterized by well developed follicles and relatively few large corpora lutea, whereas the ovaries of rats with implants containing no prolactin had large corpora lutea

TABLE IV

EFFECTS OF A PROLACTIN IMPLANT INTO THE MEDIAN EMINENCE ON PITUITARY
PROLACTIN CONCENTRATION AND HYPOTHALAMIC PIF CONTENT[a]

Treatment[c]	AP[b] weight (mg)	AP prolactin concentration (IU/100 mg)	PIF content (AP prolactin released *in vitro*)
Intact controls (13)	8.1 ± 0.2	2.36 ± 0.50	1.77 ± 0.30
Intact prolactin-implanted (10)	6.2 ± 0.4	1.32 ± 0.20	0.81 ± 0.14
OVX controls (6)	11.3 ± 0.6	3.31 ± 0.23	1.09 ± 0.40
OVX, prolactin-implanted (6)	9.5 ± 0.5	2.35 ± 0.56	0.32 ± 0.15

[a] After Clemens and Meites (1968).
[b] AP = anterior pituitary.
[c] OVX = ovariectomy; ( ) = number of rats.

characteristic of pseudopregnancy. In addition, the prolactin implants produced marked mammary gland regression. A similar reduction in pituitary prolactin levels after median eminence prolactin implants was observed by Mishkinsky *et al.* (1969). Human growth hormone, which has some intrinsic prolactin activity, also was shown to decrease serum prolactin levels when implanted into the median eminence of female rats (Voogt *et al.*, 1971). Pituitary GH levels were also reduced.

2. *Implants during Pseudopregnancy and Pregnancy*

The inhibitory feedback of prolactin on its own secretion was a useful tool to explore the importance of prolactin in maintaining pseudopregnancy and pregnancy. Chen *et al.* (1968) showed that a single implant of prolactin in the median eminence shortened the duration of pseudopregnancy whereas implants of LH and FSH were ineffective. They also reported that a prolactin implant was capable of preventing formation of deciduomata in pseudopregnant rats.

Implants of prolactin in the median eminence inhibited pregnancy (Clemens *et al.*, 1969a). In order to be totally effective, the implant had to be made during the first 6 days of pregnancy. Implants placed after day 6 were relatively ineffective. From these results it appeared that pituitary prolactin secretion was needed only for the first 6 days of pregnancy. The ability of prolactin to maintain pregnancy in the rat apparently is due to stimulation of progesterone secretion by the ovary, since prolactin implants on day 4 of pregnancy resulted in regression of the corpora lutea of pregnancy. Pregnancy could be maintained in implanted animals by daily injection of 2 mg of progesterone, but when progesterone treatment was withdrawn on day 12, pregnancy was terminated in all cases by day 15 (Table V).

Presumably pituitary prolactin secretion is no longer required by day 12

TABLE V

EFFECTS OF A PROLACTIN IMPLANT ON DAY 4 AND DAILY PROGESTERONE
INJECTIONS ON DAYS 4-11 ON MAINTENANCE OF PREGNANCY[a]

Treatment	No. of rats pregnant on day 11	No. of rats pregnant on day 15, after withdrawal of progesterone on day 12
Cocoa butter implant + 2 mg progesterone daily	6	6
Prolactin-cocoa butter implant + 2 mg progesterone daily	6	0

[a] From Clemens et al. (1969a).

to maintain pregnancy although ovarian progesterone is essential. At this stage of pregnancy ovarian secretion of progesterone apparently is regulated by placental luteotropin. These results have been confirmed recently by Spies and Clegg (1971), with the additional observation that prolactin may be capable of inhibiting its own secretion by acting *directly* on the pituitary. However, Nicoll (1971) concluded on the basis of *in vitro* experiments that prolactin does not act directly on the pituitary to inhibit its own secretion, and our own results (Sud and Meites, 1969) are in agreement with those of Nicoll (1971).

3. Implants during Lactation

Marked inhibition of lactation was observed when prolactin was implanted into the median eminence of lactating rats (Clemens et al., 1969b). When lactating female rats received prolactin-cocoa butter implants on day 4 postpartum, lactation as assessed by litter weight gains was seriously impaired. Table VI shows the effects of prolactin implants alone or in combination with other hormones on litter weight gains and mammary gland weights. The combination of prolactin and ACTH was more effective than prolactin alone. This is in agreement with other studies showing that adrenal steroids are necessary for lactation. In addition to the inhibitory effects on lactation, the prolactin implant produced regression of the corpora lutea of lactation and resumption of estrous cycles. The latter suggests that the prolactin implant resulted in increased gonadotropin secretion.

4. Prolactin Implants during the Prepubertal Period and Their Effects on LH and FSH Secretion

The "short loop" feedback of prolactin on its own secretion also can influence the secretion of LH and FSH. An example of this is the advancement of puberty in rats by prolactin implants in the median eminence or

TABLE VI

EFFECTS OF HORMONE IMPLANTS IN THE MEDIAN EMINENCE ON LITTER
WEIGHT GAINS AND MAMMARY GLAND WEIGHTS

Group and treatment	Average weight gain (gm) of 6 pups on designated days post implantation			Average mammary gland weight 5 days after implantation (gm)
	2 Days	5 Days	7 Days	
1. Controls, cocoa butter	12.8 ± 1.4^a (11)	40.4 ± 2.7^a (11)	70.7 ± 6.2^a (5)	2.67 ± 0.12^a (6)
2. Prolactin + cocoa butter	3.9 ± 0.4^b (14)	18.8 ± 3.5^b (14)	32.6 ± 5.9^b (9)	1.96 ± 0.16^b (5)
3. Prolactin, ACTH + cocoa butter	1.3 ± 0.2^c (9)	8.7 ± 3.6^c (9)	16.9 ± 7.0^b (3)	1.42 ± 0.14^c (6)
4. Prolactin, GH + cocoa butter	3.0 ± 0.5^b (7)	19.5 ± 3.3^b (7)	28.9 ± 6.1^b (7)	—
5. Prolactin + cholesterol pellet	8.8 ± 1.9^a (10)	35.1 ± 3.2^a (10)	71.0 ± 5.9^a (5)	2.71 ± 0.11^a (5)

Note: After Clemens et al. (1969b). ( ) = No. rats.
^{a,b,c} Values having different superscripts are significantly different from each other, $P < 0.05$.

by injections of prolactin (Clemens et al., 1969c). In this study, prolactin implants were placed in the median eminences of 21-day-old rats. Table VII shows that such implants advanced puberty by 6 days (group 1) when compared with implants of small amounts of other anterior pituitary hormones reported to be present in the amount of NIH prolactin implanted (group 2), and with subcutaneous prolactin implants (group 3). Neither of the latter two treatments had any influence on the age of

TABLE VII

EFFECTS OF IMPLANTING HORMONES IN THE MEDIAN EMINENCE (ME) OR
SUBCUTANEOUSLY ON THE ONSET OF PUBERTY IN FEMALE RATS[a]

Group and treatment	No. of rats	Av. age at onset of puberty (days)
1. Prolactin implant in ME	18	31.6 ± 1.9^b
2. Prolactin impurities implant in ME	18	38.2 ± 2.1
3. Subcutaneous prolactin implant (same amount as in 1.)	7	39.1 ± 2.0

[a] After Clemens et al. (1969c).
[b] $P < 0.01$.

TABLE VIII

EFFECTS OF IMPLANTS IN THE MEDIAN EMINENCE ON ANTERIOR PITUITARY FSH
CONCENTRATION AND UTERINE WEIGHT[a]

Treatment	FSH concentration as $\mu g/mg$ gland	λ^c	Uterine weight (mg)
Cholesterol (11)[d]	50.6 (35.9–71.3)[d]	0.136	26.1 ± 2.1
Cholesterol + prolactin (13)	Undetectable		61.1 ± 4.8[b]

[a] After Voogt et al. (1969).
[b] $P < 0.002$.
[c] λ = Index of precision.
[d] ( ) = No. of rats. Mean and 95% confidence limit.

onset of puberty. Voogt et al. (1969) reported that implants of prolactin in the median eminence evoked a highly significant release of FSH (Table VIII). Rats were given median eminence implants of prolactin at 21 days of age and were killed on day 26. We believe that this increase in FSH and probably in LH secretion as a result of prolactin treatment (Voogt and Meites, 1971) is responsible for the advancement of puberty. Injections of prolactin beginning at 21 days of age also hastened the onset of puberty by 6–7 days.

Voogt and Meites (1971) demonstrated that an implant of prolactin in the median eminence of pseudopregnant rats approximately doubled the serum levels of LH and FSH (Table IX). These implants also produced follicular growth in the ovaries, stimulated uterine development, and induced atrophy of the mammary glands. Thus, it appears quite clear that inhibition of prolactin secretion results in increased LH and FSH secretion.

TABLE IX

EFFECT OF MEDIAN EMINENCE IMPLANTATION OF PROLACTIN IN PSEUDOPREGNANT
RATS ON SERUM LH AND FSH[a]

Treatment	No. of rats	LH conc. as ng/ml serum[b,c]	FSH conc. as ng/ml serum[d]
Cocoa butter	24	109.2 ± 5.2	199.4 ± 34.4
Prolactin	25	226 ± 31.9[e]	385.9 ± 62.7[f]

[a] After Voogt and Meites (1971).
[b] Mean ± SE.
[c] Reference preparation = NIAMD-LH-RP-1.
[d] Reference preparation = NIAMD-FSH-RP-1.
[e] $P < 0.005$.
[f] $P < 0.05$.

5. Mechanism of Action of Prolactin Implant
on Prolactin Secretion

The mechanism(s) of action of implants in the median eminence is not entirely clear at this time. It is probable that inhibition of prolactin secretion by prolactin implants is mediated by an increase in PIF secretion by the brain. Elevated hypothalamic PIF levels were noted by Chen et al. (1967) in rats with pituitary tumor transplants and by Clemens and Meites (1968) in normal cycling and in ovariectomized rats, although Voogt and Meites (1971) observed no change in PIF content after prolactin implantation in pseudopregnant rats.

Evidence that supports the hypothesis that prolactin inhibits its own secretion by acting on hypothalamic catecholamines was reported by Fuxe and Hokfelt (1971). They demonstrated that prolactin injections into rats markedly activated the tuberoinfundibular *dopaminergic* neurons. It appears therefore that prolactin acts via the hypothalamus to increase dopaminergic neuron activity, resulting in increased release of PIF into the portal vessels and inhibition of prolactin release. The increased dopaminergic activity probably also explains why prolactin is capable of stimulating LH and FSH secretion. Dopamine injections into the third ventricle of rats were observed to elevate LRF and FRF levels in the hypothalamopituitary portal circulation, and to increase LH and FSH in the blood (Kamberi et al., 1970).

D. Effects of Prolactin on Hypothalamic
Unitary Activity

It is well known that hormones can modify the electrical activity of the central nervous system. Changes in both single and multiple unit activity have been reported by several workers (Beyer et al., 1967; Komisaruk et al., 1967; Ramirez et al., 1967; Sawyer et al., 1968; Steiner et al., 1969; Terasawa et al., 1969). All these studies were performed in anesthetized animals, and none were concerned with prolactin.

Utilizing methods of recording single unit activity in conscious animals, Clemens et al. (1971b) observed the presence of prolactin responsive neurons in the rabbit hypothalamus. The term "responsive" is used in preference to "sensitive" since these neurons changed their firing rates after prolactin infusion, although they may be part of a projection field from some other locus in the brain which is sensitive to prolactin. Therefore, this study could not localize any pathways. However, it did reveal two different populations of neurons that responded to prolactin. One group demonstrated an increased firing rate after prolactin administration (50 μg of NIH ovine prolactin by intravenous cannula), and the other

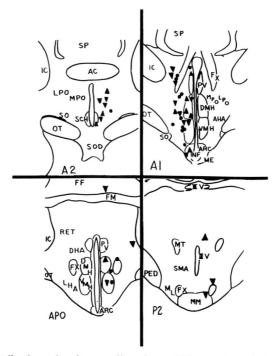

Fig. 12. Distribution of unit recording sites within the hypothalamus. Triangles with apices upward indicate increases; triangles with apices downward indicate decreases; and circles represent no change in firing rate after prolactin administration. Abbreviations: AC, anterior commissure; AHA, anterior hypothalamic area; A1, anterior 1.0 mm; A2, anterior 2.0 mm; APO, anterior posterior O; ARC, periventricular arcuate nucleus; DHA, dorsal hypothalamic area; DMH, dorsomedial hypothalamic nucleus; FF, fimbria of fornix; FM, foramen of Munro; FX, fornix; IC, internal capsule; INF, infundibulum; LHA, lateral hypothalamic area; ME, median eminence; ML, lateral mammillary nucleus; MM, medial mammillary nucleus; MPO, medial preoptic area; MT, mammillothalamic tract; OT, optic tract; P2, posterior 2.0 mm; PED, basic pedunculi; PV, paraventricular nucleus; RET, nucleus reticularis; SCH, supra chiasmatic nucleus; SMA, supra mammillary area; SO, supraoptic nucleus; SOD, diffuse supraoptic nucleus; SP, septum; VMH, ventromedial hypothalamic nucleus; IIIV, 3rd ventricle. After Clemens et al. (1971b).

group showed a decrease. As shown in Fig. 12, these neurons were rather diffuse in location. This seems to indicate that these locations are in the projection field of one or two central loci that are sensitive to prolactin feedback. In terms of PIF dynamics, it is possible that the population of neurons that showed increased firing rates after prolactin infusion were normally active in stimulating PIF release, and the ones showing decreases in firing rates diminished PIF release. Alternatively, it is possible that cells that decrease their firing rate are normally responsible for increasing release of a prolactin releasing factor (PRF). However, these hypotheses are quite speculative, and it remains to be determined whether alterations in hypothalamic neuronal firing rates following prolactin administration are characteristic of the "short loop" feedback system.

E. Possible Physiological Significance

The negative feedback of prolactin on its own secretion is probably a major mechanism for controlling prolactin secretion. Pituitary and blood levels of prolactin in animals generally are very low during most of pregnancy. It is possible that these low levels of pituitary prolactin secretion during pregnancy are due in part to the negative feedback exerted by placental lactogen on the hypothalamus. Preliminary results indicate that an implant of HPL in the median eminence of the rat decreases serum prolactin (Shaar and Meites, 1971). It also is possible that the fall after the initial abrupt rise in blood prolactin produced by the suckling stimulus or administration of certain drugs is due to the "short loop" feedback exerted by the initial high levels of circulating prolactin. This feedback of prolactin appears to be very powerful, since prolactin implants in the hypothalamus appear to counteract all the physiological processes dependent on prolactin in the rat. In contrast, inhibition of FSH, LH, TSH, and ACTH secretion appear to be regulated primarily by target organ hormone feedback. LH or FSH implants into the median eminence do not block ovulation or alter estrous cycles, and TSH and ACTH implants have not been shown to shut off thyroid and adrenal cortical functions. The physiological significance of the increase in release of LH and FSH produced by a prolactin implant in the median eminence is not clear at this time, but is yet another example of the reciprocal relationship between prolactin and gonadotropin secretion seen under many physiological conditions.

VI. Direct Effects of Some Hormones and Drugs on Prolactin Secretion

Some hormones and drugs can act directly on the anterior pituitary to increase or decrease pituitary prolactin secretion without the intervention of the hypothalamus. This has been demonstrated under *in vitro* conditions, where the anterior pituitary was cultured or incubated together with a hormone or drug in a physiological medium.

Early work by Desclin (1950) suggested that estrogen might be able to directly promote pituitary prolactin release, as indicated by persistent luteal activity and stimulation of mammary growth after injecting estrogen into hypophysectomized rats with a pituitary graft underneath the kidney capsule. Later, Chen *et al.* (1970) showed that injections of estradiol benzoate into hypophysectomized rats with a pituitary graft underneath the kidney capsule increased serum prolactin levels (see Fig. 4). However, in such an animal preparation, the possibility cannot be ruled out that part of the action of the estrogen was mediated via the hypothalamus, by decreasing hypothalamic release of PIF into the systemic circulation. More conclusive evidence that estrogen can directly stimulate the pituitary was provided by Nicoll and Meites (1962), who reported that incorporation of 0.5 µg of estradiol into the medium of organ cultures of rat anterior pituitary resulted in significant increases in prolactin release. Nicoll and Meites (1964) subsequently confirmed these observations, and showed that concentrations of 0.05 and 0.5 µg per milliliter of medium stimulated prolactin release, whereas a concentration of 2.0 µg/ml had no significant effect. This agrees with *in vivo* work showing that low or moderate doses of estrogen are more effective than high doses for increasing pituitary and serum prolactin levels in ovariectomized rats (Chen and Meites, 1970a). Since systemic administration of estrogen results in a reduction in hypothalamic PIF, it can be concluded that estrogen *in vivo* acts both by a direct action on the pituitary and via the hypothalamus to promote prolactin secretion. Progesterone, testosterone, cortisol, and corticosterone have no direct effect on pituitary prolactin release *in vitro* (Nicoll and Meites, 1964), but these steroids can produce small increments in prolactin secretion when administered *in vivo*, by reducing hypothalamic PIF levels.

Incorporation of 0.1 µg of thyroxine or triiodothyronine per milliliter of medium to an organ culture of rat anterior pituitary, significantly increased prolactin release (Nicoll and Meites, 1963), demonstrating a direct action of thyroid hormones on pituitary prolactin cells. Cohere *et al.* (1964) also reported that thyroxine and estrogen stimulated development of the endoplasmic reticulum of prolactin cells of rat pituitary tissue *in vitro*. There is considerable evidence that thyroidectomy decreases and that administration of thyroid hormones promote prolactin release *in vivo* (see Meites, 1966). *In vivo* injections of thyroxine into rats were found not to alter hypothalamic PIF activity, suggesting that the thyroid hormones stimulate prolactin secretion only by a direct action on the anterior pituitary.

In addition to estrogen and thyroid hormones, several drugs have been demonstrated to directly influence pituitary prolactin secretion. Incubation of several doses of ergocornine with rat anterior pituitary for a period of 12 hours, resulted in marked inhibition of prolactin release and accumulation of prolactin in the pituitary (Lu and Meites, 1971b). Ergocornine also prevented an increase in prolactin release when estradiol

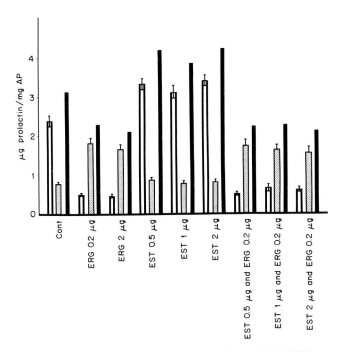

FIG. 13. Direct effects of ergocornine (ERG) and estradiol (EST) on release of prolactin by rat pituitary *in vitro*. Incubation period was 12 hours. Note that ERG inhibited release of prolactin in medium (□) and promoted accumulation of prolactin in pituitary (☒). EST increased release of prolactin, and ERG inhibited this action of EST. Total in medium and pit (■). After Lu *et al.* (1971).

was present in the incubation medium (Fig. 13). Injections of ergocornine into rats also partially or completely inhibited stimulation of prolactin release by estrogen and prevented enlargement of the pituitary. In addition to its direct action on the pituitary, ergocornine was shown to increase hypothalamic PIF activity in rats (Wuttke *et al.*, 1971a), indicating that it acts both via the hypothalamus and directly on the pituitary to depress prolactin secretion. It also is of interest that ergocornine has been reported to stimulate dopamine receptors in the median eminence (Hokfelt and Fuxe, 1971), which would result in an increase in PIF release. Because of the remarkable effects of ergot drugs on all parameters of prolactin functions, the effects of these drugs are dealt with more fully in Section VII.

Sodium pentobarbital has been shown to inhibit pituitary prolactin release when injected into rats (Wuttke and Meites, 1970b), and this was confirmed by Wakabayashi *et al.* (1971). For the first 30 minutes after injection of the drug, there was an increase in serum prolactin, but this was followed by a prolonged decrease in serum prolactin levels. In a subsequent publication, Wuttke *et al.* (1971b) presented evidence that the brief rise in serum prolactin was due to a reduction in hypothalamic PIF, and that the prolonged fall in serum prolactin was the result of a direct action of the drug on the pituitary. The latter was demonstrated by incubating rat anterior pituitary tissue with a small amount of sodium pentobarbital and observing inhibition of prolactin release. Thus sodium pentobarbital appears to decrease hypothalamic PIF activity and to inhibit pituitary prolactin release directly. Upon injection the direct inhibitory effect of the drug on prolactin release appears to predominate after a brief stimulatory action.

The possible direct effects of other hormones and drugs on prolactin release remain to be evaluated. Mention already has been made that relatively large doses of catecholamines have been reported to inhibit rat pituitary prolactin release *in vitro* directly (MacLeod, 1969; Birge *et al.*, 1970), but smaller doses were shown to stimulate prolactin release *in vitro* (Koch *et al.*, 1970). It is doubtful that these direct effects of the catecholamines are of physiological significance. Vasopressin, oxytocin, insulin, and bradykinin apparently have no direct effect on pituitary prolactin release *in vitro* (Meites *et al.*, 1963). The direct stimulatory effects of synthetic TRH reported on release of prolactin by rat pituitary tumor cells require further study (Tashjian *et al.*, 1971). As indicated elsewhere, our laboratory has not been able to observe increased prolactin release when synthetic TRH was added to an incubation system containing pituitary halves from normal rats or slices of tissue from rat pituitary tumors (Lu *et al.*, 1972). The *in vivo* release of prolactin in human subjects given synthetic TRH (Jacobs *et al.*, 1971) may be mediated by some indirect mechanism.

VII. Effects of Ergot Derivatives on Prolactin Secretion

A. Structural Types That Inhibit Prolactin

Early reports by Nordskog (1946) and Nordskog and Clark (1945) indicated that animals fed ergotoxin demonstrated reproductive failure and agalactia. Later, Tindal (1956) reported that ergotamine inhibited lactation and attributed this effect to the general toxicity of the compound. Ergotoxin was shown to be composed of 3 peptide-containing ergot alkaloids: ergocornine, ergocryptine, and ergocristine. Recently these compounds have been shown to be potent prolactin inhibitors (Nagasawa and Meites, 1970; Wuttke *et al.*, 1971a; Lu *et al.*, 1971).

We have performed extensive studies on the structural relations of ergot derivatives to their ability to inhibit prolactin secretion (Clemens

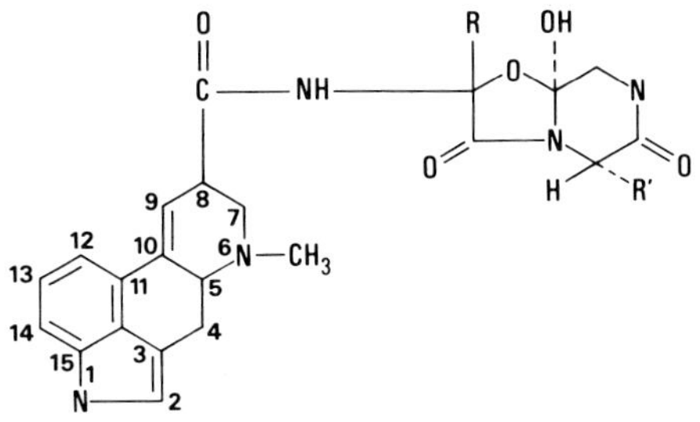

R = CH(CH$_3$)$_2$ CH(CH$_3$)$_2$ CH(CH$_3$)$_2$ CH$_3$

R' = CH(CH$_3$)$_2$ CH$_2$–C$_6$H$_5$ CH$_2$–CH(CH$_3$)$_2$ CH$_2$–C$_6$H$_5$

ERGOCORNINE   ERGOCRISTINE   ERGOCRYPTINE   ERGOTAMINE

FIG. 14. Generalized structure for the peptide-containing ergot alkaloid molecule. Note that the differences between the 4 compounds listed reside in R and R'.

et al., 1971c). Ergocornine, ergocryptine, and ergocristine inhibited prolactin secretion to the same degree, while ergotamine was not nearly as effective. The structures of these compounds are shown in Fig. 14.

In our studies a total dose of 10 μg of each of the ergot derivatives was administered to male rats by intraperitoneal injection. Serum prolactin levels were measured by radioimmunoassay 1 hour later. Table X shows serum prolactin levels from rats treated with these derivatives. Interestingly, ergotamine was not as potent as any of the ergotoxin constituents, whereas ergocorninine, a simple isomer of ergocornine, was inactive. It appears from these results that the configuration of the peptide side chain may be important for the prolactin-inhibiting activity

TABLE X

EFFECTS OF VARIOUS PEPTIDE-CONTAINING ERGOT ALKALOIDS ON
PROLACTIN SECRETION IN MALE RATS[a]

Treatment	No. of rats	Serum prolactin levels ng/ml[b]
Controls, 10% ethanol vehicle	10	31.4 ± 3.4
Ergocornine	10	5.9 ± 0.3 ($P < 0.001$)[c]
Ergocorninine	10	29.5 ± 2.9 NS
Dihydroergocornine	10	11.3 ± 1.0 ($P < 0.001$)
Ergocryptine	10	8.5 ± 0.4 ($P < 0.001$)
Dihydroergocryptine	10	5.6 ± 0.5 ($P < 0.001$)
Ergotamine	10	17.5 ± 0.9 ($P < 0.05$)
Ergocristine	10	6.8 ± 0.5 ($P < 0.001$)

[a] Clemens *et al.* (1971c).
[b] Expressed as NIAMD prolactin RP-1.
[c] Probability using Student's *t* test, treated vs. control. NS = not significant.

TABLE XI
Effects of Simple Ergot Derivatives on Prolactin Secretion

Structure	Name	R	R'	% Inhibition of prolactin
(I) – (III)	(I) Lysergic acid	H	C—OH	0
	(II) dl-N-(9,10-Didehydro-6-methyl-8α-ergolinyl) formamide	H	NHC—H	76
	(III) N-dl-$trans$-(2-Hydroxycyclopentyl)-d-lysergic acid amide	H	(2-hydroxycyclopentyl amide)	58
(IV) – (VI)	(IV) Agroclavine	H	CH₃	45
	(V) 8,9-Didehydro-6,8-dimethylergoline propionitrile	CN—(CH₂)₂—	CH₃	0
	(VI) Elymoclavine	H	CH₂OH	71
(VII), (VIII)	(VII) 6-Methyl-8β-ergolineacetonitrile	H	CH₂CN	86
	(VIII) 8β-(Chloromethyl)-6-methylergoline	H	CH₂Cl	45

of the compounds. Synthesis of peptides similar to the ergocornine side chain revealed that the complex peptide side chain itself could not inhibit prolactin and probably does not resemble PIF.

Examination of simpler ergot derivatives revealed that compounds as simple as agroclavine, with only a methyl group as a side chain at position 8, possessed prolactin inhibiting activity. Interestingly, lysergic acid was unable to inhibit prolactin, demonstrating that something other than a carboxyl group had to be present as a side chain. On the other hand, lysergic acid diethylamide (LSD) is a potent inhibitor of prolactin (Quadri and Meites, 1971a). Table XI shows a number of simple ergot derivatives that have prolactin inhibiting activity.

Apparently a compound can have many different substituents at R' and retain prolactin-inhibiting activity. If substituents (R) are added to the indole nitrogen, the derivative is not active. In addition, 9–10 dihydrogenated compounds also can inhibit prolactin secretion. Thus, it appears that there are several different structural types of ergot derivatives that are capable of inhibiting prolactin secretion.

B. EFFECTS ON PITUITARY SIZE

Ergocornine has been shown to decrease pituitary weight in rats. It is especially effective in counteracting the increase in pituitary weight in overiectomized rats treated with estradiol (Lu et al., 1971). A simpler ergot derivative, 6-methyl-8β-ergolineacetonitrile, also is capable of causing a marked reduction in pituitary weight (Table XII).

The decrease in pituitary weight and serum prolactin levels indicates that some ergot derivatives have the ability to decrease the number of prolactin cells in the pituitary. This has been demonstrated in a recent study on the effects of ergot drugs on pituitary tumor growth (Quadri

TABLE XII

EFFECTS OF 6-METHYL-8β-ERGOLINEACETONITRILE ON SERUM PROLACTIN LEVELS AND PITUITARY WEIGHT

Treatment	No. of rats	Average pituitary weight (gm)	Serum prolactin levels ng/ml[a]
Control, corn oil	4	6.0 ± 0.4	29.1 ± 1.8
6-Methyl-8β-ergolineacetonitrile, 0.6 mg	4	4.6 ± 0.2^b	5.4 ± 0.3^c

[a] Expressed as nanograms of NIAMD-rat prolactin RP-1 per milliliter.
[b] $P < 0.05$.
[c] $P < 0.001$.

et al., 1972). The pituitary tumor cells were greatly decreased in number, and many of the cells that remained were enlarged and cornified.

C. EFFECTS ON MAMMARY TUMORS AND LACTATION

The ability of ergot drugs to inhibit prolactin makes them of particular interest in the treatment of mammary tumors. Studies have shown that treatments that increase prolactin secretion result in enhanced tumor growth (Clemens *et al.*, 1968; Welsch *et al.*, 1969; Welsch and Meites, 1969) whereas ergot derivatives decrease prolactin secretion and result in decreased tumor growth (Nagasawa and Meites, 1970; Cassell *et al.*, 1971; Heuson *et al.*, 1970; Stahelin *et al.*, 1971). Yanai and Nagasawa (1971) reported that ergocryptine suppressed the growth of hyperplastic alveolar nodules in mice, and Singh *et al.* (1972) observed that ergocornine decreased growth of a transplanted mammary tumor in BALB female mice. The effects of injecting ergocornine and ergocryptine for 4 weeks into rats with DMBA-induced mammary tumors are shown in Fig. 15. Ergot drugs also appear to be able to prevent the induction of mammary tumors by DMBA (Clemens and Shaar, 1972). Table XIII shows that ergocornine treatment for 11 days before and 5 days after DMBA treatment significantly inhibited tumor induction. These results suggest that breast cancer in women may be diminished by prophylactic

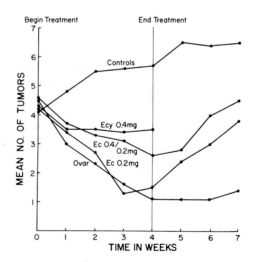

FIG. 15. Inhibition of growth in number of DMBA-induced mammary tumors by ergocornine (Ec) and ergocryptine (Ecy). Note resumption of tumor growth after cessation of Ec treatment at the end of 4 weeks. Ovar = ovariectomized. From Cassell *et al.* (1971).

TABLE XIII
EFFECT OF INITIAL TREATMENT WITH ERGOCORNINE SALTS ON DEVELOPMENT
OF DMBA-INDUCED MAMMARY TUMORS IN RATS

Group and treatment	No. of rats	No. of rats with tumors[b]	Total No. of tumors	Mean latency period (days)
1. Controls, corn oil	20	10	12	56.2 ± 4.0
2. Ergocornine methansulfate, 0.4 mg	19	2	2	56.0
3. Ergocornine hydrogenmaleate, 0.4 mg	19	1	1	63.0

[a] From Clemens and Shaar (1972).
[b] Five months after DMBA treatment.

treatment with nontoxic prolactin inhibitors, provided, of course, that prolactin is important for breast cancer development in women.

Clemens and Shaar (1972) have shown that a variety of ergot compounds are capable of inhibiting lactation. Table XIV shows the effects of a number of these agents on lactational performance of female rats as assessed by litter weight gains. Most of the ergot alkaloids markedly suppressed lactation as indicated by loss of litter weight when compared to the litters of the control group. The treated lactating mother rats lost weight, but in most cases the loss was less than 5% of body weight. The ergonovine-treated animals also lost weight, but the litters gained weight, indicating no direct relationship between weight loss of the lactating female and lactational performance in this study. All treated rats exhibited lowered serum prolactin levels. Much of the body weight loss can be accounted for by reduced weight of the mammary glands (Table XV). Lutterbeck et al. (1971) recently reported that 2-Br-ergocryptine treatment terminated galactorrhea in human subjects. Their study provides indirect evidence that ergot alkaloids can inhibit prolactin secretion in humans.

D. MECHANISMS OF ACTION

The first study demonstrating a possible mechanism of action was that of Wuttke et al. (1971a), who reported that ergot drugs can act on the hypothalamus to increase PIF activity. It was also shown by Lu and Meites (1971b) and Malven and Hoge (1971) that ergocornine can act directly on the pituitary to inhibit prolactin release. The above findings were confirmed recently by Clemens and Shaar (1972). Table XVI shows the effects of ergocornine on prolactin secretion in rats with 2 pituitary

TABLE XIV

EFFECTS OF VARIOUS ERGOT ALKALOIDS ON MATERNAL BODY WEIGHT, LITTER
WEIGHT AND SERUM PROLACTIN LEVELS OF
POSTPARTUM LACTATING FEMALE RATS

Treatment groups	No. of animals	Mean net body wt. gain (gm)	Mean net litter wt. gain (gm)	Mean serum prolactin levels (ng/ml)
I. Control—corn oil, 0.1 mg/day	16	$+12.7 \pm 1.8$	$+50.3 \pm 2.5^a$	56.3 ± 6.9
II. Ergocornine hydrogenmalienate, 0.5 mg	8	-3.8 ± 2.7^b	-2.3 ± 8.0^b	11.6 ± 2.6^b
III. Ergocornine hydrogenmalienate, 1.0 mg	8	-13.4 ± 4.2^b	-9.2 ± 3.3^b	12.4 ± 2.6^b
IV. Ergonovine maleate, 4.0 mg	8	-4.8 ± 4.1^b	$\pm 20.8 \pm 4.3^b$	15.3 ± 1.7^b
V. Dihydroergocornine, 1.0 mg	8	-6.0 ± 2.5^b	-4.0 ± 7.3^b	12.9 ± 3.1^b
VI. Ergotamine tartrate, 4.0 mg	9	-9.1 ± 4.7^b	-4.7 ± 6.9^b	28.4 ± 8.3^c
VII. Ergocryptine, 0.5 mg	6	-22.8 ± 4.5^b	-10.7 ± 4.9^b	13.2 ± 7.3^b

^{a} Mean $\pm$ SE.
^{b} Significantly different from control value ($P < 0.001$).
^{c} Significantly different from control value ($P < 0.02$).

homografts beneath the kidney capsule. Ergocornine treatment (2.5 mg/ kg for 2 days) reduced the prolactin levels to values usually found in hypophysectomized rats. The low levels of prolactin found in hypophysectomized rats apparently are due to nonspecific binding with serum proteins. Lu and Meites (1971b) suggested that release of prolactin was prevented by ergocornine, since the pituitary showed accumulation of prolactin. Electron micrographs of pituitaries of rats treated with ergot derivatives showed an increase in prolactin granules (Figs. 16 and 17). Thus, ergot alkaloids may act by preventing prolactin release from the granules contained in prolactin-secreting cells (Smith and Clemens, 1972).

VIII. EFFECTS OF BRAIN STIMULATION AND STEROID
ENVIRONMENT ON PROLACTIN RELEASE

Quinn and Everett (1967) produced delayed pseudopregnancy in rats by electrical stimulation of the dorsomedial–ventromedial hypothalamus.

TABLE XV

Effect of Ergocornine Hydrogenmalienate on Mammary Gland Weight

Treatment group	No. of animals	Mean body wt. gain (gm)	Mean litter wt. gain (gm)	Mean serum prolactin levels (ng/ml)	Mean mammary tissue wt. (gm)
I. Corn oil (control), 0.1 ml/day	6	$+3.0 \pm 0.8$	$+45.6 \pm 4.5$	43.2 ± 12.5^a	12.8 ± 0.7
II. Ergocornine hydrogenmalienate, 0.5 mg	6	-13.2 ± 2.0	-18.2 ± 7.4	4.9 ± 0.3^b	4.9 ± 0.4^c

[a] Mean $\pm$ SE.
[b] Significantly different from control value ($P < 0.02$).
[c] Significantly different from control value ($P < 0.001$).

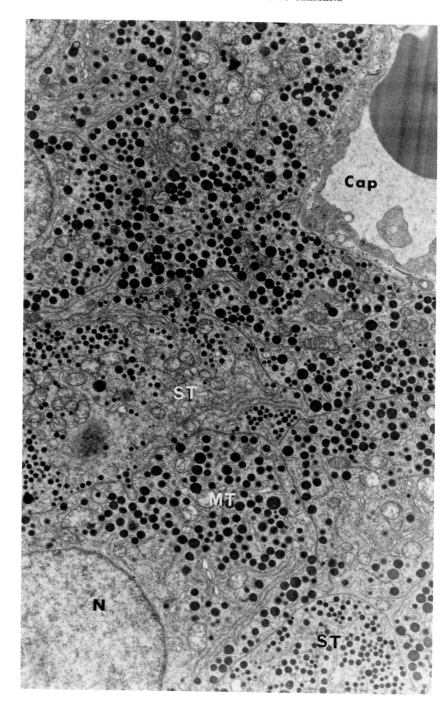

TABLE XVI

EFFECTS OF ERGOCORNINE HYDROGENMALIENATE ON HYPOPHYSECTOMIZED FEMALE
RATS WITH PITUITARY HOMOGRAFTS BENEATH THE KIDNEY CAPSULE[a]

Treatment group[a]	No. of animals	Mean serum prolactin levels (ng/ml)
I. Control, hypox + 2 AP transplants + 0.1 ml corn oil/day	10	54.2 ± 5.0[c]
II. Hypox + 2 AP transplants + 0.5 mg ergocornine hydrogenmalienate/day	9	7.3 ± 0.4[d]
III. Hypox alone + 0.1 ml corn oil/day	10	8.7 ± 0.5[e]

[a] From Clemens and Shaar (1972).
[b] Hypox = hypophysectomy; AP = anterior pituitary.
[c] Mean ± SE.
[d] Significantly different from control value ($P < 0.001$).
[e] Significantly different from value of group II ($P < 0.05$).

The stimulus presumably activated a PIF-inhibiting mechanism. Clemens
et al. (1971a) reported that electrochemical stimulation of the medial
basal hypothalamus in urethan-anesthetized rats resulted in increased
blood prolactin levels. They also showed that electrochemical stimulation
of the preoptic area caused a small, but significant decrease in blood
prolactin levels (Table XVII).

Tindal and Knaggs (1969) attempted to trace the ascending pathways
in the brain responsible for prolactin release. The lactogenic response
of the mammary glands were rated and used as an index of prolactin
release. In their study, monopolar electrodes were bilaterally implanted
into the brain, and the stimulating current was passed between the electrodes. They reported that in the midbrain the prolactin release path
lies in the lateral tegmentum. These conclusions hardly seem warranted
in view of the stimulation technique used. Since current was passed between the two electrodes, all the neurons between the two electrodes
were subjected to the stimulation current. Therefore, the pathway could
be medial rather than lateral. The pathway appears to be located

FIG. 16. A group of six mammotrophic cells (MT) and two somatotrophs (ST)
from the anterior pituitary of an adult female rat given 0.6 mg of ergocornine daily
for 10 days. These cells contain a massive number of mature ovoid secretion granules,
600–800 mμ in size. MT cells in a control estrous or lactating rat usually contain a
limited number of mature secretion granules. × 10,000. See Smith and Farquhar
(1966).

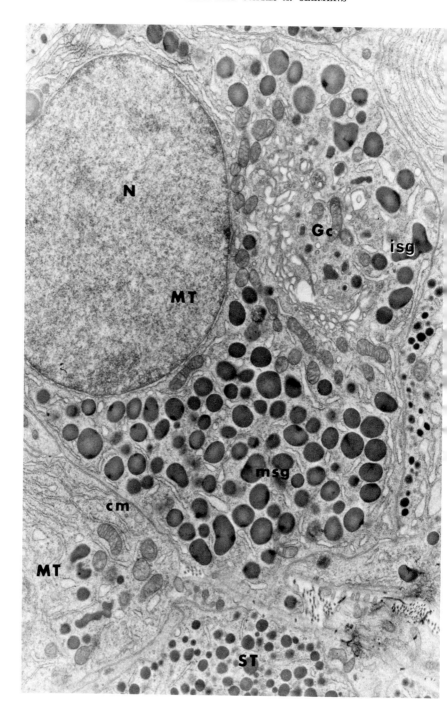

TABLE XVII

EFFECTS IN RATS OF ELECTROCHEMICAL STIMULATION OF THE PREOPTIC AREA
(POA) AND MEDIAL BASAL HYPOTHALAMUS (MBH)
ON PLASMA PROLACTIN LEVELS[a]

Area stimulated and hormone	Control level (ng/ml)[c]	0.5-Hour level (ng/ml)
MBH prolactin (7)[d]	6.92 ± 0.6[b]	21.7 ± 3.1 $(P < 0.001)$
POA prolactin (23)	9.6 ± 1.4	6.2 ± 0.6 $(P < 0.01)$

[a] After Clemens et al. (1971a).
[b] Mean ± SE.
[c] Expressed as nanograms of NIAMD prolactin RP-1 per milliliter.
[d] ( ) = Number of rats.

medially at the level of the posterior hypothalamus. In a subsequent study, Tindal and Knaggs (1970) reported that the prolactin release pathway ascended through the lateral hypothalamus and appeared to be associated with orbitofrontal cortex projections to the medial preoptic area. The exact sequence of pathways that the suckling induced stimulus for prolactin release takes between these forebrain structures is not clear at this time.

The proper steroid environment appears to be needed for prolactin release in response to certain stimuli. Clemens et al. (1971b) found that electrochemical stimulation of the median eminence–arcuate area was unable to cause prolactin release when placed 10 days after ovariectomy or in ovariectomized rats treated with 4 mg of progesterone. Both the surgical stress of sham stimulation and electrical stimulation of this area induced prolactin release in ovariectomized rats treated with 2 μg of estradiol benzoate. In animals treated with 2 μg of estradiol benzoate and 4 mg of progesterone, sham stimulation was ineffective whereas true

FIG. 17. A representative mammotroph from an ergocornine-treated rat. These cells show the typical morphological features of a functioning cell, producing and packaging hormone into secretion granules for discharge. There is sufficient rough endoplasmic reticulum (ER) to suggest some synthesis. A medial cut through the Golgi complex (Gc) shows the presence of filling images, immature secretion granules (isg), and mature secretion granules (msg). There is no evidence of granule discharge or exocytosis. Of further significance is the absence of autophagic structures and a limited number of multivesicular and dense-body-type lysosomes. The massive numbers of secretion granules contained suggest an impedence of secretion granule discharge from the cell. × 15,000. See Smith (1969); and Farquhar (1971).

TABLE XVIII

EFFECTS OF ELECTROCHEMICAL STIMULATION OF THE MEDIAN EMINENCE–ARCUATE
COMPLEX AND SHAM STIMULATION ON PROLACTIN RELEASE IN
STERIOD-TREATED OVARIECTOMIZED RATS[a]

Group and treatment	No. of rats	Prestimulation prolactin level (ng/ml)[d]	0.5-Hr poststimulation prolactin level (ng/ml)[d]
1. Corn oil + stimulation	8	7.5 ± 1.9	8.3 ± 2.0
Corn oil + sham stimulation	7	4.1 ± 0.4	4.2 ± 2.0
2. 2 μg EB[b] + stimulation	13	20.0 ± 3.8	39.4 ± 6.9[e]
2 μg EB + sham stimulation	14	19.9 ± 1.9	35.6 ± 6.1[e]
3. 4 mg PROG[c] + stimulation	10	6.0 ± 1.4	4.2 ± 0.4
4 mg PROG + sham stimulation	10	7.0 ± 2.3	5.2 ± 0.3
4. 2 μg EB + 4 mg PROG + stimulation	15	23.2 ± 3.1	71.6 ± 11.1[f]
2 μg EB + 4 mg PROG + sham stimulation	13	27.2 ± 4.5	28.7 ± 7.4

[a] From Clemens et al. (1971b).
[b] EB = estradiol benzoate.
[c] PROG = progesterone.
[d] Expressed as nanograms of NIAMD prolactin RP-1 per milliliter of serum.
[e] $P < 0.05$.
[f] $P < 0.001$, vs. prestimulation levels using Student's t test.

stimulation caused a highly significant release of prolactin. These results are shown in Table XVIII. It appears that estradiol benzoate lowered the threshold for neurons that respond to stressful stimuli, and also lowered thresholds of neurons that inhibit PIF secreting neurons. Progesterone probably raised the threshold for excitation of neurons in the CNS which are capable of eliciting prolactin release in response to stress. It also is possible that estrogen acts directly on the pituitary to amplify the effects of small changes in hypothalamic inhibiting and/or releasing factor secretion.

Wuttke and Meites (1970a) observed that electrochemical stimulation of the medial preoptic area in old constant estrous rats resulted in significant increases in serum concentration of prolactin and LH, and subsequent ovulation, whereas similar stimulation in old pseudopregnant rats produced only a small increase in serum prolactin and no rise in serum LH or ovulation. Thus an estrogen environment in the medial preoptic area favored the release of prolactin and LH in response to electrochemical stimulation, whereas a predominantly progestin environᴍent inhibited the release of the 2 hormones in response to the same stimulus.

IX. Metabolic Clearance Rate, Secretion Rate, and Half-Life of Prolactin in the Rat

Although hormone secretion by the anterior pituitary is governed by the hypothalamus and by agents that may act directly on the pituitary, the metabolic fate of prolactin after its release into the blood at least partially determines its effects on tissues it stimulates. Are pituitary hormone levels in the blood indicative of secretion rate from the pituitary or do they also reflect metabolic clearance rate? Recently Koch *et al.* (1971) determined the metabolic clearance rate, secretion rate, and half-life of prolactin in rats.

A single intravenous injection or continuous intravenous infusion of rat prolactin [131]I (H-10-10-B) was given to anesthetized (sodium pentobarbital) intact male rats and to ovariectomized, hypophysectomized, or intact female rats. The highly purified rat prolactin was labeled with ^{131}I by a standard method for radioimmunoassay (Niswender *et al.*, 1969). Blood samples were obtained at frequent intervals and the serum was measured for immunoprecipitable prolactin and for total radioactivity. The disappearance curve after a single intravenous injection of prolactin in a rat pituitary homogenate (Fig. 18), as measured by radioimmunoassay, was the same as that of ^{131}I-labeled rat prolactin, indicating that the latter was cleared from the blood in an identical manner

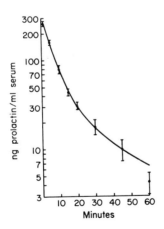

Fig. 18. Disappearance curve from serum of male rats after a single intravenous injection of 3.98 μg rat pituitary (mean and standard error from 7 rats). Note multiexponential curve. From Koch *et al.* (1971).

TABLE XIX
METABOLIC CLEARANCE RATE (MCR) AND HALF-LIFE TIME OF PROLACTIN[a]

Treatment	No. of rats	MCR (ml/min)	Half-life time (minutes)
Males, prolactin by constant infusion	6	1.3 ± 0.1[b]	—
Males, prolactin by single injection	6	1.3 ± 0.2	5.2 ± 0.6
Males, AP extract single injection	7	1.5 ± 0.1	5.8 ± 0.3
Females in estrus	6	1.3 ± 0.1	3.9 ± 0.3
Females, ovariectomized	6	1.3 ± 0.2	5.0 ± 0.6
Females, hypophysectomized	10	1.2 ± 0.0	5.2 ± 0.4

[a] After Koch et al. (1971).
[b] Mean ± SE.

to that of the endogenous hormone. Note that the disappearance curve shows the characteristics of multiexponential components.

The metabolic clearance rate (MCR), defined as the volume of blood cleared of prolactin per unit time, was 1.26 ± 0.08 ml/minute by the constant infusion method and 1.2–1.46 ml/minute by the single injection method, or an average of 1.32 ml/minute (Table XIX). The disappearance curves of the immunoprecipitable rat prolactin-^{131}I, plotted on semilogarithmic coordinates, showed the characteristics of multiexponential curves (Fig. 19). This suggests that prolactin is distributed in more than one compartment. Male rats showed similar disappearance curves. The half-life for the first exponential (first 10 minutes after injection) ranged between 3.95 and 5.76 minutes. Total serum radioactivity curves were completely different from immunoprecipitable radioactivity, reflecting the presence of free ^{131}I and nonprolactin bound radioactivity.

The secretion rate for rat prolactin (MCR × serum prolactin concentration) was found to be highest on the evening of proestrus, next highest on the evening of estrus, and about twice as high in the evening as in the morning of diestrus and metestrus. Ovariectomized females and intact male rats showed similar patterns (see Table I).

These data show that the MCR of rat prolactin is relatively constant under many physiological states, in agreement with previous reports on the MCR for LH (Kohler et al., 1968) and FSH (Coble et al., 1969) in man. Apparently the agents in the blood and tissues that metabolize prolactin are relatively constant under the conditions of these experiments. This may not necessarily be true under other physiological states.

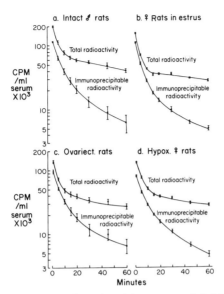

Fig. 19. Disappearance curves of total and immunoprecipitable radioactivity from serum after a single injection of prolactin-^{131}I. After Koch *et al.* (1971).

These results suggest that serum prolactin values in rats accurately reflect the secretion rate of prolactin by the pituitary during these states. The observation that the half-life of rat prolactin is only about 5 minutes differs from the reports of Grosvenor (1967), Gay *et al.* (1970), and Watson *et al.* (1971), who reported a half-life for rat prolactin of about 10 minutes. However, these workers all *assumed* that the disappearance curve of prolactin represented a single component rather than the multiple-component curves demonstrated here. More recently, Gay (1971) confirmed that the half-life time for rat prolactin was about 5 minutes.

X. Summary and Conclusions

Hypothalamic inhibition of prolactin appears to be well established in most mammalian species studied thus far, including humans. Interference with hypothalamic pathways to the anterior pituitary by appropriate hypothalamic lesions, stalk section, pituitary transplantation or by administration of certain drugs, result in augmented prolactin release. A hypothalamic PIF acts directly on the anterior pituitary to inhibit prolactin release. The particular hypothalamic neurons involved in PIF secretion and the chemistry of PIF and its mode of action on the anterior pituitary remain to be elucidated.

PIF release from the median eminence is at least partially under the regulation of biogenic amines. An increase in hypothalamic catecholamines results in increased PIF release and reduced blood prolactin levels, whereas a decrease in catecholamines results in decreased PIF release and elevated blood prolactin values. Dopamine probably is the principal catecholamine involved in this mechanism, whereas norepinephrine actually may promote prolactin release. Serotonin has been reported to increase prolactin release when injected into the third ventricle (Kamberi et al., 1971), and Lu and Meites (1971a) observed that injections of tryptophan and 5-hydroxytryptophan, both precursors of serotonin, also stimulated prolactin release. It must be emphasized that the role of specific biogenic amines on release of prolactin cannot be assessed conclusively at this time, since few of the drugs used are specific in their actions. However, there can be little doubt about the importance of biogenic amines in controlling release of prolactin and probably other pituitary hormones.

The presence of a PRF in the mammalian hypothalamus has not yet been definitely established. The ability of synthetic TRH to increase blood prolactin in human subjects (Jacobs et al., 1971; Friesen et al., 1972) and in cows (Convey, 1972) does not prove that TRH is PRF or similar to PRF, or that it acts directly on the pituitary. Convey found that TRH has no effect on release of prolactin when incubated in vitro with slices of bovine anterior pituitary, whereas LRH produced significant increases in release of LH. TRH has not been observed to increase prolactin release when a single injection is given to rats, although multi-injections for a period of 6 days increased pituitary prolactin in intact but not in thyroidectomized rats (Lu and Meites, 1971a). The latter suggests that the systemic action of TSH in promoting prolactin release may be partially mediated through the TSH-thyroid system or through other mechanisms. Claims for the existence of PRF activity in hypothalamic extracts from rats or swine require confirmation. In avian species, the presence of PRF activity in the hypothalamus appears to be well established, although the possible presence of a PIF cannot be ruled out. It is not clear why the predominant influence of the hypothalamus on prolactin secretion is inhibitory in mammals and stimulatory in birds, but prolactin may have fewer functions in mammalian than in avian species and hence may not need to be released as often as in birds.

The physiological importance of circulating prolactin in controlling secretion of pituitary prolactin remains to be elucidated. The inhibitory action of prolactin on its own secretion by the pituitary appears to be exerted via hypothalamic mechanisms, by increasing dopaminergic and

PIF activities. Although all anterior pituitary hormones have been reported to be capable of inhibiting release of their respective hormones, only implants of prolactin in the median eminence have been observed to inhibit all the major actions of prolactin in the rat. GH, like prolactin, also has no target tissues that produces hormones to inhibit pituitary GH secretion. GH injections into monkeys (Sakuma and Knobil, 1970) and implants of GH in the median eminence of rats (Katz et al., 1969; Voogt et al., 1971) decreased pituitary GH levels. The latter investigators also found a decrease in hypothalamic GHRF activity after implanting GH in the median eminence, suggesting that this is the mechanism by which GH decreases pituitary GH release. The high levels of blood prolactin found in patients with galactorrhea or of GH in patients with acromegaly suggests that elevated circulating levels of these two

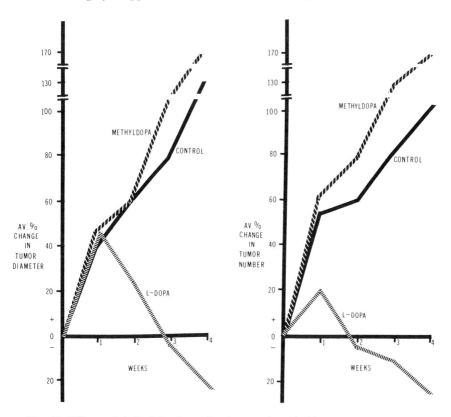

Fig. 20. Effects of daily injections of L-dopa and methyldopa on average percent change in tumor diameter (left) and average percent change in tumor number (right). Note decrease in both parameters beginning 1 week after an increased dose of L-dopa was given (after Quadri and Meites, 1971b).

hormones may not be capable of inhibiting pituitary secretion under all conditions.

The ability of many drugs to either increase or depress prolactin release suggests a useful approach for controlling the secretion and functions of prolactin in the organism. Thus ergocornine (Wuttke and Meites, 1971) and iproniazid (Gelato and Meites, 1971) have been used to demonstrate that the role of prolactin during the estrous cycle of the rat is to induce luteolysis of the old crop of corpora lutea during each cycle. Similar observations recently were made in the mouse by use of ergocornine (Grandison and Meites, unpublished observations). Ergot drugs, L-dopa, iproniazid, LSD, and pargyline were found to inhibit growth of mammary tumors in rats, whereas methyldopa, reserpine, and haloperidol increased growth of these tumors, providing evidence of the importance of prolactin for growth of these tumors (see Meites et al., 1972). The effects of L-dopa and methyldopa on growth of carcinogen-induced mammary tumors in rats are shown in Fig. 20. Ergot drugs also inhibited growth of pituitary tumors in rats (Quadri et al., 1972). L-dopa (Turkington, 1971) and 2-Br-α-ergocryptine (Lutterbeck et al., 1971) successfully inhibited galactorrhea in human subjects. It is possible therefore, that some drugs can be utilized for treating certain types of breast and pituitary tumors in human patients. Drugs may provide the same possibilities for regulating the secretion and functions of other pituitary hormones.

ACKNOWLEDGMENTS

Work from the laboratory of J. Meites was aided by NIH grants AM-04784 and CA-10771, The Michigan Agricultural Experiment Station, and a grant from the Eli Lilly Company.

REFERENCES

Amenomori, Y., and Meites, J. (1970). Proc. Soc. Exp. Biol. Med. 134, 492.
Amenomori, Y., Chen, C. L., and Meites, J. (1970). Endocrinology 86, 506.
Anden, N. E., Butcher, S. G., Carrodi, H., Fuxe, K., and Ungerstedt, U. (1970). Eur. J. Pharmacol. 11, 303.
Averill, R. L. W. (1969). Neuroendocrinology 5, 121.
Benson, G. K., and Folley, S. J. (1956). Nature (London) 117, 700.
Bern, H. A., and Nicoll, C. S. (1968). Recent Progr. Horm. Res. 24, 681.
Beyer, C., Ramirez, V. D., Whitmoyer, D. I., and Sawyer, C. H. (1967). Exp. Neurol. 18, 313.
Birge, C. A., Jacobs, L. S., Hammer, C. T., and Daughaday, W. H. (1970). Endocrinology 86, 120.
Boot, L. M. (1969). "Induction by Prolactin of Mammary Tumors in Mice." North-Holland Publ., Amsterdam.
Brodie, B. B., Spector, S., and Shore, P. A. (1959). Pharmacol. Rev. 11, 548.
Bryant, G. D., and Greenwood, F. C. (1968). Biochem. J. 109, 831.
Bryant, G. D., and Greenwood, F. C. (1972). In "Lactogenic Hormones" (G. E. W. Wolstenholme and J. Knight, eds.), p. 197. Livingstone, London.

Carlsson, A., and Lindquist, M. (1963). *Acta Pharmacol. Toxicol.* **20**, 140.

Carlsson, A., Dahlstrom, A., Fuxe, K., and Hillarp, N. A. (1965). *Acta Pharmacol. Toxicol.* **22**, 270.

Cassell, E. E., Meites, J., and Welsch, C. W. (1971). *Cancer Res.* **31**, 1051.

Chen, C. L., and Meites, J. (1969). *Proc. Soc. Exp. Biol. Med.* **131**, 576.

Chen, C. L., and Meites, J. (1970a). *Endocrinology* **86**, 503.

Chen, C. L., and Meites, J. (1970b). Unpublished data.

Chen, C. L., Minaguchi, H., and Meites, J. (1967). *Proc. Soc. Exp. Biol. Med.* **126**, 317.

Chen, C. L., Voogt, J. L., and Meites, J. (1968). *Endocrinology* **83**, 1273.

Chen, C. L., Amenomori, Y., Lu, K. H., Voogt, J. L., and Meites, J. (1970). *Neuroendocrinology* **6**, 220.

Clark, R. H., and Baker, B. L. (1964). *Science* **143**, 375.

Clark, R. H., and Meites, J. (1971). Unpublished data.

Clemens, J. A., and Meites, J. (1968). *Endocrinology* **82**, 878.

Clemens, J. A., and Meites, J. (1971). *Neuroendocrinology* **7**, 249.

Clemens, J. A., and Shaar, C. J. (1972). *Endocrinology* **89** (in press).

Clemens, J. A., Welsch, C. W., and Meites, J. (1968). *Proc. Soc. Exp. Biol. Med.* **127**, 969.

Clemens, J. A., Sar, M., and Meites, J. (1969a). *Proc. Soc. Exp. Biol. Med.* **130**, 628.

Clemens, J. A., Sar, M., and Meites, J. (1969b). *Endocrinology* **84**, 868.

Clemens, J. A., Minaguchi, H., Storey, R., Voogt, J. L., and Meites, J. (1969c). *Neuroendocrinology* **4**, 150.

Clemens, J. A., Amenomori, Y., Jenkins, T., and Meites, J. (1970a). *Proc. Soc. Exp. Biol. Med.* **132**, 561.

Clemens, J. A., Gallo, R. V., Whitmoyer, D. I., and Sawyer, C. H. (1970b). *Brain Res.* **25**, 371.

Clemens, J. A., Shaar, C. J., Kleber, J. W., and Tandy, W. A. (1971a). *Exp. Brain Res.* **12**, 250.

Clemens, J. A., Shaar, C. J., Tandy, W. A., and Roush, M. E. (1971b). *Endocrinology* **89**, 1317.

Clemens, J. A. *et al.* (1971c). Unpublished data.

Coble, Y. D., Kohler, P. O., Cargille, C. M., and Ross, G. T. (1969). *J. Clin. Invest.* **48**, 359.

Cohere, G., Bousquet, J., and Meunier, J. M. (1964). *C. R. Soc. Biol.* **158**, 1056.

Convey, E. M. (1972). Personal communication.

Coppola, J. A. (1968). *J. Reprod. Fert., Suppl.* **4**, 35.

Cross, B. A. (1961). *In* "Milk: The Mammary Gland and its Secretion" (S. K. Kon and A. T. Cowie, eds.), Vol. 1, p. 229. Academic Press, New York.

Danon, A., Dikstein, S., and Sulman, F. G. (1963). *Proc. Soc. Exp. Biol. Med.* **114**, 366.

Desclin, L. (1950). *Ann. Endocrinol. (Paris)* **11**, 656.

De Voe, W. F., Ramirez, V. D., and McCann, S. M. (1966). *Endocrinology* **78**, 158.

Dickerman, E., and Meites, J. (1971). *Excerpta Med. Found. Int. Congr. Ser.* **236**, 11 (abstr.).

Donoso, A. O., Bishop, W., Fawcett, C. P., Krulich, L., and McCann, S. M. (1971). *Endocrinology* **89**, 774.

Everett, J. W. (1954). *Endocrinology* **54**, 685.

Everett, J. W., and Quinn, D. L. (1966). *Endocrinology* **78**, 141.

Farquhar, M. G. (1971). *In* "Subcellular Organization and Function in Endocrine

Tissues" (H. Heller and K. Lederis, eds.), p. 1. Cambridge Univ. Press, London and New York.

Frantz, A. G., and Kleinberg, D. L. (1970). *Science* **170,** 745.

Frantz, A. G., Kleinberg, D. L., and Noel, G. L. (1972). *Recent Progr. Horm. Res.* **28** (in press).

Friesen, H. G. (1971). Unpublished data.

Friesen, H. G. (1972). *Recent Progr. Horm. Res.* **28** (in press).

Friesen, H. G., Belanger, C., Guyda, H., and Hwang, P. (1972). *In* "Lactogenic Hormones" (G. E. B. Wolstenholme and J. Knight, eds.), p. 83. Livingstone, London.

Fuxe, K. (1964). *Z. Zellforsch. Mikrosk. Anat.* **61,** 710.

Fuxe, K., and Hokfelt, T. (1969). *In* "Frontiers in Neuroendocrinology" (W. F. Ganong and L. Martini, eds.), p. 47. Oxford Univ. Press, London and New York.

Fuxe, K., and Hokfelt, T. (1971). *In* "The Hypothalamus" (L. Martini, M. Motta, and F. Fraschini, eds.), p. 123. Academic Press, New York.

Gay, V. L. (1971). Private communication.

Gay, V. L., Midgley, A. R., Jr., and Niswender, G. (1970). *Fed. Proc., Fed. Amer. Soc. Exp. Biol.* **29,** 1880.

Gelato, M., and Meites, J. (1971). Unpublished data.

Glick, S. M. (1969). *In* "Frontiers in Neuroendocrinology" (W. F. Ganong and L. Martini, eds.), p. 141. Oxford Univ. Press, London and New York.

Grandison, L., and Meites, J. (1972). Unpublished data.

Grosvenor, C. E. (1965). *Endocrinology* **77,** 1037.

Grosvenor, C. E. (1967). *Endocrinology* **80,** 195.

Grosvenor, C. E., and Turner, C. W. (1958). *Endocrinology* **63,** 535.

Grosvenor, C. E., McCann, S. M., and Nallar, M. D. (1964). *Proc. 46th Meet. Endocrine Soc.* p. 96.

Grosz, H. J., and Rothballer, A. B. (1961). *Nature (London)* **190,** 349.

Halasz, B. (1962). *J. Endocrinol.* **25,** 147.

Haun, C. K., and Sawyer, C. H. (1960). *Endocrinology* **67,** 270.

Heuson, J. C., Gaver, C. W., and Legros, N. (1970). *Eur. J. Cancer* **6,** 353.

Hokfelt, T., and Fuxe, K. (1971). *In* "Brain-Endocrine Interaction" (K. M. Knigge, D. E. Scott, and A. Weindl, eds.), p. 181. Karger, Basel.

Horn, A. S., and Snyder, S. (1971). *Proc. Nat. Acad. Sci. U. S.* **68,** 2325.

Innes, I. R., and Nickerson, M. (1970). *In* "The Pharmacological Basis of Therapeutics" (L. S. Goodman and A. Gilman, eds.), 4th ed., p. 478. Macmillan, New York.

Jacobs, L. S., Snyder, P. J., Wilber, J. F., Utiger, R. D., and Daughaday, W. H. (1971). *J. Clin. Endocrinol.* **33,** 996.

Jaffe, R. B., and Midgley, A. R., Jr. (1971). *Proc. 53rd Meet. Endocrine Soc.* XXX.

Janssen, P. A. J., Niemegeers, C. J. E., Schellekens, K. H. L., Dresse, A., Lenaerts, F. M., Pinchard, A., Schaper, W. K. A., Van Nueten, J. M., and Verbruggen, F. J. (1968). *Arzneim.-Forsch.* **3,** 261.

Johke, T. (1970). *Endocrinol. Jap.* **17,** 393.

Johke, T., Fuse, H., and Oshima, M. (1971). *Jap. J. Zootech. Sci.* **42,** 173.

Kamberi, I. A., Mical, R. S., and Porter, J. C. (1970). *Endocrinology* **87,** 1.

Kamberi, I. A., Mical, R. S., and Porter, J. C. (1971). *Endocrinology* **88,** 1288.

Karg, H., and Schams, D. (1970). *In* "Lactation" (I. R. Falconer, ed.), p. 141. Butterworth, London.

Katz, S. H., Molitch, M., and McCann, S. M. (1969). *Endocrinology* **85,** 725.

Koch, Y., Lu, K. H., and Meites, J. (1970). *Endocrinology* **87**, 673.
Koch, Y., Chow, Y. F., and Meites, J. (1971). *Endocrinology* **89**, 1303.
Kohler, P. O., Ross, G. T., and Odell, W. D. (1968). *J. Clin. Invest.* **47**, 38.
Komisaruk, B. R., McDonald, P. G., Whitmoyer, D. I., and Sawyer, C. H. (1967). *Exp. Neurol.* **19**, 494.
Komoto, K., and Bern, H. A. (1971). *Proc. Soc. Exp. Biol. Med.* **137**, 807.
Koprowski, J. A. *et al.* (1972). Unpublished data.
Kordon, C. (1966). Thesis, University of Paris, Paris.
Kragt, C. L., and Meites, J. (1965). *Endocrinology* **76**, 1169.
Krulich, L., Quijada, M., and Illner, P. (1971). *Proc. 53rd Meet. Endocrine Soc.* p. A-83.
Kwa, H. G., and Verhofstad, F. (1967). *J. Endocrinol.* **39**, 455.
Lu, H. G., and Meites, J. (1971a). Unpublished observations.
Lu, K. H., and Meites, J. (1971b). *Proc. Soc. Exp. Biol. Med.* **137**, 480.
Lu, K. H., Amenomori, Y., Chen, C. L., and Meites, J. (1970). *Endocrinology* **87**, 667.
Lu, K. H., Koch, Y., and Meites, J. (1971). *Endocrinology* **89**, 229.
Lu, K. H., Shaar, C., Kortright, K., and Meites, J. (1972). *Endocrinology.* In press.
Lutterbeck, P. M., Pryor, J. S., Varga, L., and Winer, R. (1971). *Brit. Med. J.* **3**, 228.
Lyons, W. R. (1937). *Cold Spring Harbor Symp. Quant. Biol.* **5**, 198.
MacLeod, R. M. (1969). *Endocrinology* **85**, 916.
MacLeod, R. M., Smith, M. C., and DeWitt, G. W. (1966). *Endocrinology* **79**, 1149.
Malven, P. V., and Hoge, W. R. (1971). *Endocrinology* **88**, 445.
Markee, J. E., Sawyer, C. H., and Hollinshead, W. H. (1948). *Recent Progr. Horm. Res.* **2**, 117.
Meites, J. (1962). *Proc. Int. Pharmacol. Meet., 1st, 1961* Vol. 1, p. 151.
Meites, J. (1966). *In* "Neuroendocrinology" (L. Martini and W. F. Ganong, eds.), Vol. 1, p. 669. Academic Press, New York.
Meites, J. (1967). *Arch. Anat. Microsc. Morphol. Exp.* **56**, Suppl. 3–4, 516.
Meites, J. (1970). *In* "Hypophysiotropic Hormones of the Hypothalamus: Assay and Chemistry" (J. Meites, ed.), p. 261. Williams & Wilkins, Baltimore, Maryland.
Meites, J., and Nicoll, C. S. (1966). *Annu. Rev. Physiol.* **28**, 57.
Meites, J., and Turner, C. W. (1948). *Mo., Agr. Exp. Sta., Res. Bull.* **415**.
Meites, J., and Turner, C. W. (1950). *In* "Hormone Assay" (C. W. Emmens, ed.), p. 237. Academic Press, New York.
Meites, J., Talwalker, P. K., and Nicoll, C. S. (1960). *Proc. Soc. Exp. Biol. Med.* **103**, 298.
Meites, J., Nicoll, C. S., and Talwalker, P. K. (1963). *Advan. Neuroendocrinol., Proc. Symp., 1961* p. 238.
Meites, J., Lu, K. H., Wuttke, W., Welsch, C. W., Nagasawa, H., and Quadri, S. K. (1972). *Recent Progr. Horm. Res.* **28** (in press).
Minaguchi, H., and Meites, J. (1967). *Endocrinology* **80**, 603.
Minaguchi, H., Clemens, J. A., and Meites, J. (1968). *Endocrinology* **82**, 555.
Mishkinsky, J., Khazen, K., and Sulman, F. G. (1968). *Endocrinology* **82**, 611.
Mishkinsky, J., Nir, I., and Sulman, F. G. (1969). *Neuroendocrinology* **5**, 48.
Mizuno, H., Talwalker, P. K., and Meites, J. (1964). *Proc. Soc. Exp. Biol. Med.* **115**, 604.
Munson, P. L. (1963). *Advan. Neuroendocrinol., Proc. Symp., 1961* p. 427.

Nagasawa, H., and Meites, J. (1970). *Proc. Soc. Exp. Biol. Med.* **135**, 469.
Neill, J. D., Freeman, M. E., and Tillson, S. A. (1971). *Endocrinology* **89**, 1448.
Nicoll, C. S. (1971). *In* "Frontiers in Neuroendocrinology" (L. Martini and W. F. Ganong, eds.), p. 291. Oxford Univ. Press, London and New York.
Nicoll, C. S., and Meites, J. (1962). *Endocrinology* **70**, 272.
Nicoll, C. S., and Meites, J. (1963). *Endocrinology* **72**, 544.
Nicoll, C. S., and Meites, J. (1964). *Proc. Soc. Exp. Biol. Med.* **117**, 579.
Nicoll, C. S., Talwalker, P. K., and Meites, J. (1960). *Amer. J. Physiol.* **198**, 1103.
Nicoll, C. S., Fiorindo, R. P., McKenee, C. T., and Parsons, J. A. (1970). *In* "Hypophysiotropic Hormones of the Hypothalamus: Assay and Chemistry" (J. Meites, ed.), p. 115. Williams & Wilkins, Baltimore, Maryland.
Niswender, G. D., Chen, C. L., Midgley, A. R., Jr., Meites, J., and Ellis, S. (1969). *Proc. Soc. Exp. Biol. Med.* **130**, 793.
Nordskog, A. W. (1946). *Amer. J. Vet. Res.* **7**, 490.
Nordskog, A. W., and Clark, R. T. (1945). *Amer. J. Vet. Res.* **6**, 107.
Nyback, H., and Sedvall, G. (1968). *J. Pharmacol. Exp. Ther.* **162**, 294.
Parsons, J. A. (1970). *J. Physiol. (London)* **210**, 973.
Pasteels, J. L. (1961). *C. R. Acad. Sci.* **253**, 2140.
Quadri, S. K., and Meites, J. (1971a). *Proc. Soc. Exp. Biol. Med.* **137**, 1242.
Quadri, S. K., and Meites, J. (1971b). Unpublished data.
Quadri, S. K., Lu, K. H., and Meites, J. (1972). *Science* **176**, 417.
Quinn, D. L., and Everett, J. W. (1967). *Endocrinology* **80**, 155.
Ramirez, V. D., Komisaruk, B. R., Whitmoyer, D. I., and Sawyer, C. H. (1967). *Amer. J. Physiol.* **212**, 1376.
Ratner, A., Talwalker, P. K., and Meites, J. (1965). *Endocrinology* **77**, 315.
Raud, H. R., Kiddy, C. A., and Odell, W. D. (1971). *Proc. Soc. Exp. Biol. Med.* **136**, 689.
Reece, R. P., and Turner, C. W. (1937). *Mo., Agr. Exp. Sta., Res. Bull.* **266**.
Ruf, K. *et al.* (1970). Unpublished data.
Sakuma, M., and Knobil, E. (1970). *Endocrinology* **86**, 890.
Sar, M., and Meites, J. (1967). *Neuroendocrinology* **4**, 25.
Sawyer, C. H., Markee, J. E., and Townsend, B. F. (1949). *Endocrinology* **44**, 18.
Sawyer, C. H., Kawakami, M., Meyerson, B., Whitmoyer, D. I., and Lilley, J. J. (1968). *Brain Res.* **10**, 213.
Schally, A. V., Kastin, A. J., Locke, W., and Bowers, C. Y. (1967). *In* "Hormones in Blood" (C. H. Gray and A. L. Bacharach, eds.), 2nd rev. ed., Vol. 1, p. 492. Academic Press, New York.
Schneider, H. P. G., and McCann, S. M. (1970). *Endocrinology* **86**, 1127.
Sgouris, J. T., and Meites, J. (1953). *Amer. J. Physiol.* **175**, 319.
Shaar, C. J., and Meites, J. (1971). Unpublished data.
Singh, D. V., Meites, J., Halmi, L., Kortwright, K. H., and Brennan, M. J. (1972). *J. Nat. Cancer Inst.* (in press).
Sinha, Y. N., and Tucker, H. A. (1968). *Proc. Soc. Exp. Biol. Med.* **128**, 84.
Smith, R. (1969). *Ann. N. Y. Acad. Sci. U. S.* **166**, Art. 2, 525.
Smith, R., and Clemens, J. A. (1972). Unpublished observations.
Smith, R., and Farquhar, M. (1966). *J. Cell Biol.* **31**, 319.
Spies, H. G., and Clegg, M. T. (1971). *Neuroendocrinology* **8**, 205.
Stahelin, H., Burckhardt-Vischer, B., and Fluckiger, E. (1971). *Experientia* **27**, 915.
Steiner, F. A., Ruf, K., and Akert, K. (1969). *Brain Res.* **12**, 74.
Sud, S. C., and Meites, J. (1969). Unpublished data.

Talwalker, P. K., Ratner, A., and Meites, J. (1963). *Amer. J. Physiol.* **205**, 213.

Tashjian, A. H., Barowsky, N. J., and Jensen, D. K. (1971). *Biochem. Biophys. Res. Commun.* **43**, 516.

Terasawa, E., Whitmoyer, D. I., and Sawyer, C. H. (1969). *Amer. J. Physiol.* **217**, 1119.

Tindal, J. S. (1956). *J. Endocrinol.* **14**, 268.

Tindal, J. S., and Knaggs, G. S. (1969). *J. Endocrinol.* **45**, 111.

Tindal, J. S., and Knaggs, G. S. *J. Endocrinol.* **48**, xxxii.

Turkington, R. W. (1971). *Proc. Cent. Soc. Clin. Res.* **44**, 44.

Valverde, C., and Chieffo, V. (1971). *Proc. 53rd Meet., Endocrine Soc., San Francisco,* p. 84.

Vogt, M. (1954). *J. Physiol. (London)* **123**, 451.

Voogt, J. L., and Meites, J. (1971). *Endocrinology* **88**, 286.

Voogt, J. L., Clemens, J. A., and Meites, J. (1969). *Neuroendocrinology* **4**, 157.

Voogt, J. L., Chen, C. L., and Meites, J. (1970). *Amer. J. Physiol.* **218**, 396.

Voogt, J. L., Clemens, J. A., Negro-Vilar, A., Welsch, C. W., and Meites, J. (1971). *Endocrinology* **88**, 1363.

Wakabayashi, I., Arimura, A., and Schally, A. V. (1971). *Proc. Soc. Exp. Biol. Med.* **137**, 1189.

Watson, J. T., Krulich, L., and McCann, S. M. (1971). *Endocrinology* **89**, 1412.

Welsch, C. W., and Meites, J. (1969). *Cancer* **23**, 601.

Welsch, C. W., Negro-Vilar, A., and Meites, J. (1968a). *Neuroendocrinology* **3**, 238.

Welsch, C. W., Sar, M., Clemens, J., and Meites, J. (1968b). *Proc. Soc. Exp. Biol. Med.* **129**, 817.

Welsch, C. W., Clemens, J. A., and Meites, J. (1969). *Cancer Res.* **29**, 1541.

Welsch, C. W., Nagasawa, H., and Meites, J. (1970). *Cancer Res.* **30**, 2310.

Welsch, C. W., Amenomori, Y., and Meites, J. (1971a). *Experientia* **27**, 11.

Welsch, C. W., Squiers, M. D., Cassell, E. E., Chen, C. L., and Meites, J. (1971b). *Amer. J. Physiol.* **221**, 1714.

Wurtman, R. J. (1970). *In* "Hypophysiotropic Hormones of the Hypothalamus: Assay and Chemistry" (J. Meites, ed.), p. 184. Williams & Wilkins, Baltimore, Maryland.

Wuttke, W., and Meites, J. (1970a). Unpublished data.

Wuttke, W., and Meites, J. (1970b). *Proc. Soc. Exp. Biol. Med.* **135**, 648.

Wuttke, W., and Meites, J. (1971). *Proc. Soc. Exp. Biol. Med.* **137**, 988.

Wuttke, W., and Meites, J. (1972). *Endocrinology* (in press).

Wuttke, W., Cassell, E. E., and Meites, J. (1971a). *Endocrinology* **88**, 737.

Wuttke, W., Gelato, M., and Meites, J. (1971b). *Endocrinology* **89**, 1191.

Yanai, R., and Nagasawa, H. (1971). *Experientia* **26**, 649.

Yoshinaga, K., Hawkins, R. A., and Stocker, J. F. (1970). *Endocrinology* **85**, 103.

Comparative Endocrinology of Gestation

I. JOHN DAVIES AND KENNETH J. RYAN

*Department of Obstetrics and Gynecology, University of California, San Diego,
School of Medicine, La Jolla, California*

I. INTRODUCTION

A. GENERAL CONSIDERATIONS

The comparative endocrinology of pregnancy is a broad field, and it is advantageous to consider it under headings that represent separate functional units. Three endocrine systems can be defined on the basis of their function in relationship to the physiology of pregnancy: (1) preimplantation, (2) postimplantation, and (3) metabolic-homeostatic. These are discrete, but interrelated systems, and each has an essential role in mammalian reproduction.

The preimplantation endocrine system (Table I) controls gametogenesis, sexual behavior, ovulation, conception, and implantation. For

TABLE I

PREIMPLANTATION ENDOCRINE SYSTEM

Hormone	Primary origin	Primary function
FSH	Anterior pituitary	Tropic to follicle
LH	Anterior pituitary	Ovulation; tropic to corpus luteum
Estrogen	Ovarian follicle or corpus luteum	Tropic to reproductive tract
Progesterone	Corpus luteum	Tropic to reproductive tract

many nonmammalian vertebrates, a "preimplantation" system has sufficed to accomplish fertilization of the ovum and its expulsion into an environment that is suitable for the subsequent development of the embryo. It is from a "preimplantation" system that postimplantation endocrine activity can be assumed to have evolved. This connection is readily apparent in the simplest mammalian systems, in which the hormones of both the preimplantation phase and the postimplantation period are essentially the same.

In the preimplantation endocrine system a high degree of neuroendocrine integration is readily apparent, and it can be stated with confidence that the preimplantation phase of reproduction is controlled by the central nervous system, by both neural and neuroendocrine mechanisms. This has relevance to our understanding of the control of the postimplantation endocrine system.

The postimplantation endocrine system (Table II) is necessary for the

TABLE II

POSTIMPLANTATION ENDOCRINE SYSTEM

Hormone	Primary source	Primary function
LH	Anterior pituitary	Tropic to corpus luteum
Chorionic gonadotropin	Placenta	Replaces LH
Estrogen	Ovary or placenta	Tropic to reproductive tract
Progesterone	Ovary or placenta	Tropic to reproductive tract; uterine quiescence
Chorionic somatomammotropin	Placenta in man	Metabolic effects
Chorionic thyrotropin	Placenta in man	Tropic to thyroid
Oxytocin	Posterior pituitary	Completion of parturition; lactation
Prolactin	Anterior pituitary	Lactation
Relaxin	Ovary	Facilitate parturition

maintenance of pregnancy, the accomplishment of parturition, and the nursing of the newborn. As indicated above, this phase of reproduction is related to the preimplantation period, and remains linked to it via the corpus luteum and its associated hormones. While the same hormones may participate in both systems, the functions of the hormones in the postimplantation phase are, for the most part, unique to pregnancy, and in this sense can be said to be pregnancy specific. In its simplest form, this system looks much like a prolonged version of the luteal phase of the preimplantation period. The preimplantation corpus luteum becomes the corpus luteum of pregnancy, and the specificity is perhaps as much quantitative as qualitative. In the subsequent evolution of this system, we observe increasing specificity of hormonal function, and the development of new mechanisms and new hormones. Among the most readily apparent innovations are placental gonadotropins, placental steroidogenic function, integrated fetal-placental steroid synthesis, and last, placental metabolic hormones.

The development of the postimplantation endocrine system is a central aspect of the evolution of viviparity. It is characterized by: (1) an increasing length of gestation, (2) increasingly specific endocrine mechanisms, (3) increasing endocrine participation by the conceptus, and (4) as we will postulate, an increasing transfer of the neuroendocrine control of gestation from the central nervous system of the mother to that of the fetus.

At one end of the developmental scale are species such as the ferret in which sterile-mating can induce a pseudopregnancy which, although there is no conceptus, is indistinguishable from true pregnancy, both in its duration and in its endocrine parameters. The control of pregnancy in these species resides in the central nervous system, and it is mediated via the pituitary-ovarian axis. At the other end of the spectrum are primates in which the maternal pituitary and ovaries can be dispensed with a short time after implantation, their gestational endocrine function having been replaced by the endocrine activity of the fetus and placenta.

The metabolic-homeostatic endocrine system (Table III) is not primarily a part of reproductive function. However, it must provide for the adaptation of the maternal organism to the changes imposed by gestation. This system, in maintaining control of the internal environment, must permit, and perhaps facilitate, the reproductive process.

Some aspects of the relationship of this system to gestation are directly related to pregnancy-specific phenomena. Examples of this are the secretion by the placenta of thyrotropic and somatomammotropic hormones. Other relationships which are less direct include changes induced by elevated levels of steroid hormones. Examples of this are increased

TABLE III

METABOLIC-HOMEOSTATIC ENDOCRINE SYSTEM

Hormone	Source	Function	Changes in human pregnancy
Somatotropin	Anterior pituitary	Growth and metabolism	Release in response to altered blood glucose blunted; augmented by chorionic somato-mammotropin
Thyrotropin	Anterior pituitary	Thyroid	Increased concentration; increased thyroid activity
Thyroxine	Thyroid	Metabolism	Increased plasma thyroxine-binding globulin
Adrenocorticotropin	Anterior pituitary	Adrenal cortex	No known change
Cortisol	Adrenal cortex	Metabolism	Increased plasma corticosteroid-binding globulin; increased unbound cortisol
Aldosterone	Adrenal cortex	Water and electrolyte balance	Increased production; elevation of renin-angiotensin system
Insulin	Pancreas	Metabolism of glucose and fat	Early, activity on glucose increased. Late, activity on glucose decreased and blood levels elevated
Catecholamines	Adrenal medulla	Homeostasis	None established
Parathormone	Parathyroid	Metabolism of calcium and phosphorus	Increased activity with pregnancy and lactation
Vasopressin	Posterior pituitary	Metabolism of water	None established
Melanocyte-stimulating hormone	Anterior pituitary	Pigmentation	Increased activity

plasma protein binding of cortisol and thyroxine which is induced by estrogen, and altered renal function which is induced by progesterone. While pregnancy requires important adaptive responses from the metabolic-homeostatic system, the mechanisms which are utilized are generally not unique to pregnancy, and metabolic-homeostatic function can be considered to be not pregnancy specific.

From the foregoing it is apparent that the comparative endocrinology of gestation is too broad an area to be reviewed in its entirety within this presentation. The subsequent discussion will be confined to the postimplantation system. Within this area, we have restricted our attention especially to those pregnancy-specific mechanisms by which gestation is maintained, and by which parturition is initiated. Consideration of the protein hormones has been largely omitted, and the discussion will focus on the two steroid hormones, estrogen and progesterone.

From the list of hormones which have been included in the pregnancy-specific system (Table II), only two can be selected as being probably essential for the maintenance of normal gestation, throughout essentially all of pregnancy, and in all species. The requirement for progesterone seems clear. There is no species in which pregnancy can be maintained to its normal completion in the absence of progesterone. The absolute necessity for estrogen is less clear-cut. In some species, animals which have been experimentally oophorectomized during pregnancy can be maintained with progesterone replacement alone, without any evident source of estrogen. Suffice it to say that optimal hormone replacement in these animals is accomplished with progesterone and estrogen together, and when progesterone alone will suffice it is usually in a short-gestation animal. In all species, estrogen is normally present during pregnancy. It has well established specific effects on the uterus, and it seems unlikely that truly normal pregnancy is possible in its absence.

The gonadotropic hormones, both from the pituitary and the placenta, have an important function in promoting the synthesis of the essential steroid hormones, estrogen and progesterone, in the ovary. A source of gonadotropin is present in all species in early pregnancy, and the universality of gonadotropin directs our attention again to the steroid hormones. The remainder of the hormones which have been included in Table II do not appear to be essential for the maintenance of pregnancy and/or the initiation of parturition in all species. Oxytocin, an interesting hormone which has very old phylogenetic origins in common with vasopressin, will be discussed briefly as it relates to the steroid hormones.

Within the broad framework of the comparative endocrinology of gestation, the central theme is the necessity for estrogens and progesterone in all species, and the major comparative data relate to the relative amounts, sources, and actions of these hormones in different species.

Discussion of the maintenance of pregnancy will be undertaken separately from consideration of the initiation of parturition. We believe that failure to make this distinction in the past has led to some confusion, and perhaps erroneous reasoning. For example, the failure of progesterone administration to prevent parturition in some species has been taken as evidence against the importance of progesterone in the maintenance of pregnancy. While the termination of pregnancy could be the result of the removal of supportive factors, this is not necessarily so. We will consider the maintenance of pregnancy first, and then we will turn our attention to the initiation of parturition.

B. NOMENCLATURE

The following trivial names and abbreviations have been used:

Trivial name	Systematic name
ACTH	Adrenocorticotropin
Aldosterone	11β,21-Dihydroxy-3,20-dioxopregn-4-en-18-al
Androstenedione	Androst-4-ene-3,17-dione
11β-OH-androstenedione	11β-Hydroxyandrost-4-ene-3,17-dione
16α-OH-androstenedione	16α-Hydroxyandrost-4-ene-3,17-dione
Cholesterol	Cholesta-5-en-3β-ol
Cortisol	11β,17α,21-Trihydroxypregn-4-ene-3,20-dione
Dehydroepiandrosterone	3β-Hydroxyandrost-5-en-17-one
Dexamethasone	9α-Fluoro-16α-methyl-11β,17α,21-trihydroxy-1,4-pregnandiene-3,20-dione
16α-OH-Dehydroepiandrosterone	3β,16α-Dihydroxyandrost-5-en-17-one
Epitestosterone	17α-Hydroxyandrost-4-en-3-one
Equilen	3-Hydroxyestra-1,3,5(10),7-tetraen-17-one
Equilenin	3-Hydroxyestra-1,3,5(10),6,8-pentaen-17-one
Estradiol-17α	Estra-1,3,5(10)-triene-3,17α-diol
Estradiol-17β	Estra-1,3,5(10)-triene-3,17β-diol
Estriol	Estra-1,3,5(10)-triene-3,16α,17β-triol
Estrone	3-Hydroxyoestra-1,3,5(10)-trien-17-one
16α-OH-estrone	3,6α-Dihydroxyoestra-1,3,5(10)-trien-17-one
FSH	Follicle-stimulating hormone
LH	Luteinizing hormone
Pregnanediol	5β-Pregnane-3α,20α-diol
Pregnenolone	3β-Hydroxypregn-5-en-20-one
Progesterone	Pregn-4-ene-3,20-dione
6β-OH-progesterone	6β-Hydroxypregn-4-ene-3,20-dione
20-αOH-progesterone	20α-Hydroxypregn-4-en-3-one
20-βOH-progesterone	20β-Hydroxypregn-4-en-3-one
Testosterone	17β-Hydroxyandrost-4-en-3-one

II. THE MAINTENANCE OF PREGNANCY

A. PROGESTERONE

1. General Considerations

In all viviparous animals, progesterone is necessary for the sequence of events leading to conception, and, with some qualification in regard to the armadillo and the guinea pig, progesterone is essential for implantation as well (Amoroso and Finn, 1962; Deanesly, 1971). The corpus luteum, which is the source of progesterone prior to implantation, continues to serve this function throughout pregnancy in many animals. In other species, the placenta secretes progesterone which supplants that of the corpus luteum, to a greater or lesser degree, during pregnancy. This discussion will consider the role of progesterone in the maintenance of pregnancy following placentation.

More than 50 years ago, Allen and Corner (1929, 1930) demonstrated the essential requirement for progesterone (Allen, 1930; Heckel and Allen, 1938) in the maintenance of pregnancy in the rabbit. In reviewing the subject twenty years later, Reynolds (1949) concluded: "While the evidence for an inhibitory action of progesterone upon the myometrium of the rabbit and several other species is conclusive, a divergent group of data exists for the rat, mouse, and guinea pig. Unfortunately for our understanding of the situation, the greater number of results do not support the view that progesterone inhibits or inactivates the human myometrium." Some uncertainty concerning the role of progesterone in the maintenance of pregnancy remains. Csapo (1956, 1969) and others (Kumar, 1967; Kuriyama, 1961; Marshall, 1962) have supported the "progesterone-block" hypothesis. Kao (1967) denies its validity, even in the rabbit. On the basis of electrophysiological data, he concludes that the progesterone-block hypothesis is incompatible with fundamental principles of the ionic theory of excitation. Porter (1969, 1970) has been unable to influence uterine activity in the pregnant guinea pig by progesterone administration, and he has concluded that progesterone is not a myometrial inhibitor in the pregnant guinea pig. Administered progesterone is also largely ineffectual in human beings, and the proposed myometrium-inhibiting role of progesterone in human pregnancy is based largely on inference from the animal data. While the matter cannot be unequivocally resolved at this time, an appraisal from a comparative viewpoint may provide some perspective.

2. Uterine Accommodation of the Conceptus

a. *Corpus Luteum–Placenta Interrelationship.* It is useful to categorize species according to whether abortion is inevitable following oophorectomy or whether, after a certain period of gestation, pregnancy can continue in the absence of the ovary (Tables IV and V). It should be appreciated, however, that such a division into two groups is somewhat arbitrary. It may be more correct physiologically to consider the species as a spectrum in transition from corpus luteum to placental dependence.

There are species, such as the goat, in which the requirement for the corpus luteum is absolute and placental progesterone synthesis appears to be totally absent (Blom and Lyngset, 1971; Linzell and Heap, 1968).

TABLE IV

Oophorectomy-Intolerant Mammals

Species	Approximate length of gestation (days)	Regression of corpora lutea before term	Key references
Opossum	12.5	No	Amoroso and Finn (1962)
Hamster	16	No	Amoroso and Finn (1962)
Mouse	20	No	Amoroso and Finn (1962)
Rat	22	No	Amoroso and Finn (1962)
Rabbit	31	No	Amoroso and Finn (1962)
Ferret	42	No	Hammond and Marshall (1930)
Pig	114	No	Amoroso and Finn (1962)
Armadillo	120[a]	No	Hamlett (1935) Amoroso and Finn (1962)
Goat	151	No	Amoroso and Finn (1962)

[a] 3.5–4 months of delayed implantation; 4 months of postimplantation gestation.

The rat has generally been considered to be "oophorectomy-intolerant." However, if oophorectomy is done after day 13, an increasing percentage of fetuses are retained as the time of castration is moved closer to term. When oophorectomy is done on day 18, 90% of the fetuses can be retained until full term, 22 days (Amoroso and Finn, 1962; Csapo and Wiest, 1969). The guinea pig is considered to be an "oophorectomy-tolerant" species. However, in the earliest observations, the significance

TABLE V

Oophorectomy-Tolerant Mammals

Species	Approximate length of gestation (days)	Earliest successful oophorectomy	Regression of corpora lutea before term	Key references
Cat	63	49	Yes	Amoroso and Finn (1962)
Dog	63	Late	Yes	Courrier (1945)
Guinea pig	68	40	No	Amoroso and Finn (1962)
Sheep	144	55	Yes	Amoroso and Finn (1962)
Macaca mulatta	166	25	—	Amoroso and Finn (1962)
Baboon	175	—	Yes	Kriewaldt and Hendrickx (1968)
Human	267	40	Yes	Amoroso and Finn (1962)
Cow	280	207	No	Amoroso and Finn (1962) Courrier (1945)
Horse	330	170	Yes	Amoroso and Finn (1962)

of litter size was noted. While guinea pig litters normally range from 1 to 4, those oophorectomized animals which carried their pregnancies to term were those with only 1 or 2 fetuses (Haterius, 1936; Herrick, 1928; Nelson, 1934). In sheep (Fylling, 1970a; Linzell and Heap, 1968), cows (Erb et al., 1967), and guinea pigs (Heap and Deanesly, 1966), all of which are also "oophorectomy-tolerant," the ovarian contribution to circulating progesterone is substantial until quite late in pregnancy. In primates, throughout most of pregnancy, the corpus luteum is dispensable and the placenta is the only important source of circulating progesterone (Diczfalusy and Borell, 1961; Henry et al., 1938; Neill et al., 1969).

There may be important differences in progesterone physiology depending on whether the hormone is synthesized at an extrauterine site or in the placenta. If, in some species, ovarian and placental mechanisms are operating simultaneously, and in varying degree, overly simplistic interpretation of experimental observations might be misleading.

b. Uterine Contractile Activity. Species in which the corpus luteum is required to maintain pregnancy have been useful experimentally because they lend themselves to the classical endocrinological approach of organ-extirpation and hormone replacement. The rabbit and the rat have been most thoroughly studied, and in these two species it is most firmly established that the essential role of progesterone in pregnancy is to inhibit uterine contractility, thereby facilitating accommodation of the conceptus.

Any potential untoward effect of progesterone deprivation on the endometrium is obscured by the more prominent changes in myometrial activity. In castrate pregnant rabbits, the quantity of progesterone required to maintain pregnancy is at least 5-fold that which is necessary for endometrial proliferation (Heckel and Allen, 1938). In sterile-mated, pseudopregnant rabbits, 1 or 2 corpora lutea are sufficient for endometrial proliferation. However, if blastocysts are transplanted into the uteri of these pseudopregnant animals which have only 2 corpora lutea, 95% of the blastocysts are expelled into the vagina. With 4 corpora lutea, half the blastocysts are retained and, with 8 corpora lutea, almost 90% are retained (C. E. Adams, 1965). These experiments point to an inverse relationship between progesterone and uterine expulsive activity.

Pencharz and Long (1933) observed that hypophysectomy of the pregnant rat resulted in apparent crushing-to-death of the fetuses in utero. Selye et al. (1935) made the same observation in oophorectomized rats. These findings have been substantiated by others (Zeiner, 1943). The direct recording of intrauterine pressure in the rat has confirmed the association between oophorectomy, pressure, and fetal damage (Csapo, 1969).

The most graphic experiment was done in the rabbit by Courrier (1941). In a rabbit which was 19 days pregnant, he slit the uterine horn and delivered one fetus in its intact sac into the peritoneal cavity, retaining the placental attachment. The two remaining fetuses were left in the uterus, and the doe was oophorectomized. At repeat laparotomy on day 28, the fetus which had been exteriorized from the uterus into the peritoneal cavity was healthy and growing normally. The other two fetuses had died shortly after the initial operation, and had been extruded through a rupture in the uterine wall.

c. *Uterine Volume.* Closely related to these findings associating progesterone deprivation with uterine contractile activity are observations relating to uterine volume. The results of the blastocyst-transplantation experiments described above suggest a relationship between the quantity of luteal tissue and uterine capacity in rabbits. In oophorectomized pregnant rabbits, maintained on suboptimal doses of progesterone, the animals with small liters will carry the pregnancy longer than those with larger litters (Csapo and Lloyd-Jacob, 1962).

The significance of litter size in the oophorectomized guinea pig was indicated above. In the guinea pig, if the contents of one uterine horn are removed and replaced with wax dummies which are similar in size to the fetuses in the intact horn, the dummies are delivered prematurely prior to the fetuses. However, if the volume of the dummies is reduced to 25% of that of the fetuses in the intact horn, the dummies are retained and delivered following the contents of the intact horn at term (Schofield, 1966).

In the rat, oophorectomy alone prior to day 14 invariably terminates the pregnancy. However, if oophorectomy is accompanied by removal of all the fetuses except one, leaving the placentas *in situ,* the remaining fetus can be carried to term (Haterius, 1936).

d. *Electromechanical Effects.* The extensive literature dealing with the electrochemical and mechanical effects of progesterone on myometrium cannot be discussed in detail. The observations are pertinent to this discussion inasmuch as measurement of these effects has been utilized as a tool to observe the local influence of the placenta on the myometrium. The weight of evidence indicate that progesterone inhibits the contractile activity of myometrial strips, including both spontaneous activity and that induced by oxytocin. This inhibition of mechanical activity is associated with alteration of the electrical characteristics of the cell membrane including hyperpolarization, diminished generation of spontaneous action potentials, and, perhaps most importantly, diminished ability to propagate an action potential. The findings have been qualitatively similar, *in vitro* and *in vivo,* in the myometrium of the various species studied, including human beings (Kumar, 1967; Kuriyama, 1961; Marshall, 1962).

e. *Discussion and Conclusions.* These basic physiological observations in rats, rabbits, guinea pigs, and human beings, encompassing both "oophorectomy-intolerant" and "oophorectomy-tolerant" species, indicate that the essential role for progesterone in the maintenance of pregnancy is to effect uterine quiescence and permit physical accommodation of the conceptus. The mechanism, suppression of initiation and propagation of excitation, is a relatively fundamental biological action, and might be expected to be applicable to mammals in general.

3. The Local Effect of the Placenta

a. *General Considerations.* The suggestion that the placenta "exerts an inhibiting influence on uterine contractions" was first presented by the Dutch gynecologist de Snoo (1919). His hypothesis was based on the observation that in women with complete accidental separation of the placenta, 80% of them delivered within 24 hours, and essentially all delivered within 48 hours.

In a number of species, and by a variety of techniques, evidence has accumulated which indicates that the placenta has a local influence on the myometrium and that this influence is attributable to progesterone.

b. *Uterine Contractile Activity.* That it is possible for progesterone to exert a local effect on myometrial activity has been readily demonstrated in the bicornuate uterus of the rabbit. Progesterone injected intramniotically will suppress the contractile activity in the injected horn and prevent delivery of the fetuses. It is effective in preventing normal delivery at term in intact animals, and also in preventing premature delivery following oophorectomy or placental dislocation. The uninjected horn is not affected and delivers its contents when expected, either at term in the intact animal, or prematurely following oophorectomy or placental dislocation (Macedo-Costa and Csapo, 1959; Porter, 1968).

Similar experiments in rats also suggest a local effect of the placentas and implicate progesterone. In rats, oophorectomy accompanied by dislocation of the placentas in one horn resulted in expulsion of 85% of the dislocated fetuses, while in the intact horn 95% of the fetuses were retained. If supplemental progesterone was given, 90% of the dislocated fetuses were retained (Csapo and Wiest, 1969).

Zarrow *et al.* (1960) demonstrated a local effect of the placentas on uterine contractile activity in rabbits in which the ovaries and placentas were left intact. He removed the fetuses and substituted malleable paraffin rods. He found that the rods subsequently became shaped by constrictions which occurred approximately equidistant between neighboring placentas.

A similarly direct observation relating placental location to contractile activity was made in cows. Microballoons were implanted in the myometrium in a row from a cotyledonary site into intercotyledonary areas. Uterine activity, as measured by pressure changes in the microballoons, was proportional to the distance from the cotyledons (Gillette, 1966).

c. *Electromechanical Effects.* In a wider variety of species, it has been possible to show a local effect of the placenta by comparison of the electrochemical properties of the myometrium at the placental site with that at a nonplacental site.

Goto and Csapo (1959) found a difference in the membrane potential between placental and nonplacental myometrial strips from pregnant rabbits, and were able to abolish the difference with progesterone. Kuriyama and Csapo (1961) demonstrated in rabbit myometrial strips that an electrically elicited contractile wave, which is propagated along interplacental myometrium, is stopped when it reaches the placental site. Jung (1962) confirmed this observation in the rat uterus *in situ.* Daniel and Renner (1960), studying the cat uterus *in vitro* and *in vivo,* found the myometrium of the placental site to be lacking in spontaneous electrical activity as well as in its capacity to propagate an action potential, as compared to interplacental tissue. The difference in tissue concentrations of sodium and potassium were determined and found to correlate with the known alterations produced by progesterone in nonpregnant uteri. Kumar and his associates (Kumar, 1967; Kumar and Barnes, 1961; Kumar *et al.,* 1962) have reported that, in human myometrium, the tissue potassium, the resting membrane potential, and the tissue progesterone are higher in the myometrium overlying the placenta than in that immediately opposite to it.

d. *Placental Dislocation.* The results of the studies described above, involving placental dislocation in the rabbit and the rat, not only support the hypothesis of a local effect of placental progesterone on adjacent myometrium, but also demonstrate that the local effect is important to the activity of the uterus as a whole in retaining or expelling the conceptus. Placental dislocation results in abortion within 48 hours in rabbits (Macedo-Costa and Csapo, 1959), rats (Csapo and Wiest, 1969; Kirsch, 1938), guinea pigs (Porter, 1969), and human beings (de Snoo, 1919; Grandin and Hall, 1960). While placental separation obviously cannot be interpreted as a simple endocrinological event, it should be acknowledged that the results are consistent with the proposed myometrium-inhibiting function of the placenta.

e. *Effect of Exogenous Progesterone.* The major deterrent to the acceptance of the general applicability of the myometrium-inhibiting role of progesterone has been the inability, in some species (e.g., guinea pigs and human beings), to delay parturition with progesterone. The observed differences between species may be related to the suggested spectrum between corpus luteum dependence and placental dependence. In the mouse (Kroc *et al.*, 1959), the rat (Boe, 1938), and the rabbit (Heckel and Allen, 1938), parturition is readily prevented by progesterone. In pigs and cattle, parturition was delayed only when a highly potent synthetic progestin was used (Nellor, 1963). In sheep, the results were initially negative (Bengtsson and Schofield, 1963), but, in later experiments, a single injection at the onset of labor did delay parturition (Hindson *et al.*, 1969). In the guinea pig no effect is evident (Schofield, 1964; Porter, 1969, 1970; Zarrow *et al.*, 1963). In human beings, parturition has not been delayed (Brenner and Hendricks, 1962; Csapo *et al.*, 1966; Fuchs and Stakemann, 1960), but a limited effect on myometrial activity has been recorded when a progestin was given intravenously, intramniotically, or directly into the myometrium (Bengtsson, 1962; Hendricks *et al.*, 1961; Wood *et al.*, 1963).

f. Discussion and Conclusions. The characteristic inhibitory effects of progesterone on the myometrium have been clearly demonstrated to be greater at the placental site as compared to interplacental tissue. As will be discussed below (Section II, A, 7), the concentration of progesterone is very high in human retroplacental blood (Kumar and Barnes, 1965; Zander and von Munstermann, 1956), and the concentration of progesterone in the myometrium is highest subjacent to the placenta and diminishes progressively with increasing distance from the placenta (Kumar and Barnes, 1965; Kumar *et al.*, 1962; Zander *et al.*, 1969).

A large variety of evidence, in a wide range of species, supports the belief that placental progesterone has an important function in maintaining uterine quiescence via a locally mediated effect.

If progesterone penetrates the myometrium directly from the placenta, it is likely that it flows in the lymphatics and the interstitial fluid. The human uterus has an extremely rich lymphatic capillary bed, at least as extensive as the blood capillary bed, if not more so. These vessels increase in size in association with uterine growth during pregnancy (Maurizo and Ottaviani, 1934; Reynolds, 1949). The uterus of *Macaca mulatta* has been reported to be comparable, in this regard, to that of man (Wislocki and Dempsey, 1939).

In view of the relatively high concentration of progesterone in retroplacental blood, and the rapid destruction of progesterone in the peripheral circulation (half-life 6 minutes, Fylling, 1970b), it is possible that progesterone administered by any route other than directly into the intervillous space might not duplicate placental progesterone.

In the comparative spectrum, the extent to which a local effect of placental progesterone may have supplanted the significance of circulating progesterone of ovarian origin can only be surmised from the various extirpative experiments. It seems to be minimal in the rat and rabbit, intermediate in cattle, sheep, and guinea pigs, and of overriding importance in primates. This is the approximate order of the species in regard to the influence on uterine activity of exogenous progesterone, and it seems likely that the influence of placental progestrone is not readily duplicated by administered hormone.

4. Placental Progesterone Synthesis

a. General Considerations. Placental progesterone synthesis has been most adequately studied in human pregnancy. The secretion rate in human beings is the highest of any known species, about 290 mg per day (Van der Molen and Aakvaag, 1967). The main substrate is maternal blood cholesterol (K. Bloch, 1945; Solomon, 1960; Jaffe and Peterson, 1966; Morrison *et al.*, 1965; Ryan, 1966; Hellig *et al.*, 1969). While pregnenolone and its sulfated conjugate are readily converted to progesterone by the placenta (Pearlman *et al.*, 1954; Pion *et al.*, 1965, 1966), this is quantitatively not important (S. H. Conrad *et al.*, 1967; Younglai and Solomon, 1969). The limited *de novo* synthesis of progesterone from acetate (Van Leusden and Villee, 1965) does not appear to be physiologically significant (Hellig *et al.*, 1969). Placental progesterone production is not dependent on the fetus. There is no net secretion of progesterone from the fetus to the placenta (Harbert *et al.*, 1964), and following fetal death no important acute change in maternal blood progesterone (Lurie *et al.*, 1966) or pregnandiol excretion (Cassmer, 1959) is observed. Following fetal death, maternal blood progesterone falls slowly over a period of weeks (Wiest, 1967), suggesting a secondary effect due to the absence of the fetal–placental circulation. Placental progesterone production appears to be primarily a maternal–placental function.

b. Progesterone-Synthesizing Enzymes. The enzyme system involved in the synthesis of progesterone from cholesterol in the placenta has been investigated utilizing human tissue (Mason and Boyd, 1971; Meigs and Ryan, 1968; Morrison *et al.*, 1965). The removal of the side chain of cholesterol, to yield pregnenolone, is accomplished by a "mixed function oxidase," having an absolute requirement for molecular oxygen and reduced nicotinamide adenine dinucleotide phosphate (NADPH). The enzyme is confined to the mitochondria, and the reaction involves cytochrome P-450 and an electron transport chain composed of NADPH, a flavoprotein, and nonheme iron protein. The enzyme system is, therefore, like the cholesterol side chain-cleavage system in the adrenal cortex (Halkerston *et al.*, 1961; Simpson and Boyd, 1967ab).

Pregnenolone is converted to progesterone by a dehydrogenase and isomerase system, which is located largely in the microsomal cell fraction, and which requires nicotinamide adenine dinucleotide (NAD) as a cofactor. It is this latter reaction which has been utilized to test a variety of mammalian placentas for their capacity for progesterone synthesis.

c. Enzymatic Potential of Mammalian Placentas in Vitro. In vitro studies have demonstrated the enzymatic capacity for the conversion of pregnenolone to progesterone in the placentas of all species studied: rat (Townsend and Ryan, 1970), rabbit (Matsumoto *et al.*, 1969), cow and sheep (Ainsworth and Ryan, 1967), horse (Ainsworth and Ryan, 1969a), guinea pig (Bedwani and Marley, 1971), and 6 species of subhuman primates (Ainsworth and Ryan, 1969b; Ainsworth *et al.*, 1969; Ryan and Shinada, 1971).

d. Secretion in Vivo. The synthesis of progesterone by the rat and rabbit placentas *in vitro* is of interest. These two species have been the classical experimental models of "corpus luteum-dependent" animals, and direct measurement of progesterone in ovarian vein blood and peripheral blood (Csapo and Wiest, 1969; Grota and Eik-Nes, 1967; Hashimoto *et al.*, 1968; Wiest, 1970; Wiest *et al.*, 1968; Mikhail *et al.*, 1961) clearly indicates that essentially all of the circulating progesterone is of ovarian origin. There is indirect evidence that the rat placenta produces progesterone *in vivo* in small, but physiologically significant, quantities (Courrier and Gross, 1936; Csapo and Wiest, 1969; Selye *et al.*, 1935). There is suggestive evidence that the same may be true in the rabbit (Macedo-Costa and Csapo, 1959). The goat placenta has not been tested for progesterone synthesis *in vitro*. In this species there is a net consumption of progesterone in the pregnant uterus as determined by arteriovenous difference (Blom and Lyngset, 1971; Linzell and Heap, 1968).

In both the sheep (Basset *et al.*, 1969; Fylling, 1970a; Ronaldson, 1969) and the guinea pig (Heap and Deanesly, 1966), placental progesterone secretion *in vivo* has been established. In both of these "oophorectomy-tolerant" species, a substantial contribution to peripheral blood progesterone comes from the ovary throughout most of pregnancy. In late pregnancy, the ovarian contribution disappears and is reflected in falling blood progesterone levels. Also, in the cow, the ovary accounts for a significant portion of peripheral blood progesterone, and there is a modest decline of circulating progesterone in late pregnancy (Erb *et al.*, 1967).

In primates, the ovarian contribution to blood progesterone is significant only in early pregnancy. In *Macaca mulatta* (Neill *et al.*, 1969) and human beings (Diczfalusy and Borrell, 1961), oophorectomy during established pregnancy causes no observable decrease in progesterone production.

e. Control Mechanisms. In the ovary, progesterone synthesis and secretion are subject to complex control mechanisms (Wiest *et al.*, 1968) and, in general, ovarian progesterone secretion is curtailed before the end of pregnancy. With the possible exception of the sheep, no comparable mechanisms have been identified for the placenta.

In the oophorectomized guinea pig, the plasma progesterone concentration during the second half of gestation has been shown to correlate roughly with placental weight (Heap and Deanesly, 1966). From the general trend of plasma progesterone, it appears that the same gross correlation might be found in the oophorectomized cow, and in intact apes and human beings.

The growth of the placenta has been studied in greater depth in the rat and in human beings. In the growing rat placenta, there is a proportional increase in weight, protein content, ribonucleic acid (RNA), and deoxyribonucleic acid (DNA) until day 17. Thereafter, there is no further increase in DNA, indicating that cell replication has ceased. This conclusion is confirmed by the disappearance of observable mitotic figures and the cessation of thymidine-^{14}C incorporation. On days 18 and 19, when there is no further increase in DNA, placental weight, protein, and RNA continue to increase, indicating cellular growth and protein synthesis without nuclear replication. On days 20 and 21 (term), weight, protein, and RNA decrease proportionally (Jollie, 1964; Winick and Noble, 1966).

In the human placenta, a slowing in growth rate begins 3–4 weeks before term (Gruenwald and Minn, 1961; Hendricks, 1964). Up to about 35–36 weeks, growth is accompanied by proportional increases in protein, RNA, and DNA. At about 35–36 weeks, the increase in DNA ceases, while weight, protein, and RNA continue to increase proportionally. This growth pattern in the human placenta is quite comparable to that seen in the rat (Winick *et al.*, 1967). Therefore, in human pregnancy, the pattern of both plasma progesterone (E. D. B. Johansson, 1969) and urinary pregnanediol (Klopper and Billewicz, 1963) correspond very closely to DNA content, i.e., cell number of the placenta.

If plasma progesterone concentration accurately reflects placental synthesis in human beings, these data support the conclusion that placental progesterone synthesis is a largely autonomous process. Additional information on this subject concerning other primates is scant (Hobson, 1971; Ryan and Hopper, 1972).

The sheep is of special interest as it is the only species studied in which plasma progesterone of placental origin significantly diminishes prior to the initiation of labor (Basset *et al.*, 1969; Fylling, 1970a; Obst *et al.*, 1971; Ronaldson, 1969) and in which it might be proposed that an extrinsic control mechanism may influence placental progesterone secretion. This exception will be discussed below (Section III, F, 3). Other controlling influences might be envisioned, e.g., blood flow that delivers substrate cholesterol and oxygen, transport of cholesterol into the cell, or changes in synthetic or degradative enzymatic systems. With the possible exception of the sheep placenta, there is, at present, no substantial evidence to implicate any factor other than the growth of the placenta in the control of placental progesterone secretion.

f. Discussion and Conclusions. All placentas tested have the enzymatic capacity for the conversion of pregnenolone to progesterone. While direct evidence for *in vivo* secretion is negative in "corpus luteum-dependent" species, the possibility of some degree of physiological significance cannot be discarded at present (e.g., the physiological evidence for a local placental effect).

Mechanisms for governing placental progesterone synthesis might be anticipated, but, in general, they are not apparent. Secretion appears to be relatively autonomous, generally increasing in proportion to placental mass, or perhaps, more specifically, to DNA content. No absolute diminution of secretory activity prior to termination of pregnancy has been seen except in the sheep. Overall, while the role of placental progesterone in the maintenance of pregnancy seems well established, it appears, in most species, not to be a dynamic factor in the events leading to parturition.

5. Progesterone in the Placenta and Uterus

a. Placenta. With the notable exception of human beings, the placentas of all animals which have been studied *in vitro*, including subhuman primates, extensively metabolize progesterone to a wide variety of less active steroids (Table VI). The prominent metabolites are the ring-A reduced compounds, 5α-pregnanes in most species and 5β-pregnanes in cows and sheep. The 6β-hydroxy, 20β-hydroxy, and 20α-hydroxy compounds are minor products *in vitro*. *In vivo*, in human beings (Discfalusy, 1969), 6βOH-progesterone is formed to a limited degree, but the 20α-hydroxylase reaction is strongly in the direction of progesterone. The absence of ring-A reduction in the human placenta *in vitro*, confirmed *in vivo*, distinguishes the human placenta from all others tested. While the human placenta does not metabolize progesterone to any large extent,

TABLE VI

PROGESTERONE METABOLISM *in Vitro* BY MAMMALIAN PLACENTAS[a]

Metabolites	Species
5β-Pregnanediols, 5β-pregnanolones 5α-Pregnanediols, 5α-pregnanolones, 5α-pregnanediones	Cow, sheep Baboon, chimpanzee, orangutan, *Macaca mulatta, M. fascicularis,* squirrel monkey, horse, rat
6β-Hydroxyprogesterone	Human, baboon, chimpanzee, orangutan, *M. mulatta,* squirrel monkey
20α-Hydroxyprogesterone	Human, baboon, chimpanzee, orangutan, *M. mulatta,* *M. fascicularis,* horse, sheep, cow
20β-Hydroxyprogesterone	Horse, sheep, cow

[a]Data from Ainsworth *et al.* (1969), Ainsworth and Ryan (1967, 1969a,b), Ryan and Shinada (1971), and Townsend and Ryan (1970).

the *in vitro* studies indicate that in other species placental metabolism of progesterone to ring-A reduced compounds may be quantitatively significant.

b. Uterus. The metabolism of progesterone to a variety of compounds has been demonstrated in both the endometrium and the myometrium of the rat *in vitro* and *in vivo* (Wichmann, 1967; Wiest, 1963) and in human tissue *in vitro* (Bryson and Sweat, 1967, 1969). Ring-A reduction to 5α-pregnane compounds is prominent in both species, in addition to various hydroxylations. The rate of progesterone metabolism in the myometrium of the pregnant rat appears to be quite significant (Davies and Ryan, 1972; Wichmann, 1967).

c. Discussion and Conclusions. The biological significance of the placental metabolism of progesterone is not apparent. In the corpus luteum of the rat, metabolism of progesterone is related to the control of the rate of progesterone secretion (Wiest, 1970; Wiest *et al.*, 1968). However, no such mechanism is apparent in the placenta.

As with the placenta, the physiological significance of progesterone metabolism in the myometrium is not known. The metabolites appear to have less biological potency than progesterone, or none at all. At present, the evidence is that the biological activity of progesterone resides in the progesterone molecule itself (Wiest, 1969).

Our present concept is that progesterone is a hormone which acts rapidly and is removed from the tissue rapidly, the absence of a continuing source of hormone resulting in prompt withdrawal effects in the tissue (Davies and Ryan, 1972). In this context, the relatively rapid metabolism of progesterone in the myometrium may facilitate the control of effective tissue concentrations of the hormone.

Regardless of the biological implications of the metabolism of progesterone in placental and uterine tissues, it is certain that this clearance of hormone must be considered in the interpretation of blood concentrations and arteriovenous differences across the uterus. This is well exemplified by the goat, in which there is a net consumption of progesterone by the pregnant uterus (Blom and Lyngset, 1971; Linzell and Heap, 1968).

6. Blood Progesterone

a. *Corpus Luteum Dependent Species.* In species in which the ovary is the primary source of progesterone throughout the pregnancy, the changes in blood progesterone measured serially throughout pregnancy are qualitatively similar. In the rat (Csapo and Wiest, 1969; Grota and Eik-Nes, 1967; Hashimoto et al., 1968; Wiest, 1970; Wiest et al., 1968), rabbit (Mikhail et al., 1961), sow (Short, 1960), and goat (Blom and Lyngset, 1971; Linzell and Heap, 1968), there is a progessive rise to a peak around mid-pregnancy followed by a gradual decline to low levels at term. In some species, such as the hamster (Leavitt and Blaha, 1970), the rise may continue until later in pregnancy with an abrupt drop preceding parturition. There are no known exceptions to the overall pattern, and it may be taken as reflecting corpus luteum function in pregnancy in "oophorectomy-intolerant" species.

b. *Intermediate Species.* In the sheep, a similar pattern is observed. The peak occurs late at 130–140 days and is followed by a sharp decline. In sheep, oophorectomized at 110–125 days, there is a postoperative drop in plasma progesterone, and thereafter levels remain quite constant. The normal peak is abolished and the concentrations are less than half those found in intact animals. As was mentioned previously, however, even in the oophorectomized animals, a decline in plasma progesterone was observed in the last few days of pregnancy (Basset and Thorburn, 1969; Challis et al., 1971; Fylling, 1970a; Obst et al., 1971; Ronaldson, 1969). This is the only species studied in which the placental contribution to plasma progesterone has been observed to decline substantially before labor begins.

It should be emphasized that plasma concentrations may not accurately reflect placental synthesis. At 125 days, the plasma progesterone of the oophorectomized sheep was about half that of intact animals (Fylling, 1970a). Direct measurement of uterine vein secretion rates at this time indicated that the progesterone secretion rate of the placenta was at least 5-fold that of the ovary (Linzell and Heap, 1968).

In the cow, plasma progesterone also rises gradually until near term. During the 2 weeks preceding calving, the levels are constant, or perhaps slightly decline. In oophorectomized cows near term, the plasma progesterone is about half that of intact animals, and the same plateau or minimal decline is observed during the last 2–3 weeks (Erb *et al.*, 1967).

c. Placenta-Dependent Species. Plasma progesterone has been measured throughout pregnancy in 3 species of macaques and in human beings. The pattern in early pregnancy is similar in all 4 species. Progesterone rises to an initial peak, attributable to corpus luteum secretion. A short-lived decline is followed by a second peak attributable to placental secretion. A second decline which occurs in the macaques is seen as a plateauing in human beings at 12–14 weeks. Throughout the remainder of gestation in *M. mulatta* (Neill *et al.*, 1969), plasma progesterone is relatively low (2–4 ng/ml) and shows no upward trend. The pattern in *M. iris* and *M. radiata* (Stabenfeldt and Hendrickx, 1971) is similar. Human beings differ in that blood progesterone gradually increases from 10 weeks to about 37 weeks before plateauing, and absolute concentrations are much higher throughout. Each of the 5 individual *M. mulatta* studied showed a curious slight increase in plasma progesterone preceding parturition. In human beings studied individually, both rising and falling levels have been observed at the onset of labor (Kumar *et al.*, 1964; Yannone, 1968).

d. Discussion and Conclusions. In short-gestation species which are "corpus luteum-dependent," plasma progesterone rises during pregnancy and declines prior to parturition, and an inverse relationship between circulating progesterone and uterine activity is apparent. In some "intermediate" species, which are "oophorectomy-tolerant," we observe the same rise and fall in blood progesterone. The decline is related to diminishing corpus luteum function, and, with the exception of the sheep, placental progesterone synthesis is unabated. The relative importance of blood progesterone concentration as opposed to placental secretion in these "intermediate" species is unknown. In primates, the ovarian contribution is unimportant in the last two-thirds of pregnancy (Diczfalusy and Borrell, 1961; Neill *et al.*, 1969).

In general, it would appear that while a source of progesterone is common to the maintenance of pregnancy in all mammals, and a "withdrawal" of this source is characteristic of "corpus luteum-dependent" species, continued secretion from the placenta until term is the rule in "oophorectomy-tolerant" species.

The interpretation of blood progesterone concentrations may be complicated by many factors, e.g., placental metabolism, uterine metabolism, serum-protein binding, efficient hepatic clearance, changes in blood flow. Some of these parameters are known to change during pregnancy, and some are known to differ between species.

7. Myometrial Progesterone

Tissue Concentrations. The concentration of progesterone in the myometrium has been studied in 2 species, the rat and human beings. During the course of pregnancy in the rat, the progesterone content of the myometrium rises to a peak, and then falls, in a pattern similar to that of plasma. However, in mid-pregnancy the myometrial progesterone concentration is approximately 3-fold that of plasma. As pregnancy progresses, this differential diminishes and, at term, it has disappeared (Wiest, 1970). The timing of parturition correlates better with the concentration of progesterone in the myometrium than it does with that of plasma. The continuation of pregnancy in the oophorectomized rat, either with or without supplementary progesterone, is associated with the support of a myometrial progesterone concentration above 2 μg/100 gm. Parturition, prematurely or at term, is associated with a myometrial progesterone concentration below 2 μg/100 gm (Csapo and Wiest, 1969; Wiest, 1970).

In human beings, the concentration of progesterone in the myometrium during pregnancy is higher than that of peripheral venous blood, but not as high as that of blood from the retroplacental pool or the uterine vein (Kumar and Barnes, 1965; Zander and von Munstermann, 1956). The myometrial progesterone concentration is highest subjacent to the placenta and diminishes with increasing distance from the placenta. This gradient seems to diminish in magnitude as pregnancy progresses to term. The absolute concentration of progesterone in the myometrium varies widely between individuals throughout pregnancy, and no trend of change in mean values has been established (Kumar and Barnes, 1961, 1965; Zander et al., 1969).

In the "placenta-dependent" mammal, we have substantial evidence for a locally mediated influence of placental progesterone on the myometrium. The nature of this local relationship is not understood in depth, however it is clear that we should not assume that there must be a simple relationship between progesterone in the myometrium and progesterone concentration in the peripheral blood.

8. Cytoplasmic Progesterone-Binding Protein

a. General Considerations. Current understanding of the mechanisms by which steroid hormones act upon target tissues indicates that the binding of hormone by specific cytoplasmic "receptor" proteins is an important primary event. It is believed that the binding of the hormone by the "receptor" protein is followed by movement of the protein–steroid complex to the nucleus where alteration of cellular function is initiated (Jensen et al., 1969). The application of this concept to progesterone has been substantiated in relation to progesterone-stimulated protein synthesis in the chick oviduct (O'Malley, 1971).

Cytoplasmic "receptor" proteins have been identified in the cytoplasm of the myometrium of nonpregnant rats (Milgrom and Baulieu, 1970), rabbits (McGuire and DeDella, 1971), guinea pigs (Falk and Bardin, 1970), Macaca mulatta, and human beings (Davies and Ryan, 1971), and also in the myometrium of pregnant rats (Davies and Ryan, 1972), M. mulatta, and man (Davies and Ryan, 1971).

b. Uterine Uptake of Progesterone. As shown by Wiest (1970), the concentration of progesterone in rat myometrium in early and mid-pregnancy is 3-fold that of plasma. This differential subsequently diminishes, and at term the concentration in the myometrium is similar to that of plasma. Davies and Ryan (1972) demonstrated that radio-labeled progesterone injected into the rat in mid-pregnancy is taken up by the myometrium and that this uptake is markedly diminished at term. A "receptor" protein was identified in the cytoplasmic cell fraction, and it was shown that the binding activity of this "receptor" markedly diminished between mid-pregnancy and term.

c. Discussion and Conclusions. In "corpus luteum-dependent" species the rise and subsequent fall of plasma progesterone has been considered sufficient to explain both the maintenance of pregnancy and the initiation of parturition. These experiments suggest that the physiological effects of progesterone on target tissues may be modulated not only by variations in plasma progesterone concentration, but by changes in "receptor" protein activity.

B. ESTROGENS

1. General Considerations

Estrogens are generally believed to have an important function in mammalian gestation by virtue of a variety of anabolic and metabolic effects (McKerns, 1967; Needham and Shoenberg, 1967; Segal and Scher, 1967). Estrogen is concerned generally with the growth of the uterus, and more specifically with the synthesis of the proteins of the contractile mechanism and of enzymes concerned in energy provision. In view of this, it is somewhat surprising that pregnancy can continue in oophorectomized animals in a number of species without any evident source of estrogen.

Nevertheless, optimal hormone replacement therapy in oophorectomized animals is accomplished with a combination of estrogen and progesterone,

(Amoroso and Finn, 1962), and the presence of both hormones may be considered to be the physiological situation in all mammals.

2. Ovarian Estrogen Synthesis

In short-gestation species, estrogen synthesis is a function of the ovarian follicles. The estrogens are synthesized from acetate without the need for preformed steroid substrates. While the corpora lutea of these species make progesterone, they do not carry the sequence further to C_{19} (andro-gen) synthesis and subsequent estrogen production. The human corpus luteum is unique in having sufficient 17,20-desmolase activity for the efficient synthesis of estrogens from acetate (Savard et al., 1965).

3. Placental Estrogen Synthesis

a. General Considerations. While there is a positive relationship be-tween the normal length of gestation of different species and their capability for progesterone synthesis in the placenta, the association between long gestation and the capacity for placental estrogen synthesis is even more impressive. There is no known species with a gestational period which exceeds 70 days in which placental estrogen synthesis is not found.

b. Estrogen Synthesis in Vitro. Placentas of a variety of species have been studied in vitro to establish their enzymatic capacity for aromatiza-tion of androgen substrates (Table VII). All the placentas which pro-duced estrogens made estrone and estradiol-17β. The placentas of the goat, sheep, and cow also made estradiol-17α.

c. Estrogen Synthesis in Vivo. That the enzymatic potential for estro-gen synthesis demonstrated by the in vitro experiments is meaningful in terms of secretion in vivo is supported by a variety of indirect evidence. (1) The results correlate with the finding of estrogen in placental extracts.

TABLE VII

AROMATIZATION OF ANDROSTENEDIONE BY MAMMALIAN PLACENTAS

Species	Estrogens formed	References
Human, orangutan, squirrel monkey, *Macaca mulatta*, *M. cynomolgus*, marmoset, horse, pig	Estrone, estradiol-17β	Ainsworth et al. (1969), Ainsworth and Ryan (1966, 1969b), Ryan et al. (1961)
Sheep, cow, goat	Estrone, estradiol-17β estradiol-17α	Ainsworth and Ryan (1966), Ainsworth and Ryan (1970)
Rat, rabbit, guinea pig	None	Ainsworth and Ryan (1966), Townsend and Ryan (1970)

(2) The species variations in the epimers of estradiol correlate with the estrogens found in the urine. (3) The abrupt fall in urinary or blood estrogens following delivery of the placenta, which is well known in human beings has been observed in cows (Erb *et al.*, 1967; Mellin *et al.*, 1966; Osinga, 1970), sheep (Challis, 1971), pigs (Raeside, 1963; Fevre *et al.*, 1968; Rombauts, 1962), and goats (Challis and Linzell, 1971). In the pig, it has been shown that after both hypophysectomy and oophorectomy of the pregnant sow, the normal rising level of estrogen excretion is maintained. The same is true of the oophorectomized ewe (Rombauts *et al.*, 1967; Fevre *et al.*, 1968).

d. The Fetalplacental Unit. The concept of the fetal placental unit in human pregnancy (Diczfalusy, 1964) is well established and has been reviewed in detail elsewhere (Diczfalusy, 1969). According to this concept, the fetus and placenta form a functional unit to carry out steroid biosynthetic reactions together, which the placenta per se or the fetus per se are incapable of completing (Diczfalusy, 1964).

A central feature of this relationship is that the synthesis of estrogens

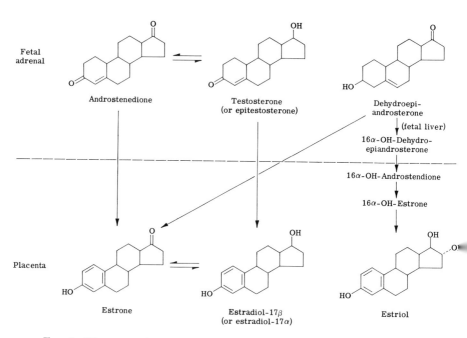

Fetal adrenal

Androstenedione   Testosterone (or epitestosterone)   Dehydroepiandrosterone

↓ (fetal liver)

16α-OH-Dehydroepiandrosterone

16α-OH-Androstendione

16α-OH-Estrone

Placenta

Estrone   Estradiol-17β (or estradiol-17α)   Estriol

Fig. 1. Diagrammatic representation of the relationships between the major estrogens in pregnancy urine and their adrenal androgen precursors. The pathways are well established for human beings. For applicability to other species, see text (Section II, B, 3, *d*).

is dependent upon the combined capabilities of the fetal adrenal and the placenta (Frandsen and Stakemann, 1963; MacDonald and Siiteri, 1965). The placenta lacks the 17,20-desmolase necessary for the conversion of C_{21} compounds (pregnenolone, progesterone) to C_{19} (androgen) estrogen precursors.

The fetal adrenal synthesizes C_{19} compounds. These androgens are transferred to the placenta, where they are aromatized to form estrogens (Fig. 1). This interdependent relationship is unique in steroid synthesis. It may be an interesting peculiarity, or it could be an important physiological mechanism. It is of great interest to know whether it might be applicable to all mammals which synthesize estrogens in the placenta.

Of all the placentas which have been tested *in vitro* (Table VII), none has been found to have the 17,20-desmolase which is essential for the conversion of pregnenolone to C_{19} estrogen precursors. When either placenta or fetal adrenal tissue separately were incubated with pregnenolone, neither tissue produced estrogen. When the two tissues mixed together were incubated with pregnenolone, estrogen was synthesized (Table VIII). The synthesis of an estrogen precursor, androstenedione, by the fetal adrenal was demonstrated *in vitro* for the pig and sheep (Table VIII), and *in vivo* in *M. mulatta* (Younglai et al., 1969). From incubations of guinea pig fetal adrenal, 11βOH-androstenedione was recovered (E. Bloch, 1969).

There is additional evidence obtained *in vivo* which indicates that the concept of the fetal-placental unit, as it applies to placental estrogen synthesis, is applicable to mammals other than man. In both the cow (Osinga, 1970) and the pig (Rombauts, 1964), an abrupt drop in urinary estrogen has been observed in association with intrauterine fetal death.

e. Urinary Estrogens. The specific estrogen compounds which have been found in pregnancy urine of various species (Table IX) are generally consistent with the results of the *in vitro* studies of placental estrogen

TABLE VIII

ESTROGEN SYNTHESIS FROM PREGNENOLONE BY COMBINATIONS OF FETAL ADRENALS AND PLACENTAS FROM SHEEP,[a] PIG,[b] AND *Macaca fascicularis*[a]

Tissue	Estrogen formed	Androstendione formed
Placenta alone	−	−
Fetal adrenal alone	−	+
Fetal adrenal plus placenta	+	−

[a] Davies et al. (1970).
[b] Ryan and Petro (1971).

TABLE IX
URINARY ESTROGENS IN PREGNANCY

Species	Estrone	17α-Estradiol	17β-Estradiol	Estriol	Reference
Pig	++++				Raeside (1963)
Goat	++++	+			Klyne and Wright (1957)
Sheep	++	++++			Fevre and Rombauts (1966)
Cow	+++	++++	+		Mellin et al. (1966)
Horse	++++	+	Trace		Bhavnani et al. (1969)
Macaca mulatta	++++		++	+	Hopper and Tullner (1967)
Baboon	++++		+	+	Merkatz and Beling (1969)
Chimpanzee	++		+	++++	Jirku and Layne (1965)
Gorilla	++		+	++++	Hopper et al. (1968)
Human	++		+	++++	Brown (1956)

synthesis. This provides additional indirect confirmation that the placenta is the important site of estrogen synthesis *in vivo*. Estrone is found in the urine of all the species studied, and it is quantitatively predominant in most species, with the noteworthy exception of apes and man. Estradiol has been found in all the species except the pig. The 17α epimer of estradiol is characteristic of the nonprimates, whereas in primates, the estradiol is the 17β epimer. Estriol has been satisfactorily demonstrated only in primates, and it is the predominant urinary estrogen only in apes and man. If the significance of estriol in human pregnancy urine can be assumed to apply to the subhuman primates, it is a reflection of 16α-hydroxylation by the fetal liver of fetal adrenal androgens, which are the precursors for placental estrogen synthesis (Fig. 1).

Ring B unsaturated estrogens, equilen and equilenin, are peculiar to horses. The biosynthetic pathway for their synthesis is not understood. Their relative physiological importance is not known, but they are quantitatively less important than estrone in the urine of the pregnant mare (Savard, 1961; Bhavnani et al., 1969).

If the increasing proportional amount of estriol is to be considered as a possible evolutionary trend, it is important to note that the large quantity of estriol is associated with a large total urinary estrogen, which includes increased absolute quantities of estrone and estradiol. Estrogens are potent hormones, biologically effective in microgram amounts. The placental production of so much estrogen, 100–200 mg/24 hours in man (Oakey, 1970), suggests the possibility of toxicity for the fetus.

Excretion of large quantities of estriol is seen in those species with higher production of estrone and estradiol. Estriol is not only a less potent estrogen, but inhibits the activity of estrone and estradiol, as measured by uterine growth stimulation in rats (Hisaw et al., 1954). As previously indicated, estriol production reflects 16α-hydroxylation by the fetal liver of estrogen precursors which would otherwise be converted to estrone and estradiol by the placenta. In addition, estrogens which reach the fetus from the placenta are extensively hydroxylated. Estrogens in the fetal circulation also are extensively sulfo-conjugated by most, if not all, fetal tissues (Diczfalusy, 1969). In human pregnancy, fetal plasma estriol levels are 10 times higher than maternal levels, and fetal estrone and estradiol are much lower than maternal concentrations (Aitken et al., 1958; Klausner and Ryan, 1964; Maner et al., 1963; Roy, 1962).

While the significance of estriol in primate pregnancy can only be surmised, it is seen in association with high production of total estrogen and appears to be one facet of a total fetal economy which limits the concentration of the potent estrogens to which the fetus is exposed.

While the absolute amounts of urinary estrogens varies markedly between species, it appears to be generally true that estrogen excretion rises progressively during pregnancy. This has been seen in the horse (Savard, 1961), cow (Erb et al., 1967; Mellin et al., 1966; Osinga, 1970), sheep (Fevre and Rombauts, 1966), goat (Challis and Linzell, 1971), and in the 4 species of subhuman primates and human beings included in Table IX. No exceptions have been identified. In the pig, goat, and sheep, a temporary decrease may be observed in late pregnancy, followed by a rapid rise until parturition.

f. Blood Estrogens. Recently developed sensitive methods for plasma estrogen determination are providing new information. As would be expected, progressively rising plasma estrogen has been found in the rat (Davies and Yen, 1971), goat (Challis and Linzell, 1971), sheep (Challis, 1971; Findlay and Cox, 1970), macaque (Davies and Yen, 1971), and human beings (Tulchinsky and Korenman, 1971). A dramatic acute rise in plasma estrogen is seen just prior to parturition in sheep and, to a lesser extent, in goats. This is not a regular occurrence in the macaque or in human beings.

g. Discussion and Conclusions. Estrogen synthesis by the placenta is found uniformly in species in which gestation exceeds 70 days. While the evidence is incomplete, it appears likely that the dependence of the placenta on estrogen precursors (androgens) from the fetal adrenal is generally applicable. The pattern of estrogen secretion appears to be one of continuous increase until parturition, and in some species there is an accelerated increase prior to parturition.

If this intepretation of the data is correct, then a mechanism has been identified by which the mammalian fetus exercises an important control in the hormonal milieu of pregnancy.

III. The Initiation of Parturition

A. General Considerations

In much of the debate concerning the role of progesterone in the maintenance of pregnancy it has been assumed that the theory of such a role for progesterone must include an explanation for the termination of gestation. It is not apparent that the two matters must necessarily be related in a direct manner. For clarity of thinking, it seems advisable to consider the two subjects separately.

B. The Corpus Luteum

The corpus luteum is essential for the initiation of gestation in all mammals, and a continuing source of progesterone is required for the accomodation of the growing conceptus. For pregnancy to continue beyond the normal luteal phase of the estrous cycle, prolongation of the life of the corpus luteum would seem to be the simplest solution. Pseudo-pregnancy, which can be elicited in a number of small animals, illustrates this mechanism. The ferret will be described as an example. In the ferret, sterile-mating with a vasectomized male induces a pseudopregnancy which is equal in length to normal pregnancy (Hammond and Marshall, 1930). The pituitary is essential for the maintenance of pregnancy and is believed to be the major source of luteotropin (McPhail, 1935). Pseudo-pregnancy can be induced by a single injection of luteotropin, and plasma progesterone levels in 30-day pregnant or pseudopregnant ferrets are equal (Carlson and Rust, 1969). Therefore, the maintenance of pregnancy appears to be a maternal neuroendocrine function.

In both the ferret and the rat, manipulation of the maternal pituitary–ovarian system in late pregnancy can interfere with the initiation of parturition. Throughout most of pregnancy, hypophysectomy results in abortion. However, hypophysectomy done just before term results in prolonged gestation in both the ferret (McPhail, 1935) and the rat (Boe, 1938; Pencharz and Long, 1933; Seyle et al., 1933). The fetuses are retained and die in utero. It has been shown in the rat that oophorectomy just before term has the same result as hypophysectomy, failure of the initiation of labor (Hain, 1934, 1935). These rats which have been oophorectomized just before term are unresponsive to oxytocin stimulation; however, injection of estrogen results in parturition in 12–24 hours (Csapo, 1969).

In 1935, Newton observed in pregnant mice when he killed the fetuses *in utero*, the placentas delivered at normal term. These experiments, and similar studies in rats (Kirsch, 1938; Selye *et al.*, 1933; Thiersch, 1960), have sometimes been interpreted as implying that the life-span of the placenta determines the length of gestation in these species. However, in 1938, Newton and Lits found that the "fetectomized" mice carried their placentas to term only if the ovaries were intact. Removal of the fetuses accompanied by oophorectomy resulted in abortion of the placentas. The same results were reported in hamsters (Klein, 1938). Therefore, these results implicate the ovaries, not the placenta, in the timing of parturition.

The experiments which have been discussed support the hypothesis of maternal neuroendocrine control of the timing of parturition in these short-gestation species, and seem to exclude any important role for the fetus and placenta in this connection.

However, this model is limited to short-gestation species. For most mammals, the question becomes, what modifications have been established to provide for longer gestation?

C. ADAPTATIONS TO LONG GESTATION

Perhaps the simplest identifiable mechanism for the extension of gestation beyond the length of pseudopregnancy is the production of placental gonadotropin. For example, this is believed to be true of the rat (Amoroso and Finn, 1962).

Species with gestational periods longer than 60 days usually secrete progesterone from the placenta in quantities sufficient to maintain pregnancy in the absence of the ovaries (Table V). In species with gestational periods longer than 151 days, this is the rule.

Placental estrogen synthesis has been found in all species in which pregnancy exceeds 70 days (Table VII). In human beings, it is well established that placental estrogen synthesis is dependent upon precursors supplied by the fetal adrenal, and evidence has been presented which indicates that this is true of mammals generally. The observations that will be reviewed in subsequent sections support the view that, in adaptation to prolonged gestation, the control of the timing of normal parturition has passed from the neuroendocrine system of the mother to that of the fetus.

D. ESTROGEN AND UTERINE CONTRACTILITY

In addition to the anabolic and metabolic effects that estrogen exerts on the uterus, it is well known to be important for the spontaneous, rhythmic, contractile activity that is characteristic of myometrium (Reynolds, 1949; Marshall, 1962). The excised uterus of a castrate or anestrus animal is inactive. Estrogen administration, prior to excision of the uterus, increases the membrane potential, initiates the spontaneous discharge of action potentials, and induces rhythmic, contractile activity. It is this estrogenized, active preparation which is inhibited by progesterone. There is a characteristic time-lag in the induction of this estrogen-induced activity *in vivo*. This probably explains the inability to demonstrate this effect of estrogen *in vitro*.

It should be noted that both the growth of the uterus and spontaneous activity can be induced in the castrate rat by uterine distension. This indicates that estrogen is not essential for these changes under all circumstances (Section III, G, 1).

There is evidence in the rat that parturition in the estrogen-deprived animal is not normal. As indicated above (Section III, B), in rats which continue pregnancy following oophorectomy 48 hours before term, parturition at the expected time does not usually occur and the fetuses eventually die *in utero*. Administration of estradiol results in delivery in 12–24 hours. In oophorectomized animals not given estrogen, those which do deliver following oophorectomy have a prolonged labor with a high fetal mortality.

Hindsen *et al.* (1969) reported the results on three ewes which were injected with 20 mg of stilbesterol 2 weeks before term. Uterine activity developed within 24 hours and two of the ewes delivered within 30 hours. In the third ewe, uterine activity increased, reached a maximum in 36 hours, and subsequently declined. In this ewe, parturition occurred normally 2 weeks later with the delivery of twins. Pierrepont *et al.* (1970) infused epitestosterone (a potential placental estrogen precursor) into a lamb fetus and successfully induced parturition.

Efforts to stimulate the contractile activity of the pregnant uterus in human beings by administration of estrogen have been largely ineffectual (Kelly, 1961; Klopper and Dennis, 1962; Martin and Menzies, 1955). Resort to large doses intravenously, and to intrauterine administration, did produce a minimal effect. The intravenous infusion of 17β-estradiol at 200–400 μg/minute to women near term elicited an increase in uterine tone and contractile activity. The cervix softened and dilated, and the uterine sensitivity to oxytocin increased (Pinto *et al.*, 1964). In a group of women who were given estriol-sulfate directly into the amniotic cavity, an increase in uterine activity, as compared to controls, was observed 5 hours after the initiation of treatment (Klopper *et al.*, 1969).

As we have discussed above in relation to progesterone, it is highly questionable whether exogenously administered steroids can substitute for hormones which are synthesized in the placenta, which is in immediate apposition to the uterine wall.

E. Estrogen : Progesterone Ratio

It is clear that progesterone and estrogen are intimately related in their cellular effects. In regard to their action on uterine tissues, physiological effects are related to the relative amounts of the two hormones. From the evidence which has been reviewed, the following generalizations might be inferred: (1) For the maintenance of pregnancy in an oophorectomized animal, there is an optimal estrogen-progesterone ratio. (2) Estrogen, over a period of time, induces spontaneous uterine activity. (3) Progesterone inhibits the generation and propagation of estrogen-induced electrocontractile activity. (4) In the physiological range, the inhibition of uterine by progesterone is not an all-or-none phenomenon, but a matter of degree which is dose-dependent.

In "corpus luteum-dependent" species, diminution of progesterone secretion prior to parturition is the rule (Section II, B, 6). The effectiveness of administered progesterone in delaying parturition supports the belief that declining progesterone secretion plays an important role in the timing of parturition.

In species in which the placenta produces progesterone, an absolute decrease in placental progesterone secretion is not usually found. In the sheep, decreasing blood progesterone during the last half of pregnancy is due largely to diminishing corpus luteum activity, although, during the week preceding parturition, placental progesterone secretion apparently falls. Also in the guinea pig and probably the cow, plasma progesterone declines in the last half of pregnancy. However, in both the oophorectomized guinea pig and the oophorectomized cow, it is seen that this decline is due entirely to decreasing corpus luteum secretion, the placental contribution being sustained until term.

In primates, corpus luteum function becomes insignificant early in pregnancy, and no fall in placental progesterone secretion is seen prior to labor. However, insofar as blood and urinary measurements reflect placental secretion, rising progesterone production is not observed during late pregnancy. The macaque maintains a low, more-or-less constant level throughout most of gestation. In human beings the progressively increasing plasma progesterone and urinary pregnanediol concentrations plateau during the last weeks of pregnancy.

As indicated above (Section II, B, 3), urinary and plasma estrogens increase progressively until parturition in all species for which we have adequate information. An acute increase shortly before parturition is evident in the goat, sheep, and cow. In primates the increase is more gradual.

Klopper and Billewicz (1963) measured urinary pregnanediol and estriol serially in pregnant women. In early pregnancy, the ratio of pregnanediol to estriol was 100:1. At 20 weeks it was 3:1. Between 20 weeks and term the ratio gradually decreased to about 1:1. He also observed an inverse correlation between estriol excretion and gestational length. Subjects with higher estriol tended to deliver earlier than those with lower estriol. This latter relationship was evident for estriol determinations done at both 20 weeks and at 38 weeks. This observation in human beings has been confirmed (Turnbull and Anderson, 1969), and the same correlation was noted in cows (Erb *et al.*, 1967). No relationship between pregnanediol excretion and gestational length is evident. The increasing estrogen:progesterone ratio described by Klopper can be related temporally to the gradually increasing uterine activity observed between mid-gestation and term (Caldeyro-Barcia, 1964; Csapo and Sauvage, 1968; Hendricks and Brenner, 1964). It might also be correlated with the rapid growth of the fetal zone of the fetal adrenal gland (the source of the estrogen precursors) between 28 weeks and term (Lanman, 1953).

In connection with the proposed relationship between estrogen:progesterone ratio and the gradual evolution of uterine activity observed in human beings, comparison with the sheep is of interest. In the sheep, we observe low levels of estrogens accompanied by relatively high progesterone throughout most of pregnancy. There is an acute rise in estrogen at term, accompanied by a fall in progesterone (Section II, A, 6 and B, 3). In contrast to primates, uterine contractile activity in the ewe cannot be detected until 12 hours before parturition, at which time rapid evolution of activity occurs, culminating in parturition (Hindson *et al.*, 1965).

A single case report of a woman with placental sulfatase deficiency, while admittedly anecdotal, is of interest (France and Liggins, 1969). This patient was found to have urinary estrogens 5% of normal values in two successive pregnancies. Enzymatic studies on the placentas from the last two pregnancies clearly defined a marked deficiency of the sulfatase enzyme which is required for hydrolysis of C_{19}-sulfate the initial step in human placental estrogen synthesis. Information is given for the last five of her pregnancies. One of these aborted at 22 weeks. Two ended at 42 weeks following intrauterine fetal death. In the last two pregnancies, attempted induction of labor at 38 weeks was ineffectual, delivery being accomplished by cesarean section. This is the only example of defective placental estrogen synthesis which has been recognized, and, therefore, the possible association between estrogen deficiency and the failure of labor to occur at the normal time cannot be established.

F. Fetal Adrenal

1. Short Gestation Species

Species such as the rat, mouse, rabbit, hamster, and ferret, which have short gestational periods, have been characterized as being largely dependent on the ovary for the steroid hormones of pregnancy. It has been suggested that the initiation of parturition in these species is primarily under maternal neuroendocrine control, the role of the fetus being largely passive (Section III, B).

The adrenal cortex of the rat fetus grows substantially between days 16 and 20 of pregnancy and is under fetal hypothalamic-pituitary stimulation. Between day 20 and parturition the adrenal ceases growth, and appears to be less active and unresponsive to ACTH. In the neonatal rat, and in the fetus *in utero* with artificially prolonged pregnancy, adrenal growth and ACTH responsiveness resume on about day 24. Therefore, in the rat, the time of parturition is apparently associated with quiescence of the fetal adrenal. The same seems to be true in the mouse and the rabbit (Jost, 1966).

2. Long-Gestation Species

a. General Considerations. Generally, species with longer gestational periods have the capacity for placental steroid synthesis. More specifically, and without exception, species in which pregnancy exceeds 70 days have been found to synthesize estrogen in the placenta. Furthermore, it seems likely that the requirement for performed C_{19} precursors is generally applicable and estrogen synthesis may be dependent on precursors of fetal origin (Section II, B, 3).

As the fetal neuroendocrine system appears to develop on a predictable timetable (Kerr *et al.*, 1969; Lanman, 1953), the hypothesis of fetal neuroendocrine control of the timing of normal parturition is attractive. It has long been recognized in animal husbandry that, in the mating of different breeds, the length of gestation was determined by both the dam and the sire, i.e., by the fetal genotype (Clegg, 1959; Holm, 1967). This correlation is seen even more dramatically in the interbreeding of different species (Table X).

b. Cattle. Prolonged pregnancy in association with a congenitally ab-

TABLE X

APPROXIMATE LENGTH OF GESTATION IN HORSE-DONKEY CROSSES[a]

Stallion × mare	340 Days
Stallion × jennet	350 Days
Jack × mare	355 Days
Jack × jennet	365 Days

[a] Derived from data of Asdell (1946).

normal calf is relatively common in inbred cattle (Holm, 1967; Kennedy, 1971). Of particular interest are two syndromes which have received systematic study. The ancestry of 30 over-term Holstein calves was traced to a single bull, and it was determined that the abnormality was due to a single autosomal recessive gene. The same cows which carried the prolonged-pregnancy calves had normal pregnancies when bred with normal bulls. The abnormal pregnancies are usually characterized by partial or complete failure of the usual signs of impending parturition such as filling of the udder, pelvic ligament relaxation, vulvar swelling, and cervical secretion. When these signs do partially appear at term, they subsequently regress, and pregnancy continues for as long as 374 days (normal term 280 days). The calves become overgrown and post-mature, but are otherwise grossly normal. The calves rarely survive vaginal delivery and, if delivered by cesarean section, even shortly after normal term, they quickly die. Prolonged survival has been obtained only by corticosteroid therapy. It has been established that the calves' adrenals secrete no 17-OH corticosteroids into the adrenal effluent and their adrenals are unresponsive to ACTH.

A different syndrome is seen in Guernsey cattle in which the fetus shows gross defects of the skull and brain. Aplasia of the adenohypophysis is a consistent finding, and the neurohypophysis may be hypoplastic. These calves all die within a few minutes of birth and are incapable of ventilating their lungs. They are hypoglycemic at birth, and postmortem findings include pituitary aplasia, adrenal and thyroid hypoplasia, and jejunal atresia. These findings are all consistent with pituitary-adrenal insufficiency.

In both these syndromes of prolonged pregnancy, the uterus is hypotonic, flaccid, and completely unresponsive to oxytocin. Determination of blood steroid levels in the cows disclosed that progesterone is maintained at mid-pregnancy values. Estrogen, which normally increases up to term in normal pregnancies, shows a peak earlier than term in these abnormal pregnancies and is declining as the time for normal parturition approaches. Estradiol infusion into the cow resulted only in fetal death.

In normal pregnant cattle, the injection of 20 mg of dexamethasone at 262–280 days (0–18 days before term) induced parturition within 56 hours. In 4 cows injected earlier, it was successful in only one (Adams, 1969; W. M. Adams and Wagner, 1969). The induction of parturition in cows with potent glucocorticoids has been confirmed by Osinga (1970).

c. *Sheep.* In ewes, syndromes of prolonged pregnancy have also been reported. They are of nongenetic origin, the primary determinant in each instance being a particular dietary plant ingested by the pregnant ewe (Holm, 1967; Kennedy, 1971). The disorder which has been most adequately studied is that which occurs in the United States in southwestern Idaho. The toxic plant is *Veratrum californicum* and the teratogen is a steroidal alkaloid, 11-deoxyjervine (cyclopamine). Ewes which ingest the plant on day 14 of gestation produce offspring with various cephalic anomalies, and pregnancy may be prolonged as much as 6–9 weeks beyond term. The anatomic description of the postterm calves is not complete. The pituitary is present but the apparent absence of hypothalamic-pituitary connections has been reported.

Prolonged pregnancy in normal sheep has been induced experimentally by fetal adrenalectomy *in utero* (Drost and Holm, 1968). In some lambs, adrenal cortical tissue regenerated, and these were born at term. When removal of the adrenals was complete, the ewe failed to show the usual changes in the udder, pelvic ligaments, and vulva at normal term (147 days) and pregnancy was prolonged up to 180 days. Fetal hypophysectomy prolonged pregnancy up to 187 days (Liggins *et al.*, 1967). In addition to hypoplasia of the fetal adrenals, thyroid, and testes, retardation of somatic growth was evident. This was especially apparent in deficient epiphyseal development (Liggins and Kennedy, 1968). Continuous infusions of cortisol (50 mg/24 hours) into lamb fetuses resulted in parturition within 5 days. Infusion of ACTH (0.1 mg/24 hours) into the fetus gave similar results. The latter premature lambs had adrenal weights comparable to mature lambs. Infusions of either cortisol or ACTH into the ewe were relatively ineffective (Halliday and Buttle, 1968; Liggins, 1968; Van Rensburg, 1967). The sheep placenta is relatively impermeable to both ACTH and cortisol (D. P. Alexander *et al.*, 1968; Bassett and Thorburn, 1969; Beitins *et al.*, 1970; Jones *et al.*, 1964).

Dexamethasone infused into the fetus (0.6–4 mg/24 hours) induced parturition. While infusion of 4.0 mg/24 hours into the ewe was ineffective, 6 mg/24 hours did result in parturition in 4 days (Adams and Wagner, 1969; Bosc, 1970; Fylling, 1971; Liggins, 1969).

Observations in normal pregnant sheep support the implications of the investigations which have been described. In the last 7–10 days of pregnancy the fetal lamb adrenals grow rapidly, doubling in weight (Comline and Silver, 1961). Associated with this rapid adrenal growth, there is a dramatic rise in corticosteroid concentration in the fetal blood (Bassett and Thornburn, 1969).

d. *Pigs.* Naturally occurring prolonged gestation has been observed in pigs, and the breeding data were indicative of a genetic disorder. Unfortunately, further information has not been obtained (Holm, 1967).

e. *Goats.* In a naturally occurring disorder of habitual abortion in Angora goats, it has been reported that the fetuses exhibit adrenal hyperplasia. It was suggested that excessive corticosteroids might have impaired placental function (Van Rensburg, 1965).

f. *Subhuman Primates.* Syndromes associated with abnormal gestational length have not been identified in subhuman primates. Extirpation experiments comparable to those in sheep have been technically difficult and hampered by postoperative abortion and fetal death *in utero*. However, fetal hypophysectomy in rhesus monkeys has been successfully accomplished and did result in prolonged gestation up to 184 days (normal 165 days) (Chez *et al.*, 1970). The adrenals of the post-term monkeys weighed one-fifth that of normal-term monkeys. The fetal zone, which is normally 80% of the adrenal at term, had regressed. The definitive cortex showed clear differentiation into 3 zones, which normally occurs after parturition, the glomerulosa layer being predominant.

g. *Human Beings. i. Anencephaly.* Human fetal–placental endocrinology has been frequently reviewed (Diczfalusy, 1969; Oakey, 1970) and will be considered here only in a comparative context. The relatively common naturally occurring abnormality in human beings which is associated with prolonged gestation is anencephaly. In these fetuses, the hypothalamus is absent. The anterior pituitary, while invariably present may be hypoplastic. The adrenal glands are small, primarily owing to premature regression of the fetal zone. The definitive cortex is also smaller than normal, and there is differentiation into three zones (Benirschke, 1956). The animal model to which anencephaly seems most closely comparable is that of the 11-deoxyjervine poisoned lambs: (1) the defect is environmentally determined (Fedrick, 1970; Richards, 1969). (2) The hypothalamic–pituitary axis is anatomically abnormal. (3) The severity of the defect is variable, some fetuses delivering spontaneously at term, while others have prolongation of pregnancy to a variable degree. In anencephaly, it has been reported that there is a strong inverse correlation between the size of the fetal adrenals and the degree of prolongation of pregnancy. Those fetuses which deliver near term may have adrenals approaching normal weight (Anderson *et al.*, 1969).

In neither the abnormal lambs nor the anencephalic fetus is there conclusive evidence of glucocorticoid deficiency. The concentration of

17-OH-corticosteroids in the cord blood of anencephalic infants is the same as the of normal infants (Nichols *et al.*, 1958). However, in contrast to sheep, cortisol readily crosses the placenta in both the macaque (Bashore *et al.*, 1970) and man (Abramovich and Wade, 1969; Migeon *et al.*, 1957), and fetal plasma cortisol is believed to be regulated by the maternal blood concentration (Bashore *et al.*, 1970; Oakey, 1970). Cortisol production rates measured on 2 newborn anencephalic infants were reported to be within the lower limit of the normal range (Kenny *et al.*, 1966). These results must be interpreted with the following qualifications: (1) By necessity, the determinations were done within 48 hours of birth when a maternal contribution to fetal plasma cortisol is present. (2) The correction for body surface area is probably prejudicial in these anencephalic infants (Naeye and Blanc, 1971). (3) Again, by necessity, the infants were selected by their prolonged survival (72 and 96 hours), while most anencephalics die during labor or shortly thereafter (Anderson *et al.*, 1969). (4) The duration of gestation is not stated. The weight of the adrenals given (for 1 infant, 620 mg) is consistent with a defect of intermediate severity (Anderson *et al.*, 1969; Frandsen and Stakemann, 1963). In view of these considerations, it is significant that the cortisol production rates in these two infants were 2 standard deviations below the normal mean, and the findings are consistent with the observed variation in severity of the adrenal hypoplasia.

The subnormal synthesis of C_{19} estrogen precursors by the adrenal of the anencephalic infant is well known. Maternal estrogen excretion is usually low (Frandsen and Stakemann, 1961, 1963), and umbilical cord blood dehydroepiandrosterone and 16α-OH-dehydroepiandrosterone concentrations are usually low (Colas *et al.*, 1964; Easterling *et al.*, 1966; France, 1971). Placental steroidogenic function is normal as indicated by normal urinary pregnanediol (Frandsen and Stakemann, 1961) and plasma progesterone (Hellig *et al.*, 1970) and intact capacity for aromatization of infused C_{19} estrogen precursors (Nakayama *et al.*, 1967).

ii. Congenital adrenal hypoplasia. Congenital adrenal hypoplasia in normocephalic infants is a rare condition, but it is being recognized with increasing frequency. It occurs in association with pituitary hypoplasia (Blizzard and Alberts, 1956; Brewer, 1957; Mosier, 1956; Roselli and Barbosa, 1965) and also as a primary adrenal defect (Migeon *et al.*, 1965; Stempfel and Engel, 1960). No association with prolonged gestation has been reported. Although precise data are not given, with the exception of one premature infant, the pregnancies are reported as being "normal term." On reviewing the case reports, it is noted that the infants have been modestly above average in weight for "normal term" at birth.

Of specific interest is a familial disorder of adrenal hypoplasia in which there is a block in the ability of the adrenal to respond to ACTH. The infant studied by Stempfel and Engel (1960), born at "full term" weighing 8.25 pounds, was found to have adrenal insufficiency without hypoaldosteronism and was subsequently shown to be completely refractory to ACTH. This infant had a previous sibling, also "full term" who died at 18 hours of age, and at necropsy no adrenal tissue could be found. Migeon et al. (1965) reported 5 surviving, but presumably similar, cases. The adrenal removed from one of these infants was small (0.35 g) with a normal glomerulosa, small fasciculata, and no discernible reticularis. Incubation of the tissue with pregnenolone resulted in the formation of cortisol and corticosterone in a ratio of 0.3, the ratio for the normal control being 15. The presence of low urinary 17-OH-corticosteroids in these infants indicates that they have some limited capacity for cortisol synthesis. There is no report concerning maternal estriol excretion in these syndromes.

While these disorders of adrenal hypoplasia are not well defined, the information which has been reported must be seriously considered in any inference drawn from the observations in domestic animals and human anencephalics concerning the possible implication of fetal corticosteroids in the initiation of parturition.

iii. Congenital adrenal hyperplasia. In considering the hypothesis that the initiation of parturition might be a function of fetal adrenal cortical activity, the question arises as to whether the important hormone might be cortisol or an estrogen precursor. Congenital adrenal hyperplasia, in which cortisol synthesis is defective and, as a consequence, androgen secretion is elevated, might be hoped to provide some insight. No abnormality in gestational length has been reported in association with these disorders. However, the quantitative aspects of the hormonal situation *in utero* are not well defined (Merkatz et al., 1969).

3. Glucocorticoids and Parturition in Ruminants

The observations in cows and sheep which have been described (Section III, F, 2) strongly implicate the hypothalamic–pituitary–adrenal system in the initiation of parturition in these species. The induction of labor with glucocorticoids in both of these species suggests that the specific stimulus for the initiation of parturition may be glucocorticosteroid secretion from the fetal adrenal. The following reservations should be considered: (1) Glucocorticoids have no evident intrinsic oxytocic properties. (2) The infusion rates of cortisol required to cause parturition in sheep fetuses are well above the secretion rate estimated for the acute rise observed in lambs preceding parturition. (3) Prior to spontaneous parturition, the concentration of blood progesterone in the ewe falls. This progesterone is produced by the placenta. The infusion of dexamethasone at a rate of 4 mg/24 hours failed to induce parturition, while 6 mg/24 hours did result in delivery. It has been reported that, while 4 mg/24 hours of dexamethasone has no effect on the concentration of blood progesterone in the pregnant ewe, 6 mg/24 hours causes a decline in progesterone concentration comparable to that preceding spontaneous parturition (Fylling, 1971). (4) The results of the pituitary and adrenal extirpation experiments, which cannot be attributed to "pharmacological doses," do not distinguish between the possible significance of glucocorticosteroid hormones and estrogen precursors. The sharp rise in cortisol concentration in fetal lamb blood which precedes parturition is associated with an equally dramatic rise in plasma estrogen in the ewe. (5) Cortisol does not appear to cross the sheep placenta; the rise in fetal blood cortisol is not reflected in maternal plasma cortisol concentrations. Therefore, it seems unlikely that this fetal cortisol reaches the intervillous blood, and therefore the myometrium. The hypothesis which best fits the sum of the available information is that glucocorticoids, in sufficient concentration, influence placental steroidogenesis.

4. *Glucocorticoids in Human Parturition*

Evidence for an association between an intact hypothalamic–pituitary–adrenal system and the timely initiation of parturition has been presented for a variety of species including the macaque and human beings. In the sheep, which is the most adequately studied of the animal species, it might be inferred that the acute rise in fetal cortisol which precedes parturition is important in the initiation of labor.

If this inference is correct for the sheep, it cannot be directly transposed to primates. In human beings and macaques, cortisol crosses the placenta to a significant degree (Section III, F, 2, *g*). The evidence indicates that the concentration of cortisol in the fetal circulation is a function of maternal plasma concentration. Increased pituitary stimulation of the fetal adrenal would result in increased secretion of both cortisol and C_{19} estrogen precursors. Unbound cortisol which was not promptly metabolized by the placenta or fetus would be largely transferred to the maternal blood. The net result of the adrenal stimulation would be augmented placental estrogen secretion. The evidence that this view is correct has been recently reviewed (Oakey, 1970). The most direct demonstration is provided by the administration of pharmacological doses of corticosteroids to pregnant women which results in a marked depression of urinary estriol excretion. The administration of metapyrone, which blocks cortisol synthesis, increases maternal estrogen excretion. ACTH, which probably does not cross the placenta at physiological concentrations, when administered to the mother in large doses, has been reported to cross the placenta and caused increased estriol excretion (Oakey, 1970).

The continuous treatment of pregnant women with large doses of potent synthetic corticosteroids has not had any predictable influence on the timing of parturition. The naturally occurring condition of maternal hypercorticism, Cushing's syndrome, can result in sustained high levels of blood cortisol. While premature labor is seen, this may be associated with rupture of the chorioamnion, and the toxic status of the fetus is evidenced by the high intrauterine and perinatal mortality (Kreines and De Vaux, 1971; Kreines et al., 1964).

G. Uterine Volume

1. Uterine Growth

The comparative aspects of uterine growth during pregnancy and the influence of the volume of the conceptus have been reviewed in detail by Reynolds (1949). It is pertinent to this discussion to emphasize the interrelationships between uterine distension, estrogen, and progesterone in providing for uterine growth and accommodation of the conceptus.

In the nonpregnant uterus, growth of the myometrium is stimulated by both estrogen and progesterone in optimal quantities. However, this response is limited both in degree and in duration. A more impressive and sustained response is elicited by artificial uterine distension, even in the castrate animal in the absence of hormones (Csapo et al., 1965; Reynolds and Kaminester, 1936). A physiological demonstration of the primary role of distension in eliciting growth of the uterus can be observed in the unilaterally pregnant rabbit (Knaus, 1929) or rat (Siegmund, 1930). The growth of the gravid horn far exceeds that of the sterile horn. A comparable demonstration is seen in human beings with extrauterine pregnancy, tubal or abdominal, in which uterine growth is very limited.

Steroid hormones have important modifying effects on the distension-growth response. Estrogen alone given to the castrate animal eliminates the growth response to distension. The effect of estrogen plus distension is limited to the response which is elicited by estrogen alone in the undistended uterus (Reynolds, 1937). With progesterone, the distension-growth response is unimpeded. Under the influence of progesterone, the myometrium is more distensible, and the degree of distension which elicits optimal growth is increased (Reynolds and Allen, 1937). While estrogen is important in stimulating the synthesis of contractile proteins and a variety of enzymes (Csapo, 1950), progesterone is more effective in stimulating uterine hypertrophy and hyperplasia (Crandall, 1938; de Mattos *et al.*, 1967; Reynolds and Allen, 1937). Maximal growth is seen in the distended uterus in the presence of both estrogen and progesterone (de Mattos *et al.*, 1967; Reynolds and Allen, 1937).

In summary, the uterus grows in response to distension, and grows optimally under the combined influence of distension, estrogen, and progesterone.

2. *Uterine Contractile Activity*

In laboratory studies of myometrial strips, it can be shown that acute stretch of the myometrium will cause an increase in action potential discharge (Kuriyama, 1961; Marshall, 1962). To define this response more precisely, the term "resting length" has been used. When an excised strip of myometrium from an "estrogenized" uterus is stretched, over a certain range, there is no increase in the resting tension of the strip. When stretched beyond a certain critical length, an increase in the resting tension of the muscle is observed. The "resting length" has been defined as the maximum length to which the muscle can be drawn without causing an increase in its resting tension. It is acute stretch beyond this "resting length" which will elicit an increase in action potential discharge. This electrical response to acute stretch is blocked by progesterone.

These experiments have been described here only to emphasize that the electrocontractile response of myometrium to stretch is a response to acute stretch and has no demonstrated relevance to chronic distension. It has been shown with myometrial strips from the cat and guinea pig (Bozler, 1941) and human beings (J. T. Conrad and Kuhn, 1967; J. T. Conrad *et al.*, 1966) that myometrium has viscoelastic properties. As indicated above, when a myometrial strip is stretched beyond its "resting length" there is, by definition, an increase in resting tension. However, if the muscle strip is maintained at this increased length, the tension progressively declines with time, and a new "resting length" is attained. An additional increase in the length of the strip will again increase the resting tension, and, again, this tension will progressively decrease with time and a new "resting length" is attained.

J. T. Conrad *et al.* (1966) have pointed out that this behavior of the myometrial strip is characteristic of viscoelastic polymers. They believe that the changes in resting tension observed in these experiments reflect the properties of the connective tissue rather than the contractile elements.

These *in vitro* observations suggest that the gradual distension of the uterus by the growing conceptus would not result in an increase in

resting tension and, therefore, no stretch-induced increase in electrocontractile activity would be anticipated. Observations *in vivo* indicate
that no increase in myometrium resting tension occurs in association with
the growth of the conceptus. Schofield and Wood (1964) examined
myometrium obtained from term pregnancies in both rabbits and human
beings. They found that the myometrium was not stretched beyond its
"resting length." Direct measurement of intrauterine pressure, which has
been utilized extensively in a variety of animals and in women, has not
shown any increase in resting pressure within the uterus in advanced
pregnancy.

In summary, there is no physiological evidence that would indicate
that the increase in uterine volume resulting from the normal growth
of the conceptus induces an increase in electrocontractile activity.

3. The Initiation of Parturition

a. Normal Gestation. Distension of the uterus by the growing conceptus, in conjunction with estrogen and progesterone, induces uterine
growth and the potential for contractile activity. Progesterone has a
specific role in blocking potential electrocontractile activity.

Reynolds (1949) concluded, "it is clear that the rate of fetal growth
is the principal condition which determines the span of gestation within
a given species." More recently it has been suggested, "clinical labor,
premature or normal, is thought to occur whenever the ratio, volume/
progesterone, increases beyond a critical value" (Csapo and Sauvage,
1968). As applied to primates and other "oophorectomy-tolerant" species,
in which there is no diminution of progesterone prior to parturition, this
view implies that the timing of normal parturition is determined by
the growth of the conceptus to a critical volume. Support for this thesis
is derived largely from: (1) observations indicating an inverse correlation between gestational length and litter size in polytocous species, (2)
observations in experimentally derived abnormal circumstances in small
animals, and (3) observations in human gestation in which the uterus
is distended beyond the normal range.

As indicated by Holm (1967), the evidence pertaining to litter size
in polytocous species does not support a primary role for uterine volume
in the timing of the initiation of normal parturition. To the contrary,
it seems significant how small is the difference in gestational length
which is observed with variations in litter size. In mice there is a small
difference in gestational length associated with a wide range in litter
size (Biggers *et al.*, 1963). Examination of the data from 34 breeds of
rabbits revealed a statistical relationship between litter size and gestational length in 12 breeds, and no apparent relationship in 22 breeds

(Wilson and Dudley, 1952). In a purebred strain of guinea pigs, the mean gestational length was 70 days when the litter size was 1, and 65 days when the litter size was 6 (Goy et al., 1957). Gestational–lengths of twin pregnancies in sheep are shorter by 0.6 day than those of singleton pregnancies (Dry, 1933; Terrill and Hazel, 1947). When twins are carried in cattle (gestation 279–283 days), the length of pregnancy is reduced by 3–6 days (M. H. Alexander, 1950; Bonadonna and Valerani, 1947; Knott, 1932; Wing, 1899). In goats, the correlation between litter size and pregnancy length falls short of statistical significance (Asdell, 1929; Hinterthur, 1933). In pigs, litter size has no influence on the length of gestation (Burger, 1952; Carmichael and Rice, 1920; Cox, 1964; I. Johansson, 1929; Joubert and Bonsma, 1952; Krizenecky, 1935; McKenzie, 1928). In ferrets, with litter sizes that varied from 5 to 13, there was no correlation between the number of young and the length of gestation (Hammond and Marshall, 1930).

In singleton pregnancies in primates, an inverse correlation between fetal weight and pregnancy length has never been reported. In *M. mulatta*, it has been documented that the opposite is true, that smaller fetuses are associated with shorter gestation and larger fetuses with longer gestation (Fujikura and Niemann, 1967).

In human beings, the positive correlation between fetal size and gestational length in singleton pregnancy is well documented (Hendricks, 1964; Thompson et al., 1968). The individual variation in fetal weight for any given length of gestation is appreciable. Two standard deviations from the mean, to include 95% of infants, encompasses a range of ±26%, e.g., at term 2400–4000 gm. The mean rate of fetal growth slows appreciably approaching term, from a maximum of about 34 gm per day at 37 weeks to about 20 gm per day at term, and continuing to fall thereafter. While the volume of the amniotic fluid varies widely between individuals (Gadd, 1966; Marsden and Huntingford, 1965), the average amount progressively decreases after 37 weeks' gestation. The mean decrease of about 15 ml/day approaches the fetal growth increment. It seems likely that, on the average, the uterine volume changes very little after 37 weeks.

b. Abnormal Gestation. It should not be assumed that factors that may be operative in abnormal situations have the same importance under normal circumstances. Premature parturition in human multiple pregnancy and in association with hydramnios have been interpreted as supporting a central role for uterine volume in the timing of normal parturition.

In the syndromes of prolonged gestation in sheep and Holstein cows (Section III, F, 2) the fetuses grow to a very large size and, yet, may be retained *in utero*. In the cows, the marked flaccidity of the uterus has been noted, and the uterus may become so large and heavy that the abdominal wall ruptures.

In human twin gestation, while the combined fetal weight reaches that of a term singleton by 32 weeks, the median time of parturition is 37 weeks (Guttmacher, 1939; Guttmacher and Kohl, 1958; Hendricks, 1966; Thompson *et al.*, 1968). The mean combined weight of twins at 37 weeks is about 5000 gm (Hendricks, 1966), and excessive amniotic fluid is common (Barry, 1958; Yordan and D'Esopo, 1955).

In hydramnios, the mean duration of gestation is also about 37 weeks (Yordan and D'Esopo, 1955). Perhaps more striking than the tendency toward early delivery is the marked uterine distension which may be observed, with fluid volumes in excess of 6 liters (Gadd, 1966).

While the relevance of these abnormal situations to normal gestation is uncertain, it is apparent that the uterus can accommodate volumes far in excess of the range which is encountered in normal pregnancy.

c. Discussion and Conclusions. Within the physiological range, the mechanisms providing for the maintenance of gestation and its timely termination accommodate wide variations in the volume of the conceptus without an important effect on the duration of pregnancy. In normal pregnancy in human beings, wide variations in fetal size are observed without evident effect on the timing of parturition. In abnormal pregnancies with gross overdistention of the uterus, the capacity of the uterus to accommodate large volumes is evident, but premature parturition is observed.

H. OXYTOCIN

While this discussion is confined primarily to gestational steroid hormones, oxytocin must be briefly discussed because of the interrelationships between the physiology of this polypeptide and the steroid hormones.

First, it may be stated generally that the "estrogenized," spontaneously active uterus responds to oxytocin stimulation, and the superimposition of progesterone, which inhibits spontaneous activity, also blocks the response to oxytocin. Second, it may also be said generally, that the uterine response to oxytocin is blocked during pregnancy, and that the evolution of spontaneous activity preceding parturition is associated with the return of oxytocin sensitivity (Caldeyro-Barcia, 1964). The association between the level of spontaneous activity and the sensitivity to oxytocin is sufficiently consistent that it is likely that both phenomena reflect the same physiological parameters in the myometrium.

On the basis of these generalizations, it seems unlikely that oxytocin can be assigned an initiating role in parturition. It becomes physiologically effective only when more fundamental changes have taken place that provide an oxytocin-sensitive uterus.

The sheep appears to be the best example of oxytocin physiology as it relates to mammalian gestation. In the nonpregnant sheep, vaginal distension induces the release of oxytocin and an elevation of pressure in the milk ducts (Debackere et al., 1961; Roberts and Share, 1968). Administration of progesterone blocks this reflex by preventing the release of oxytocin (Roberts and Share, 1969). When the ewe becomes pregnant, spontaneous uterine activity (Hindson et al., 1965), the sensitivity of the uterus to administered oxytocin (Hindson et al., 1969), and the reflex release of oxytocin following vaginal distension (Roberts and Share, 1968) are all blocked. The beginning of spontaneous uterine activity in the ewe occurs only 12 hours prior to parturition (Hindson et al., 1965). Sensitivity to oxytocin may increase prior to this time, but it is irregular and unpredictable (Hindson et al., 1969). The initiation of labor is preceded by diminishing progesterone secretion (Section II, A, 6) and is accompanied by increasing oxytocin sensitivity and a return of the oxytocin-releasing vaginal–hypothalamic reflex. In labor, injection of progesterone will consistently block the vaginal–hypothalamic reflex. When progesterone is injected very early in labor, it may abolish spontaneous activity and delay parturition up to a week. It is important to note, however, that when injected progesterone is unsuccessful in abolishing labor and preventing parturition, it still totally blocks the vaginal–hypothalamic reflex. In this situation, although there may be no diminution in recorded intrauterine pressure waves, labor is prolonged (Hindson et al., 1969).

There is evidence for the existence of a comparable vaginal or cervical oxytocin-releasing reflex, which can be blocked by progesterone, in other species, e.g., the rat (Barraclough and Cross, 1963), rabbit (Schofield, 1969), and goat (Roberts and Share, 1970). In the goat it has been clearly demonstrated that progesterone blocks the reflex release of oxytocin in a classical, logarithmic dose-response manner (Roberts and Share, 1970).

In the goat (Folley and Knaggs, 1965), the cow (Fitzpatrick, 1966), and human beings (Coch et al., 1965) there is a rise in plasma oxytocin to detectable levels (bioassay) in the second stage of labor, as the fetus is expelled.

In summary, it is well established that oxytocin is important postpartum in lactation. In at least some subprimate species, it seems likely that oxytocin may facilitate parturition, especially in the expulsive phase. The available evidence indicates that both the reflex release of oxytocin and the oxytocin sensitivity of the myometrium are dependent upon a decrease, absolute or relative, of progesterone. The role of oxytocin in parturition, therefore, is probably of a secondary nature and relates to the completion of parturition rather than to initiation.

In primates, in which there is no consistent change in plasma progesterone prior to parturition, and in which no striking vaginal–hypothalamic reflex is evident, oxytocin appears to be of minimal importance prior to expulsion of the fetus. The development of a sensitive radioimmunoassay for oxytocin may be expected to provide more definitive information.

IV. Discussion and Speculation

A. General Considerations

In the comparative study of gestation, a primary objective is to identify those features that may be characteristic of mammals in general. We would infer that those aspects which have general applicability are likely to be of fundamental importance. To be distinguished from fundamental mammalian mechanisms are variations peculiar to a particular group or species. Only to the extent to which this distinction can be accomplished can we intelligently apply the diverse observations in animals to an improved understanding of human reproduction.

Having been given the liberty of speculation, we will attempt to establish a model which is applicable to mammals generally, and then to construct 3 representative, species-specific models for the rat, the sheep, and human beings.

B. General Model

Uterine muscle is dependent on estrogen for growth and for its maintenance in a physiological state. This physiological state is one of spontaneous, rhythmic electrochemical excitation, which is propagated through the muscle, resulting in rhythmic contraction. In the intact uterus, the anatomical organization of the tissue translates the contractile activity into expulsive force. Progesterone alters the cellular electrochemical physiology so as to suppress the initiation and propagation of excitation, and thereby maintains uterine quiescence and viscoelasticity. Estrogen and progesterone together facilitate the effect of distension of the uterus by the conceptus in causing growth of the uterus.

The effects of estrogen and progesterone are variable in degree in a dose-dependent manner, and the effects of the two hormones are intimately interrelated at the intracellular level. Optimal relative quantities of estrogen and progesterone facilitate the maintenance of pregnancy. Species with relatively high concentrations of one hormone have high concentrations of both. Preceding parturition, an increase in the estrogen-progesterone ratio is observed which may be either gradual or abrupt. In species for which we have adequate information, no exception is apparent.

Blood hormone levels will not always accurately reflect effective tissue concentrations. Modifying factors which are apparent include site of production, blood flow, plasma-protein binding, vascular permeability, cell-membrane transport, cytoplasmic "receptor" activity, and the complexities of the intracellular economy. The opportunities for hormone interaction and modifying factors are manifold.

In distinction to the effects of estrogen and progesterone, which are considered primary, examples of potential secondary modifying factors might include myometrial distension, oxytocin, cortisol, prostaglandins and catecholamines.

The predictability and relative precision of the timing of parturition for a given species or strain is impressive. It is our hypothesis that the timing of parturition is a neuroendocrine function. In short-gestation species this refers to the maternal hypothalamic–pituitary–ovarian system, in what can be viewed figuratively as an extension of the estrous cycle. In long gestation species, this function is adopted by the fetal hypothalamus as part of its genetically programmed development, and mediated via the pituitary–adrenal system. The final common pathway in both short-gestation and long-gestation species is the elevation of the effective myometrial estrogen:progesterone ratio.

C. Species-Specific Models

1. Rat

The rat is an example of short gestation species in which pregnancy is primarily under maternal hypothalamic–hypophyseal–ovarian control. Plasma progesterone, of ovarian origin, rises to a mid-pregnancy peak, and then falls prior to parturition. Plasma estrogen rises progressively until parturition. The changes in both progesterone and estrogen secretion contribute to the marked elevation of estrogen:progesterone ratio preceding parturition. Parturition, which fails to occur in the absence of the ovaries or pituitary, can be initiated by estrogen injection. Conversely, parturition can be prevented in the intact animal by progesterone injection.

In addition, secondary factors are identifiable. The decrease in myometrial progesterone concentration preceding parturition is greater than would be anticipated from the decline in plasma levels. This is related to a diminution in myometrial cytoplasmic "receptor" activity.

Placental gonadotropins, and possibly placental progesterone, are additional supportive factors.

2. Sheep

Gestation is relatively long, and hormonal control is adopted by the fetus. The ovarian contribution to blood progesterone concentration, while substantial, is nonessential during two-thirds of pregnancy. Progesterone synthesized in the placenta, in addition to appearing in the circulation, probably also reaches the myometrium directly from intervillous blood through interstitial channels. The falling concentration of blood progesterone preceding parturition primarily reflects the disappearance of the ovarian contribution, but probably a decrease in placental secretion also occurs.

Estrogen, which is synthesized in the placenta, is dependent on C_{19} precursors of fetal adrenal origin. Near term, the fetal adrenals grow rapidly under hypothalamic-pituitary stimulation. This results in an abrupt increase in placental estrogen synthesis. The associated rapid increase in estrogen-progesterone ratio is associated with rapid evolution of uterine activity leading to parturition.

In association with the preparturient stimulation of the fetal adrenals, a marked rise in fetal blood cortisol occurs. It is possible that this cortisol suppresses placental progesterone synthesis. There are many other potential mechanisms for the interaction of cortisol with estrogen and progesterone.

In the sheep, distension of the upper vagina elicits a reflex release of oxytocin. This reflex is blocked in the hypothalamus by progesterone. The preparturient diminution in progesterone secretion probably facilitates parturition through this secondary mechanism.

3. Human Beings

The human model, on initial appraisal, appears to be less dramatic than the sheep. Progesterone secretion, a function of the placenta, rises progressively until a few weeks before term and then plateaus. The influence of progesterone on the myometrium is primarily locally mediated, and the erratic variations in blood concentrations in the same individual are probably not meaningful. Estrogen secretion by the placenta rises progressively throughout pregnancy, and the rate of increase is maintained, or perhaps accelerated, during the last third of gestation. This pattern is a reflection of the rapid growth of the fetal adrenals, especially the fetal zone, which is observed during this period. The growth of the fetal zone of the adrenal is dependent on fetal hypothalamic-pituitary stimulation. The local effect on the uterus of placental estrogen is probably important as has been suggested for progesterone. The increase in the estrogen:progesterone ratio is more gradual in women than in sheep, and this is reflected in the gradual evolution of uterine activity.

Secondary factors are less apparent in human beings than in the sheep. While marked overdistension of the uterus in some abnormal conditions is associated with premature labor, an influence of fetal size on the initiation of parturition is not seen within the physiological range.

The increasing uterine activity during active labor which is seen is not satisfactorily encompassed by this model. With the current development of sensitive assays it will be possible to reassess the possible role of a cervical-pituitary-oxytocin reflex in facilitating the completion of parturition in women.

D. Conclusion

These models are not offered as an explanation of the control of gestation, but as a working hypothesis, imperfect and incomplete. The hypothesis is, however, consistent with the accumulated observations in mammalian gestation, and it is hoped that it will provide a valid basis for further investigation.

Acknowledgments

Original research quoted from this laboratory was supported by grants from the U. S. Public Health Service HD 05613-02, Rockefeller Foundation, United Cerebral Palsy, and the Ford Foundation.

REFERENCES

Abramovich, D. R., and Wade, A. P. (1969). *J. Obstet. Gynaecol. Brit. Commonw.* **76**, 610.

Adams, C. E. (1965). *J. Endocrinol.* **31**, xxix.

Adams, W. M. (1969). *J. Amer. Vet. Med. Ass.* **154**, 261.

Adams, W. M., and Wagner, W. C. (1969). *J. Amer. Vet. Med. Ass.* **154**, 1396.

Ainsworth, L., and Ryan, K. J. (1966). *Endocrinology* **79**, 875.

Ainsworth, L., and Ryan, K. J. (1967). *Endocrinology* **81**, 1349.

Ainsworth, L., and Ryan, K. J. (1969a). *Endocrinology* **84**, 91.

Ainsworth, L., and Ryan, K. J. (1969b). *Steroids* **14**, 301.

Ainsworth, L., and Ryan, K. J. (1970). *Steroids* **16**, 553.

Ainsworth, L., Daenen, M., and Ryan, K. J. (1969). *Endocrinology* **84**, 1421.

Aitken, E. H., Preedy, J. R. K., Eton, B., and Short, R. V. (1958). *Lancet* **ii**, 1096.

Alexander, D. P., Britton, H. G., James, V. H. T., Nixon, D. A., Parker, R. A., Wintour, E. M., and Wright, R. D. (1968). *J. Endocrinol.* **40**, 1.

Alexander, M. H. (1950). *J. Dairy Sci.* **33**, 337.

Allen, W. M. (1930). *Amer. J. Physiol.* **92**, 174.

Allen, W. M., and Corner, G. W. (1929). *Amer. J. Physiol.* **88**, 340.

Allen, W. M., and Corner, G. W. (1930). *Proc. Soc. Exp. Biol. Med.* **27**, 403.

Amoroso, E. C., and Finn, C. A. (1962). *In* "The Ovary" (S. Zuckerman, ed.), Vol. 1, p. 451. Academic Press, New York.

Anderson, A. B. M., Laurence, K. M., and Turbull, A. C. (1969). *J. Obstet. Gynecol. Brit. Commonw.* **76**, 196.

Asdell, S. A. (1929). *J. Agr. Sci.* **19**, 382.

Asdell, S. A. (1946). "Patterns of Mammalian Reproduction." Cornell Univ. Press (Comstock), Ithaca, New York.

Barraclough, C. A., and Cross, B. A. (1963). *J. Endocrinol.* **26**, 339.

Barry, A. P. (1958). *Obstet. Gynecol.* **11**, 667.

Bashore, R. A., Smith, F., and Gold, E. (1970). *Nature (London)* **228**, 774.

Bassett, J. M., and Thorburn, G. D. (1969). *J. Endocrinol.* **44**, 285.

Bassett, J. M., Oxborrow, T. J., Smith, I. D., and Thorburn, G. D. (1969). *J. Endocrinol.* **45**, 449.

Bedwani, J. R., and Marley, P. B. (1971). *J. Reprod. Fert.* **26**, 343.

Beitins, I. Z., Kowarski, A., Shermeta, D. W., De Lemos, R. A., and Migeon, C. J. (1970). *Pediat. Res.* **4**, 129.

Bengtsson, L. P. (1962). *Acta Obstet. Gynecol. Scand.* **41**, 124.

Bengtsson, L. P., and Schofield, B. M. (1963). *J. Reprod. Fert.* **5**, 423.

Benirschke, K. (1956). *Obstet. Gynecol.* **8**, 412.

Bhavnani, B. R., Short, R. V., and Solomon, S. (1969). *Endocrinology* **85**, 1172.

Biggers, J. D., Curnow, R. N., Finn, C. A., and McLaren, A. (1963). *J. Reprod. Fert.* **6**, 125.

Blizzard, R. M., and Alberts, M. (1956). *J. Pediat.* **48**, 782.

Bloch, E. (1969). *Steroids* **13**, 589.

Bloch, K. (1945). *J. Biol. Chem.* **157**, 661.

Blom, A. K., and Lyngset, O. (1971). *Acta Endocrinol. (Copenhagen)* **66**, 471.

Boe, F. (1938). *Acta Pathol. Microbiol. Scand. Suppl.* **26**, 1.

Bonadonna, T., and Valerani, L. (1947). *Zootec. Vet* **1**, 129 and 274; *Anim. Breed. Abstr.* **15**, 174 (1947).

Bosc, M. J. (1970). *C. R. Acad. Sci.* **270**, 3127.

Bozler, E. (1941). *J. Cell. Comp. Physiol.* **18**, 385.

Brenner, W. E., and Hendricks, C. H. (1962). *Amer. J. Obstet. Gynecol.* **83**, 1094.

Brewer, D. B. (1957). *J. Pathol. Bacteriol.* **73**, 59.

Brown, J. B. (1956). *Lancet* **1**, 704.

Bryson, M. J., and Sweat, M. L. (1967). *Endocrinology* **81**, 729.

Bryson, M. J., and Sweat, M. L. (1969). *Endocrinology* **84**, 1071.

Burger, J. F. (1952). *Onderstepoort J. Vet. Res., Suppl.* **2**, 1.

Caldeyro-Barcia, R. (1964). *In* "Muscle" (W. M. Paul *et al.,* eds.), p. 317. Pergamon, Oxford.

Carlson, I. H., and Rust, C. C. (1969). *Endocrinology* **85**, 623.

Carmichael, W. J., and Rice, J. B. (1920). *Ill., Agr. Exp. Sta., Bull.* **226**.

Cassmer, O. (1959). *Acta Endocrinol. (Copenhagen), Suppl.* **45**, 1.

Challis, J. R. G. (1971). *Nature (London)* **229**, 208.

Challis, J. R. G., and Linzell, J. L. (1971). *J. Reprod. Fert.* **26**, 401.

Challis, J. R. G., Harrison, F. A., and Heap, R. B. (1971). *J. Reprod. Fert.* **25**, 306.

Chez, R. A., Hutchinson, D. L., Salazar, H., and Mintz, D. H. (1970). *Amer. J. Obstet. Gynecol.* **108**, 643.

Clegg, M. T. (1959). *In* "Reproduction in Domestic Animals" (H. H. Cole and P. T. Cupps, eds.), 1st ed., Vol. 1, p. 509. Academic Press, New York.

Coch, J. A., Brovetto, J., Cabot, H. M., Fielitz, C. A., and Caldeyro-Barcia, R. (1965). *Amer. J. Obstet. Gynecol.* **91**, 10.

Colas, A., Heinrichs, W. L., and Tatum, H. J. (1964). *Steroids* **3**, 417.

Comline, R. S., and Silver, M. (1961). *J. Physiol. (London)* **156**, 424.

Conrad, J. T., and Kuhn, W. (1967). *Amer. J. Obstet. Gynecol.* **97,** 154.

Conrad, J. T., Kuhn, W. K., and Johnson, W. L. (1966). *Amer. J. Obstet. Gynecol.* **95,** 254.

Conrad, S. H., Pion, R. J., and Kitchin, J. D., III. (1967). *J. Clin. Endocrinol. Metab.* **27,** 114.

Courrier, R. (1941). *C. R. Soc. Biol.* **135,** 820.

Courrier, R. (1945). "Endocrinologie de la Gestation." Masson, Paris.

Courrier, R., and Gross, G. (1936). *C. R. Soc. Biol.* **121,** 1517.

Cox, D. F. (1964). *J. Reprod. Fert.* **7,** 405.

Crandall, W. R. (1938). *Anat. Rec.* **72,** 195.

Csapo, A. (1950). *Amer. J. Physiol.* **162,** 406.

Csapo, A. (1956). *Amer. J. Anat.* **98,** 273.

Csapo, A. (1969). *Ciba Found. Study Group* [*Pap.*] **34,** 13.

Csapo, A., and Lloyd-Jacob, M. A. (1962). *Amer. J. Obstet. Gynecol.* **83,** 1073.

Csapo, A., and Sauvage, J. (1968). *Acta Endocrinol. (Copenhagen)* **47,** 181.

Csapo, A., and Wiest, W. G. (1969). *Endocrinology* **85,** 735.

Csapo, A., Erdos, T., de Mattos, C. R., Gramss, E., and Moscowitz, C. (1965). *Nature (London)* **207,** 1378.

Csapo, A., de Sousa-Filho, M. B., de Souza, J. C., and de Souza, O. E. (1966). *Fert. Steril.* **17,** 621.

Daniel, E. E., and Renner, S. A. (1960). *Amer. J. Obstet. Gynecol.* **80,** 229.

Davies, I. J., and Ryan, K. J. (1971). Unpublished data.

Davies, I. J., and Ryan, K. J. (1972). *Endocrinology* **90,** 507.

Davies, I. J., and Yen, S. S. C. (1971). Unpublished data.

Davies, I. J., Ryan, K. J., and Petro, Z. (1970). *Endocrinology* **86,** 1457.

Deanesly, R. (1971). *J. Reprod. Fert.* **26,** 391.

Debackere, M., Peters, G., and Tuyttens, N. (1961). *J. Endocrinol.* **22,** 321.

de Mattos, C. E. R., Kempson, R. L., Erdos, T., and Csapo, A. (1967). *Fert. Steril.* **18,** 545.

de Snoo, K. (1919). *Ned. Tijdschr. Geneesk.* **2,** 306.

Diczfalusy, E. (1964). *Fed. Proc., Fed. Amer. Soc. Exp. Biol.* **23,** 791.

Diczfalusy, E. (1969). *In* "The Foeto-Placental Unit" (A. Pecile and C. Finzi, eds.), p. 65. Exerpta Medica Found., Amsterdam.

Diczfalusy, E., and Borell, U. (1961). *J. Clin. Endocrinol. Metab.* **21,** 1119.

Drost, M., and Holm, L. W. (1968). *J. Endocrinol.* **40,** 293.

Dry, F. W. (1933). *N. Z. J. Agr.* **47,** 386.

Easterling, W. E., Jr., Simmer, H. H., Dignam, W., Frankland, M. V., and Naftolin, F. (1966). *Steroids* **8,** 157.

Erb, R. E., Gomes, W. R., Randel, R. D., Estergreen, V. L., Jr., and Frost, O. L. (1967). *J. Dairy Sci.* **51,** 420.

Falk, R. J., and Bardin, C. W. (1970). *Endocrinology* **86,** 1059.

Fedrick, J. (1970). *Ann. Hum. Genet.* **34,** 31.

Fevre, J., and Rombauts, P. (1966). *Ann. Biol. Anim., Biochim., Biophys.* **6,** 165.

Fevre, J., Leglise, P. C., and Rombauts, P. (1968). *Ann. Biol. Anim., Biochim., Biophys.* **8,** 225.

Findlay, J. K., and Cox, R. I. (1970). *J. Endocrinol.* **46,** 281.

Fitzpatrick, R. J. (1966). *In* "The Pituitary Gland" (G. W. Harris and B. T. Donovan, eds.), Vol. 3, p. 453. Butterworths, London.

Folley, S. J., and Knaggs, G. S. (1965). *J. Endocrinol.* **33,** 301.

France, J. T. (1971). *Steroids* **17,** 697.

France, J. T., and Liggins, G. C. (1969). *J. Clin. Endocrinol. Metab.* **29,** 138.

Frandsen, V. A., and Stakemann, G. (1961). *Acta Endocrinol. (Copenhagen)* **38,** 383.

Frandsen, V. A., and Stakemann, G. (1963). *Acta Endocrinol. (Copenhagen)* **43,** 184.

Fuchs, F., and Stakemann, G. (1960). *Amer. J. Obstet. Gynecol.* **79,** 172.

Fujikura, T., and Niemann, W. H. (1967). *Amer. J. Obstet. Gynecol.* **97,** 76.

Fylling, P. (1970a). *Acta Endocrinol. (Copenhagen)* **65,** 273.

Fylling, P. (1970b). *Acta Endocrinol. (Copenhagen)* **65,** 284.

Fylling, P. (1971). *Acta Endocrinol. (Copenhagen)* **66,** 289.

Gadd, R. L. (1966). *J. Obstet. Gynaecol. Brit. Commonw.* **73,** 11.

Gillette, D. D. (1966). *Amer. J. Physiol.* **211,** 1095.

Goto, M., and Csapo, A. (1959). *J. Gen. Physiol.* **43,** 455.

Goy, R. W., Hoar, R. M., and Young, W. C. (1957). *Anat. Rec.* **128,** 747.

Grandin, D. J., and Hall, R. E. (1960). *Amer. J. Obstet. Gynecol.* **79,** 237.

Grota, L. J., and Eik-Nes, K. B. (1967). *J. Reprod. Fert.* **13,** 83.

Gruenwald, P., and Minn, H. N. (1961). *Amer. J. Obstet. Gynecol.* **82,** 312.

Guttmacher, A. F. (1939). *Amer. J. Obstet. Gynecol.* **38,** 277.

Guttmacher, A. F., and Kohl, S. G. (1958). *Obstet. Gynecol.* **12,** 528.

Hain, A. M. (1934). *Quart. J. Exp. Physiol.* **24,** 101.

Hain, A. M. (1935). *Quart. J. Exp. Physiol.* **24,** 101.

Halkerston, I. D. K., Eichhorn, J., and Hechter, O. (1961). *J. Biol. Chem.* **236,** 374.

Halliday, R., and Buttle, H. R. L. (1968). *J. Endocrinol.* **41,** 447.

Hamlett, G. W. D. (1935). *Quart. Rev. Biol.* **10,** 432.

Hammond, J., and Marshall, F. H. A. (1930). *Proc. Roy. Soc., Ser. B* **105,** 607.

Harbert, G. M., Jr., McGaughey, H. S., Jr., Scoggin, W. A., and Thornton, W. M. (1964). *Obstet. Gynecol.* **23,** 314.

Hashimoto, I., Henricks, D. M., Anderson, L. L., and Melampy, R. M. (1968). *Endocrinology* **82,** 333.

Haterius, H. O. (1936). *Amer. J. Physiol.* **114,** 399.

Heap, R. B., and Deanesly, R. (1966). *J. Endocrinol.* **34,** 417.

Heckel, G. P., and Allen, W. A. (1938). *Amer. J. Obstet. Gynecol.* **35,** 131.

Hellig, H., Lefebre, Y., Gattereau, D., and Bolte, E. (1969). *In* "The Foeto-Placental Unit" (A. Pecile and C. Finzi, eds.), p. 152. Exerpta Med. Found., Amsterdam.

Hellig, H., Gattereau, D., Lefebvre, Y., and Bolte, E. (1970). *J. Clin. Endocrinol. Metab.* **30,** 624.

Hendricks, C. H. (1964). *Obstet. Gynecol.* **24,** 357.

Hendricks, C. H. (1966). *Obstet. Gynecol.* **27,** 47.

Hendricks, C. H., and Brenner, W. E. (1964). *Amer. J. Obstet. Gynecol.* **90,** 485.

Hendricks, C. H., Brenner, W. E., Sabel, R. A., and Kerenyi, T. (1961). *In* "Progesterone" (A. C. Barnes, ed.), p. 53. Brook Lodge Press, Kalamazoo, Michigan.

Henry, J. S., Venning, E. H., and Browne, J. S. L. (1938). *In* "New International Clinics," Vol. 4, Ser. 48, p. 67. Lippincott, Philadelphia, Pennsylvania (cited by Reynolds, 1949).

Herrick, E. H. (1928). *Anat. Rec.* **39,** 193.

Hindson, J. C., Schofield, B. M., Turner, C. B., and Wolff, H. S. (1965). *J. Physiol. (London)* **181,** 560.

Hindson, J. C., Schofield, B. M., and Ward, W. R. (1969). *J. Endocrinol.* **43,** 207.

Hinterthur, W. (1933). *Zuechtungskunde* **8,** 55; *Anim. Breed. Abstr.* **1,** 24.

Hisaw, F. L., Velardo, J. T., and Goolsby, S. M. (1954). *J. Clin. Endocrinol. Metab.* **14**, 1134.

Hobson, B. M. (1971). *Advan. Reprod. Physiol.* **5**, 67.

Holm, L. W. (1967). *Advan. Vet. Sci.* **11**, 159.

Hopper, B. R., and Tullner, W. M. (1967). *Steroids* **9**, 517.

Hopper, B. R., Tullner, W. M., and Gray, C. W. (1968). *Proc. Soc. Exp. Biol. Med.* **129**, 213.

Jaffe, R. B., and Peterson, E. P. (1966). *Steroids* **5**, 37.

Jensen, E. V., Numata, M., Smith, S., Suzuki, T., Brecher, P. I., and De Sombre, E. R. (1969). *Develop. Biol., Suppl.* **3**, 151.

Jirku, H., and Layne, D. S. (1965). *Steroids* **5**, 37.

Johansson, E. D. B. (1969). *Acta Endocrinol. (Copenhagen)* **61**, 609.

Johansson, I. (1929). *Z. Tierzuecht. Zuechtungsbiol.* **15**, 49.

Jollie, W. P. (1964). *Amer. J. Anat.* **114**, 161.

Jones, I. C., Jarret, I. G., Vinson, G. P., and Potter, K. (1964). *J. Endocrinol.* **29**, 211.

Jost, A. (1966). *Recent Progr. Horm. Res.* **22**, 541.

Joubert, D. M., and Bonsma, J. C. (1957). *S. Afr. J. Sci.* **53**, 340.

Jung, H. (1962). *J. Obstet. Gynaecol. Brit. Commonw.* **69**, 1040.

Kao, C. Y. (1967). *In* "Cellular Biology of the Uterus" (R. M. Wynn, ed.), p. 386. Appleton, New York.

Kelly, J. V. (1961). *Amer. J. Obstet. Gynecol.* **82**, 1207.

Kennedy, P. C. (1971). *Fed. Proc., Fed. Amer. Soc. Exp. Biol.* **30**, 110.

Kenny, F. M., Preeyasombat, C., Spaulding, J. S., and Migeon, C. J. (1966). *Pediatrics* **37**, 960.

Kerr, G. R., Kennan, A. L., Waisman, H. A., and Allen, J. R. (1969). *Growth* **33**, 201.

Kirsch, R. E. (1938). *Amer. J. Physiol.* **122**, 86.

Klausner, D. A., and Ryan, K. J. (1964). *J. Clin. Endocrinol. Metab.* **23**, 445.

Klein, M. (1938). *Proc. Roy. Soc., Ser. B* **125**, 348.

Klopper, A. I., and Billewicz, W. (1963). *J. Obstet. Gynaecol. Brit. Commonw.* **70**, 1024.

Klopper, A. I., and Dennis, K. J. (1962). *Brit. Med. J.* **2**, 1157.

Klopper, A. I., Dennis, K. J., and Farr, V. (1969). *Brit. Med. J.* **2**, 786.

Klyne, W., and Wright, A. A. (1957). *Biochem. J.* **66**, 92.

Knaus, H. H. (1929). *Muenchen. Med. Wochenschr.* **76**, 404 (cited by Reynolds, 1949).

Knott, J. C. (1932). *J. Dairy Sci.* **15**, 87.

Kreines, K., and De Vaux, W. D. (1971). *Pediatrics* **47**, 516.

Kreines, K., Perrin, E., and Salzer, R. (1964). *J. Clin. Endocrinol. Metab.* **24**, 75.

Kriewaldt, F. H., and Hendrickx, A. G. (1968). *Lab. Anim. Care* **18**, 361.

Krizenecky, J. (1935). *Akad. Zemed.* **10**, 351.

Kroc, R. L., Steinetz, B. G., and Beach, V. L. (1959). *Ann. N. Y. Acad. Sci.* **75**, 942.

Kumar, D. (1967). *In* "Cellular Biology of the Uterus" (R. M. Wynn, ed.), p. 449. Appleton, New York.

Kumar, D., and Barnes, A. C. (1961). *Amer. J. Obstet. Gynecol.* **82**, 736.

Kumar, D., and Barnes, A. C. (1965). *Amer. J. Obstet. Gynecol.* **92**, 717.

Kumar, D., Barnes, A. C., and Goodno, J. A. (1962). *Amer. J. Obstet. Gynecol.* **84**, 1207.

Kumar, D., Ward, E. F., and Barnes, A. C. (1964). *Amer. J. Obstet. Gynecol.* **90**, 1360.

Kuriyama, H. (1961). *Ciba Found. Study Group* [Pap.] **9**, 51.

Kuriyama, H., and Csapo, A. I. (1961). *Amer. J. Obstet. Gynecol.* **82**, 592.

Lanman, J. A. (1953). *Medicine (Baltimore)* **32**, 389.

Leavitt, W. W., and Blaha, G. C. (1970). *Biol. Reprod.* **3**, 353.

Liggins, G. C. (1968). *J. Endocrinol.* **44**, 323.

Liggins, G. C. (1969). *J. Endocrinol.* **45**, 515.

Liggins, G. C., and Kennedy, P. C. (1968). *J. Endocrinol.* **40**, 371.

Liggins, G. C., Kennedy, P. C., and Holm, L. W. (1967). *Amer. J. Obstet. Gynecol.* **98**, 1080.

Linzell, J. L., and Heap, R. B. (1968). *J. Endocrinol.* **41**, 433.

Lurie, A. O., Reid, D. E., and Villee, C. A. (1966). *Amer. J. Obstet. Gynecol.* **96**, 670.

McGuire, J. L., and DeDella, C. (1971). *Endocrinology* **88**, 1099.

McKenzie, F. F. (1928). *Mo., Agr. Exp. Sta., Res. Bull.* **118**, 1.

McKerns, K. W. (1967). *In* "Cellular Biology of the Uterus" (R. M. Wynn, ed.), p. 71. Appleton, New York.

McPhail, M. R. (1935). *Proc. Roy. Soc. Ser. B* **117**, 34.

MacDonald, P. C., and Siiteri, P. K. (1965). *J. Clin. Invest.* **44**, 465.

Macedo-Costa, L., and Csapo, A. (1959). *Nature (London)* **184**, 144.

Maner, F. D., Saffan, B. D., Wiggins, R. A., Thompson, J. D., and Preedy, J. R. K. (1963). *J. Clin. Endocrinol. Metab.* **23**, 445.

Marsden, D., and Huntingford, P. J. (1965). *J. Obstet. Gynaecol. Brit. Commonw.* **72**, 65.

Marshall, J. M. (1962). *Physiol. Rev.* **42**, 213.

Martin, R. H., and Menzies, D. N. (1955). *J. Obstet. Gynaecol. Brit. Commonw.* **62**, 256.

Mason, J. I., and Boyd, G. S. (1971). *Eur. J. Biochem.* **21**, 308.

Matsumoto, K., Yamone, G., Endo, H., Kotoh, K., and Okano, K. (1969). *Acta Endocrinol. (Copenhagen)* **61**, 577.

Maurizio, E., and Ottaviani, G. (1934). *Ann. Ostet. Ginecol.* **56**, 1251.

Meigs, R. A., and Ryan, K. J. (1968). *Biochim. Biophys. Acta* **165**, 476.

Mellin, T. N., Erb, R. E., and Estergreen, V. L., Jr. (1966). *J. Anim. Sci.* **25**, 955.

Merkatz, I. R., and Beling, C. G. (1969). *J. Reprod. Fert., Suppl.* **6**, 129.

Merkatz, I. R., New, M. I., Peterson, R. E., and Seaman, M. P. (1969). *J. Pediat.* **75**, 977.

Migeon, C. J., Bertrand, J., and Wall, P. E. (1957). *J. Clin. Invest.* **36**, 1350.

Migeon, C. J., Kowarski, A., Snipes, C. A., Kenney, F. M., Spaulding, J. S., Finkelstein, J. W., and Blizzard, R. M. (1965). *J. Pediat.* **67**, 934.

Mikhail, G., Noall, M. W., and Allen, W. M. (1961). *Endocrinology* **69**, 504.

Milgrom, E., and Baulieu, E. E. (1970). *Endocrinology* **87**, 276.

Morrison, G., Meigs, R. A., and Ryan, K. J. (1965). *Steroids, Suppl.* **2**, 177.

Mosier, H. D. (1956). *J. Pediat.* **48**, 633.

Naeye, R. L., and Blanc, W. A. (1971). *Arch. Pathol.* **91**, 140.

Nakayama, T., Arai, K., Yanaihara, T., Tabei, T., Satoh, K., and Nagatomi, K. (1967). *Acta Endocrinol. (Copenhagen)* **55**, 369.

Needham, D. M., and Shoenberg, C. F. (1967). *In* "Cellular Biology of the Uterus" (R. M. Wynn, ed.), p. 291. Appleton, New York.

Neill, J. D., Johansson, E. D. B., and Knobil, E. (1969). *Endocrinology* **84**, 45.

Nellor, J. E. (1963). *Physiologist* **6**, 244.
Nelson, W. O. (1934). *Endocrinology* **18**, 33.
Newton, W. H. (1935). *J. Physiol. (London)* **84**, 196.
Newton, W. H., and Lits, J. J. (1938). *Anat. Rec.* **72**, 333.
Nichols, J., Lescure, O. L., and Migeon, C. J. (1958). *J. Clin. Endocrinol. Metab.* **18**, 444.
Oakey, R. E. (1970). *Vitam. Horm. (New York)* **28**, 1.
Obst, J. M., Seamark, R. F., and McGowan, C. J. (1971). *J. Reprod. Fert.* **26**, 259.
O'Malley, B. W. (1971). *N. Engl. J. Med.* **284**, 370.
Osinga, A. (1970). Doctoral Thesis, Communications Agricultural University Wageningen, The Netherlands.
Pearlman, W. H., Cerceo, E., and Thomas, M. (1954). *J. Biol. Chem.* **208**, 231.
Pencharz, R. I., and Long, J. A. (1933). *Amer. J. Anat.* **53**, 117.
Pierrepont, C. G., Anderson, A. B. M., Griffiths, K., and Turnbull, A. C. (1970). *Biochem. J.* **118**, 901.
Pinto, R. M., Votta, R. A., Montuori, E., and Baleiron, H. (1964). *Amer. J. Obstet. Gynecol.* **88**, 759.
Pion, R. J., Jaffe, R. B., Eriksson, G., Wiqvist, N., and Diczfalusy, E. (1965). *Acta Endocrinol. (Copenhagen)* **48**, 234.
Pion, R. J., Conrad, S. H., and Wolf, B. J. (1966). *J. Clin. Endocrinol. Metab.* **26**, 225.
Porter, D. G. (1968). *J. Reprod. Fert.* **15**, 437.
Porter, D. G. (1969). *Ciba Found. Study Group* **34**, 79.
Porter, D. G. (1970). *J. Endocrinol.* **46**, 425.
Raeside, J. I. (1963). *J. Reprod. Fert.* **6**, 427.
Reynolds, S. R. M. (1937). *Proc. Soc. Exp. Biol. Med.* **36**, 453.
Reynolds, S. R. M. (1949). "Physiology of the Uterus." Hafner, New York.
Reynolds, S. R. M., and Allen, W. M. (1937). *Anat. Rec.* **69**, 481.
Reynolds, S. R. M., and Kaminester, S. (1936). *Amer. J. Physiol.* **116**, 510.
Richards, I. D. G. (1969). *Brit. J. Prev. Soc. Med.* **23**, 218.
Roberts, J. S., and Share, L. (1968). *Endocrinology* **83**, 272.
Roberts, J. S., and Share, L. (1969). *Endocrinology* **84**, 1076.
Roberts, J. S., and Share, L. (1970). *Endocrinology* **87**, 812.
Rombauts, P. (1962). *Ann. Biol. Anim., Biochim., Biophys.* **2**, 151.
Rombauts, P. (1964). *C. R. Acad. Sci.* **258**, 5257.
Rombauts, P., Terqui, M., and Fevre, J. (1967). *Proc. Int. Congr. Horm. Steroids, 2nd, 1966* Abstracts, p. 283.
Ronaldson, J. W. (1969). *Aust. J. Exp. Biol. Med. Sci.* **47**, 679.
Roselli, A., and Barbosa, L. T. (1965). *Pediatrics* **35**, 70.
Roy, E. J. (1962). *J. Obstet. Gynaecol. Brit. Commonw.* **64**, 196.
Ryan, K. J. (1966). *Amer. J. Obstet. Gynecol.* **96**, 676.
Ryan, K. J., and Hopper, B. R. (1972). *Primatology* (in press).
Ryan, K. J., and Petro, Z. (1971). Unpublished data.
Ryan, K. J., and Shinada, T. (1971). Unpublished data.
Ryan, K. J., Benirschke, K., and Smith, O. W. (1961). *Endocrinology* **69**, 613.
Savard, K. (1961). *Endocrinology* **68**, 411.
Savard, K., Marsh, J. M., and Rice, B. F. (1965). *Recent Progr. Horm. Res.* **21**, 285.
Schofield, B. M. (1964). *J. Endocrinol.* **30**, 347.
Schofield, B. M. (1966). *Mem. Soc. Endocrinol.* **14**, 221.
Schofield, B. M. (1969). *J. Endocrinol.* **43**, 673.
Schofield, B. M., and Wood, C. (1964). *J. Physiol. (London)* **175**, 125.

Segal, S. J., and Scher, W. (1967). In "Cellular Biology of the Uterus" (R. M. Wynn, ed.), p. 114. Appleton, New York.

Selye, H., Collip, J. B., and Thompson, D. L. (1933). Proc. Soc. Exp. Biol. Med. 30, 589.

Selye, H., Collip, J. B., and Thompson, D. L. (1935). Endocrinology 19, 151.

Short, R. V. (1960). J. Reprod. Fert. 1, 61.

Siegmund, H. (1930). Arch. Gynaekol. 140, 583.

Simpson, E. R., and Boyd, G. S. (1967a). Eur. J. Biochem. 2, 275.

Simpson, E. R., and Boyd, G. S. (1967b). Biochem. Biophys. Res. Commun. 28, 945.

Solomon, S. (1960). In "The Placenta and Foetal Membranes" (C. A. Villee, ed.), p. 201. Williams & Wilkins, Baltimore, Maryland.

Stabenfeldt, G. H., and Hendrickx, A. G. (1971). Anat. Rec. 169, 437.

Stempfel, R. S., Jr., and Engels, F. L. (1960). Pediatrics 57, 443.

Terrill, C. E., and Hazel, L. N. (1947). J. Vet. Res. 8, 66.

Thiersch, J. B. (1960). Congenital Anomalies, Ciba Found. Symp. p. 270.

Thompson, A. M., Billewicz, W. Z., and Hytten, F. E. (1968). J. Obstet. Gynaecol. Brit. Commonw. 75, 903.

Townsend, L., and Ryan, K. J. (1970). Endocrinology 87, 151.

Tulchinsky, D., and Korenman, S. G. (1971). J. Clin. Invest. 50, 1490.

Turnbull, A. C., and Anderson, A. B. M. (1969). Ciba Found. Study Group [Pap.] 34, 106.

Van Der Molen, H. J., and Aakvaag, A. (1967). In "Hormones in Blood" (C. H. Gray and A. L. Bacharach, eds.), 2nd rev. ed., Vol. 2, p. 221. Academic Press, New York.

Van Leusden, H. A., and Villee, C. A. (1965). Steroids 6, 31.

Van Rensburg, S. J. (1965). J. S. Afr. Vet. Med. Ass. 36, 491.

Van Rensburg, S. J. (1967). J. Endocrinol. 38, 83.

Wichmann, K. (1967). Acta Endocrinol. (Copenhagen), Suppl. 116, 1.

Wiest, W. G. (1963). Endocrinology 73, 310.

Wiest, W. G. (1967). Steroids 10, 279.

Wiest, W. G. (1969). Ciba Found. Study Group [Pap.] 34, 56.

Wiest, W. G. (1970). Endocrinology 87, 43.

Wiest, W. G., Kidwell, W. R., and Balogh, K., Jr. (1968). Endocrinology 82, 844.

Wilson, W. K., and Dudley, F. J. (1952). J. Genet. 50, 384.

Wing, H. H. (1899). N. Y., Agr. Exp. Sta., Ithaca, Bull. 162.

Winick, M., and Noble, A. (1966). Nature (London) 212, 34.

Winick, M., Coscia, A., and Noble, A. (1967). Pediatrics 39, 248.

Wislocki, G. B., and Dempsey, E. W. (1939). Anat. Rec. 75, 341.

Wood, C., Elstein, M., and Pinkerton, J. H. M. (1963). J. Obstet. Gynaecol. Brit. Commonw. 70, 839.

Yannone, M. E. (1968). Amer. J. Obstet. Gynecol. 101, 1054.

Yordan, E., and D'Esopo, D. A. (1955). Amer. J. Obstet. Gynecol. 70, 266.

Younglai, E. V., and Solomon, S. (1969). In "Foetus and Placenta" (A. Klopper and E. Diczfalusy, eds.), p. 249. Blackwell, Oxford.

Younglai, E. V., Stern, M., Ling, W., Leung, K., and Solomon, S. (1969). In "The Foeto-Placental Unit" (A. Pecile and C. Finzi, eds.), p. 190. Exerpta Med. Found., Amsterdam.

Zander, J., and von Münstermann, A. M. (1956). Klin. Wochenschr. 34, 944.

Zander, J., Holzmann, K., von Münstermann, A. M., Runnebaum, B., and Sieber,

W. (1969). *In* "The Foeto-Placental Unit" (A. Pecile and C. Finzi, eds.), p. 162. Exerpta Med. Found., Amsterdam.

Zarrow, M. X., Wilson, E. D., Coldwell, A. L., Yochim, J., and Sawin, P. B. (1960). *Fert. Steril.* **11**, 370.

Zarrow, M. X., Anderson, N. C., and Callantine, M. R. (1963). *Nature (London)* **198**, 690.

Zeiner, F. N. (1943). *Endocrinology* **33**, 239.

Hormonal Changes in Pathological Pregnancy

HUBERTUS A. VAN LEUSDEN

University Department of Obstetrics and Gynecology, St. Radboud Ziekenhuis,
Nijmegen, The Netherlands

I. Introduction

A. Scope

Normal human pregnancy is accompanied by impressive hormonal changes. Tremendous insight has been gained, especially in the last decade. The idea put forward by Diczfalusy to consider the fetoplacental unit as an integrated functional unit has proved to be extremely fruitful for research. The enormous amount of data concerning endocrine functions of the human placenta and fetoplacental unit has been discussed in a number of reviews of varying scope and detail (Diczfalusy and Troen, 1961; Fuchs, 1962; Ryan, 1962; Diczfalusy, 1964; Eik-Nes and Hall, 1965; Mitchell, 1967; Klopper, 1968, 1969, 1970; Diczfalusy and Mancuso, 1969; Solomon and Younglai, 1969; Van Leusden, 1969, 1972a). Especially noteworthy is the book edited by Klopper and Diczfalusy (1969), in which inter alia the assessment of placental function in clinical practice is discussed. The emphasis in the present review will be placed on the findings in pathological pregnancy.

Information from animals may be transferred to humans only with considerable caution. Therefore, in this review the work to be considered for the most part will be that which has been conducted with human material. Those hormones will be reviewed that have been shown to be produced predominantly by or within the fetoplacental unit. Data concerning the maternal metabolism of estrogens and progesterone will be considered only as and when it affects the subject under review. It will be assessed whether or not HCG, HPL, estrogens, and progesterone, or their metabolites change in different categories of early and late pathologic pregnancy. Early pathological pregnancy comprises abortion, molar pregnancy, and choriocarcinoma. Late pathological pregnancy includes inter alia abdominal pregnancy, congenital defects of the fetus, multiple pregnancy, hypertension, Rh isoimmunization, disturbed carbohydrate metabolism, prematurity, and postmaturity. Closely related to the subjects of prematurity and postmaturity is the onset of labor.

In the different kinds of pathological pregnancy, hormonal studies have been carried out measuring excretion, levels in the plasma, placental tissue, and amniotic fluid, and umbilical arterial and venous blood concentrations. Secretion rates of several hormones have been determined. Dynamic tests have been devised involving infusion of various steroid precursors into the maternal circulation or into the amniotic fluid with measurement of the urinary excretion of metabolic products. Incubation experiments have been performed with placental minces and homogenates in the presence of labeled precursors. Much insight has also been provided by the study of experiments of nature, such as anencephalic monsters and hydatidiform mole pregnancy, where the fetus is absent.

Problems of variability, practical usefulness, and the prognostic value of hormone determinations in pathological pregnancy are of paramount importance. The question whether or not dissociation of fetoplacental pathology occurs very often is crucial. Isolated disturbances within the fetoplacental unit bring about specific hormonal alterations. On the other hand, specific alterations of hormone excretion do not always point to localized lesions within the fetoplacental unit.

B. NOMENCLATURE

The following trivial names of steroids and abbreviations are used in this review.

Trivial name	Systematic name
ACTH	Adrenocorticotropic hormone
Aldosterone	Pregn-4-ene-18,21-diol-11β,18-epoxy-3,20-dione
Androstenedione	Androst-4-ene-3,17-dione
16-Oxoandrostenediol	3β,17β-Dihydroxyandrost-5-en-16-one
Cholesterol	Cholesta-5-en-3-ol
Corticosterone	11β,21-Dihydroxypregn-4-ene-3,20-dione
Cortisol	11β,17α,21-Trihydroxypregn-4-ene-3,20-dione
Dexamethasone	9α-Fluoro-16α-methylprednisolone
Dydrogesterone	9β,10α-Pregna-4,6-diene-3,20-dione
DHA(S)	3β-Hydroxyandrost-5-en-17-one (sulfate)
16α-OH-DHA	3β,16α-Dihydroxyandrost-5-en-17-one
Estetrol	Estra-1,3,5(10)-triene-3,15α,16α,17β-tetrol
Estradiol	Estra-1,3,5(10)-triene-3,17β-diol
11-Dehydro-17α-hydroxyestradiol	Estra-1,3,5(10),11-tetraene-3,17α-diol
Estriol	Estra-1,3,5(10)-triene-3,16α,17β-triol
15α-OH-Estriol	Estra-1,3,5(10)-triene-3,15α,16α,17β-tetrol
Estrone	3-Hydroxyestra-1,3,5(10)-trien-17-one
16α-OH-estrone	3,16α-Dihydroxy-estra-1,3,5(10)-triene-17-one
HCG	Human chorionic gonadotropin
HPL	Human placental lactogen
Pregnanediol	3α,20α-Dihydroxy-5β-pregnane
Pregnanetriol	3α,17α,20α-Trihydroxy-5β-pregnane

(Continued)

Trivial name	Systematic name
Pregnanolone	3α-Hydroxy-5β-pregnan-20-one
Pregnenolone	3β-Hydroxypregn-5-en-20-one
16α-OH-pregnenolone	3β,16α-Dihydroxypregn-5-en-20-one
Progesterone	Pregn-4-ene-3,20-dione
16α-OH-progesterone	16α-Hydroxy-pregn-4-ene-3,20-dione
16β-OH-progesterone	16β-Hydroxypregn-4-ene-3,20-dione
17α-OH-progesterone	17α-Hydroxypregn-4-ene-3,20-dione
PSR	Progesterone secretion rate
Retroprogesterone	9β,10α-Pregn-4-ene-3,20-dione
Testosterone	17β-Hydroxyandrost-4-en-3-one
THE	3α,17α,21-Trihydroxy-5β-pregnane-11,20-dione
THF	3α,11β,17α,21-tetrahydroxy-5β-pregnan-20-one

II. HUMAN CHORIONIC GONADOTROPIN

A. INTRODUCTION

1. *Immunological Methods and Biological Assays*

Several immunological methods have been described for the detection of HCG. These laboratory tests include hemagglutination inhibition (Wide and Gemzell, 1960), complement fixation (Brody and Carlström, 1960), gel precipitation (McKean, 1960), and latex agglutination inhibition (Little, 1962). The development of these assay techniques has thoroughly transformed the field of HCG assay; the determination of HCG has become less time-consuming and more reliable. Sensitivity, specificity, accuracy, precision, and practicability of HCG determinations have been reviewed by Brody (1969a).

Extraction, purification, physicochemical, and biochemical properties of HCG have been reviewed by Brody (1969a), Hellema (1971), and Saxena (1971). These authors also discussed the problem whether or not normal and tumor HCG are identical, the biological properties of HCG, and its antigenic properties.

Immunological techniques measure a spectrum of "gonadotropins" different from that detected by biological methods (e.g., Hobson and Wide, 1964). Immunoassays can give rather different results from those obtained with the earlier biological methods (e.g., Daniëlsson, 1965; Toaff *et al.*, 1965). However, agreement between immunoassay and biological assay for HCG has been established (e.g., Haskins, 1967). Therefore, previous findings from biological tests cannot be applied to the immunological tests without further investigation. Both can be useful, as the trend of values obtained by biological tests is usually the same as that obtained by immunoassay.

Urinary HCG (MW about 30,000) probably has several antigenic sites (Wide, 1967), but these may not be the same as the biologically important parts of the molecule. In the second trimester of normal pregnancy, an "immunologically active" (I) but "biologically inactive" (B) HCG has been separated from urinary HCG with both activities (Hobson and Wide, 1964). The B:I ratio (Section II, B, 2) changes as pregnancy progresses.

2. Normal Pregnancy

The determination of HCG excretion above 1000 IU per liter is now a well established routine pregnancy test. The repeated finding of excretion below 1000 IU/liter in the first 80–100 days of pregnancy suggests intrauterine fetal death. A number of authors express HCG excretion as IU per liter, although the expression IU per 24 hours is more reliable. HCG excretion in normal pregnancy increases until day 55; after that it falls (Wilson et al., 1949; Haskins and Sherman, 1952; Behrman and Niemann, 1955a,b; Brody and Carlström, 1962a,b,c). Toward the end of pregnancy, there may be a slightly increased excretion. From week 9 of gestation onward, amniotic fluid HCG rises, reaching peak values around week 13 (Berle, 1969).

3. Renal Clearance

Renal clearance of HCG (Gastineau et al., 1949; Loraine, 1950; Johnson et al., 1968) was found to be constant throughout pregnancy. According to Loraine (1958), variations in serum and urine concentrations of HCG reflect changes in production rate and/or inactivation rather than altered renal excretion rate.

4. Fetal Metabolism

Fetal metabolism of HCG is suggested by the data of Lauritzen and Lehmann (1967) and Berle and Schultze-Mosgau (1967, 1968), who established higher HCG concentration in the umbilical vein than in the arteries. Administration of HCG to newborn infants significantly increased urinary excretion of DHA (Lauritzen and Lehmann, 1967). This rise was even more pronounced in premature infants. It was suggested (Lauritzen, 1969) that HCG is an adrenocorticoptropic hormone in the fetus, regulating the supply of fetal adrenal DHA as a precursor for the production of estrogens in the placenta. Johannisson (1968) injected ACTH and HCG into the amniotic fluid in mid-pregnancy and found similar electron microscopic effects of ACTH and HCG on the inner fetal zone of the adrenal cortex. The supply of DHA (Lauritzen, 1969), in turn, would determine the production of estriol by the fetoplacental unit. It is suggested that a feedback control mechanism might exist between estriol and HCG. Further experimentation is needed to supply evidence for the hypothesis that HCG acts like an ACTH for the fetus.

B. Abortion, Hydatidiform Mole Pregnancy, Choriocarcinoma, Ectopic Pregnancy, Luteoma of Pregnancy

1. Abortion

Rakoff (1940) has indicated the relation between serum and urinary HCG and placental function. In abortion, urinary (Szenjberg and Rabau, 1950; Rabau and Szenjberg, 1955; Hon and Morris, 1955, 1956; B. Zondek and Goldberg, 1957; P. J. Keller, 1966; Hepp, 1967; Abdul Enein and Sharman, 1967) and serum (Delfs and Jones, 1948; Delfs, 1957; Vermelin et al., 1957) levels of HCG have been reported to be low, but normal values have also been reported in unsuccessful pregnancies (J. B. Brown et al., 1970b). Hughes et al. (1964) and Baumgarten (1966) consider urinary HCG assays of no prognostic value in threatened abortion.

Brody and Carlström (1962a), using a complement fixation technique, determined the HCG concentration in the serum of patients with clinical evidence of abortion, and found that in early threatened abortion reduction of HCG levels below the normal range was invariably associated with abortion, whereas normal HCG values usually indicated a favorable outcome of the pregnancy. The same has been found in the assessment of HCG excretion per 24 hours (Van Leusden, 1972b).

Carlsson (1964), using the Wide technique, was able to confirm the prognostic value of serum HCG assays in threatened abortion. The prognostic value of serum HCG determinations has been confirmed in a large series (Brody and Carlström, 1965a; Brody, 1969a,b). Yagami and Ito (1965) found spontaneous abortion invariably in 12 women whose level of serum HCG was lower than normal. The finding that late aborters (with the expulsion of fetuses larger than 25 cm) tend to have normal serum HCG (Brody and Carlström, 1962a) and normal HCG excretion per 24 hours (Van Leusden, 1972b) is in accordance with the established fact that the etiologic mechanism in late abortion is different from that in patients with early abortion.

It may be concluded that in early threatened abortion the use of serum and urinary HCG determinations is of prognostic value. Serum and urinary HCG is of little or no prognostic value in late abortion. The etiologic mechanism of late abortion is different from that of early abortion.

2. Hydatidiform Mole Pregnancy

The quantitative relationship between urinary immunological and biological activity (B:I ratio; see Section II, A, 1) changes as pregnancy progresses (Wide and Hobson, 1967), suggesting that the two methods do not measure the same activity. Urine specimens from women with hydatidiform mole have a higher B:I ratio than specimens from women with normal pregnancies (Wide and Hobson, 1967). This difference can be used to distinguish between normal and hydatidiform mole pregnancy. The B:I ratio of the serum of pregnant women is higher than that of urine. The B:I ratios of serum from women with a hydatidiform mole and from those with a normal pregnancy are of the same magnitude. Thus, the urinary B:I ratio can be used to help diagnose hydatidiform mole pregnancy.

Yogo (1969) established different electrophoretic and chromatographic behavior of urinary HCG extracts in the third and in the tenth month of pregnancy, different again in urinary extracts from patients with hydatidiform mole or chorionepithelioma. Differences in the distribution of the gonadotropic activity in serum protein fractions of women with normal pregnancy or with trophoblastic tumors were already indicated by Reisfeld et al. (1959). Matthies and Diczfalusy (1968) reported differences in the physical properties of HCG extracts from different sources, i.e., urinary HCG from women with chorionic tumors, HCG from placental tissue, maternal plasma, and amniotic fluid in the first trimester, and also commercial preparations of HCG.

Increased HCG concentration in hydatidiform mole tissue as compared with normal placental tissue was found by Diczfalusy et al. (1958). Hobson (1955, 1958) found a higher concentration of HCG in molar tissue than in normal placental tissue of comparable age. N. Sciarra (1970) found that the HCG concentration of fluid of small hydatid vesicles is higher than that of large vesicles. Serum HCG is always much lower than small and large vesicular fluid HCG. The urinary HCG level is higher than both serum and vesicular fluid levels. These data are in accordance with the hypothesis that the hydatid fluid is a product of the trophoblastic tissue of the mole.

Increased urinary HCG in hydatidiform mole pregnancy has been well established as compared with normal pregnancies of the same duration (e.g., B. Zondek, 1929, 1942; Hamburger, 1944; Wide, 1962; Noto et al., 1964; Campbell et al., 1970). However, reported urinary HCG levels in normal and in hydatidiform mole pregnancy are scattered, and the overlap is great (e.g., Hamburger, 1944, 1958; Hobson, 1955; Hellema, 1965; Kock et al., 1965; P. J. Keller, 1966; Teoh, 1967; Campbell et al.,

1970). Furthermore, increased HCG excretion does not always indicate hydatidiform mole pregnancy, and conditions such as twin pregnancy must be excluded.

Serum levels of HCG are of importance, as in all patients with hydatidiform mole, serum HCG was abnormally elevated (Delfs, 1957; Brody and Carlström, 1962a,b,c; Yagami and Ito, 1965; Teoh, 1967). The HCG assay of serum can be employed to distinguish between a molar and a normal pregnancy, but not to differentiate between benign hydatidiform mole and choriocarcinoma (Delfs, 1959).

3. Choriocarcinoma

Careful follow-up after a molar pregnancy remains essential to ensure recognition of choriocarcinoma while it is still curable (e.g., Bagshawe et al., 1969). In about 50% of the cases, choriocarcinoma appears after a hydatidiform mole and may be diagnosed early by the persistence of HCG in blood or urine. Thus, in a series of 328 molar pregnancies Beischer et al. (1970) found an incidence of malignant sequelae of 4.3%, whereas 55% of trophoblastic malignancies followed hydatidiform moles.

Increased HCG excretion in choriocarcinoma has been well established (e.g., B. Zondek, 1929, 1935, 1937). Levels of serum HCG in 3 women with chorionepithelioma showed normal or high values (Yagami and Ito, 1965).

Choriocarcinoma of the uterus and its related trophoblastic tumors represent the only cancer that can be consistently cured with chemotherapy. Serum HCG and/or urinary HCG titers are of paramount importance in the clinical evaluation of patients with choriocarcinoma submitted to chemotherapy (Hertz et al., 1958; Brewer et al., 1964; Goldstein and Reid, 1967; Johnson et al., 1968; Yen et al., 1968).

HCG has been detected in the cerebrospinal fluid of pregnant and nonpregnant subjects with a high concentration of the hormone in the plasma and urine (Ehrhardt, 1931; B. Zondek, 1937, 1942; Mathieu, 1939; Vesell and Goldman, 1944). According to McCormick (1954) and Tashima (1965), HCG would not appear in the cerebrospinal fluid until a high threshold value equivalent to a urinary excretion rate of about 250,000 IU of HCG per day, was exceeded. In contrast herewith, Rushworth et al. (1968) and Bagshawe et al. (1969) in subjects without evidence of metastases in the central nervous system found no evidence of a threshold effect. The HCG concentration in cerebrospinal fluid, determined immunologically, is directly proportional to that in plasma. The factor of proportionality is higher in patients with intracranial metastases than in patients without metastases. Thus evidence of metastases in the brain or spinal cord may be obtained.

4. Ectopic Pregnancy

Pattillo et al. (1966) have grown throphoblastic tissue from 13 ectopic pregnancies (and 2 hydatidiform moles) in prolonged explant cultures. Persistent gonadotropin production is associated with a characteristic cell, which migrates from the explant and displays a broad and elongated form with multiple cytoplasmic projections. This cell was described originally by G. E. S. Jones et al. (1943).

HCG excretion of less than 1000 IU per liter, between 1000 and 3000 IU per liter and more than 3000 IU per liter was reported in ectopic pregnancies by Simmons and Israelstam (1968). Very low urinary HCG was found by P. J. Keller (1966), whereas Wide (1967) found usually between 200 and 10,000 IU of HCG per liter. In a careful study, Hepp et al. (1968) showed that in tubal abortion the pregnancy test failed as an indicator of trophoblastic activity, but in ruptured tubal pregnancies the HCG titer and the morphological-microscopical appearance of the trophoblast showed close agreement.

5. Luteoma of Pregnancy

In luteoma of pregnancy the augmentation of the net synthesis of Δ^4-androstene-3,17-dione by HCG has been demonstrated in vitro (Rice et al., 1969). This finding and the clinical observation of postpartum regression are compatible with the concept that HCG plays some role in the development and maintenance of this specific ovarian lesion.

C. ABDOMINAL PREGNANCY

Considerable amounts of HCG are excreted for several weeks following termination of abdominal pregnancy when the placenta is left in situ (Siegler et al., 1959; Michie et al., 1966; Hamersma and Schopman, 1967; Friedman et al., 1969).

Serum HCG remains stationary during the first week after delivery in this condition, then declines steadily from day 7 to day 64 at an almost constant rate of -14.1% per day, which corresponds to an apparent half-life of 110 hours (Kim et al., 1971). Since the half-life of HCG antigen in serum after the third postpartum day has been reported as 37.3 hours (Midgley and Jaffe, 1968), the apparent disappearance rate observed by Kim et al. (1971) is much lower and mainly reflects slowly declining production rather than metabolic clearance of the hormone.

D. Fetal Sex and Multiple Pregnancy

1. Fetal Sex

Fetal sex and maternal serum HCG level in the last trimester of pregnancy are related (Brody and Carlström, 1965a,b). Female fetuses are associated with higher HCG levels than males, which may suggest that the fetus exerts some control over placental HCG synthesis, or point to an inherent sex-determined difference in metabolic activity. However, this relation cannot be used for the diagnosis of sex because of the large scatter and overlap.

2. Multiple Pregnancy

In this condition the urinary HCG has been reported to be above or at the upper limit of the normal range (Borth et al., 1959; Haskins and Sherman, 1952; Behrman and Niemann, 1955b). Serum HCG (G. E. S. Jones et al., 1944) has been reported abnormally high or in the normal range in twin pregnancy.

E. Hypertension, Rh Isoimmunization, and
   Carbohydrate Metabolism

1. Hypertension

In patients with hypertension (BP $\geq$ 140/90 prior to pregnancy or prior to week 24 without superimposed preeclampsia), HCG excretion is in the normal range; also in cases of intrauterine fetal death HCG excretion remained in the normal range prior to or at the moment of fetal death (Aubry and Nesbitt, 1970).

In toxemia of pregnancy serum HCG has been found to be increased (G. V. Smith and Smith, 1934, 1939, 1948). However, serum HCG and urinary HCG were reported to be increased only in severe toxemia by H. C. Taylor and Scandron (1939), Loraine and Mathew (1950), and Lloyd et al. (1951). Brody (1969b), in contrast to Carlsson (1964), found increased serum HCG levels in patients with serious manifestations of toxemia.

Increased urinary HCG excretion in severe toxemia has been reported by G. V. Smith and Smith (1934, 1939, 1948) Watts and Adair (1943), Haskins and Sherman (1952), Spadoni et al. (1966), P. J. Keller (1966), Soiva et al. (1968), and Helbing et al. (1969). However, Rubin et al. (1946) described normal HCG excretion even in severe toxemia.

Serum HCG level, severity of toxemia, birth weight, and Apgar score were not found to be correlated in 178 patients with severe toxemia (Teoh and Sivasamboo, 1968), although the average HCG titers were higher than those encountered during the last trimester of normal pregnancy. In retarded intrauterine growth (with or without hypertension) abnormally low HCG excretion throughout pregnancy has been found by Bell et al. (1967).

In moderate and severe toxemia the placental tissue has a higher HCG concentration than normal placental tissue (Loraine and Mathew, 1953; Wilken et al., 1966). In mild toxemia umbilical arterial and venous HCG are the same as in normal pregnancy (Berle and Schultze-Mosgau, 1967, 1968).

2. Rh Isoimmunization

The urinary HCG excretion has been reported to be considerably increased in Rh isoimmunization (Spadoni et al., 1966; Connon, 1966), especially when hydropic placentas are present.

In cases of severely affected fetuses the serum HCG is increased (Bradbury and Goplerud, 1963; McCarthy and Pennington, 1964a).

Berle and Schultze-Mosgau (1968) and Berle (1969) reported an elevation of HCG concentration in the umbilical arteries as well as in the umbilical vein, compared to that in normal pregnancy, which may possibly be caused by an increased HCG production in the placenta. Kaivola et al. (1967) found the HCG content of the placenta in Rh isoimmunization slightly higher than normal, but the difference was statistically not significant.

The HCG content of the amniotic fluid has been reported normal (McCarthy and Pennington, 1964b) or increased (Berle, 1969) in severe erythroblastosis fetalis.

3. Carbohydrate Metabolism

Increased serum HCG as well as urinary excretion have been reported by Loraine (1956) in 33% of pregnant diabetics. White (1952) recorded increased serum concentrations in 91% of the pregnant diabetics studied. These findings may explain the (rare) occurrence of bilateral thecalutein cysts in a pregnant diabetic at term (Staffeldt, 1966). In diabetic pregnancy there is also an increased HCG concentration in the amniotic fluid and in umbilical vein blood (Berle, 1969). Increased HCG excretion has also been reported by Spadoni et al. (1966). However, P. J. Keller (1966) and Aubry and Nesbitt (1970) found normal HCG excretion in diabetics with normal outcome of pregnancy. Even in cases of fetal death in utero, the HCG excretion was within the normal range both prior to and at the time of fetal death (Aubry and Nesbitt, 1970). Loraine (1958) and Brody (1969a,b) found no relationship between HCG levels in the body fluids and the outcome of pregnancy.

It seems thus, as indicated previously by Loraine and Mathew (1950) and Loraine (1956), that the determination of HCG is of no clinical significance in pregnancy complicated by diabetes.

F. PREMATURITY AND PROLONGED PREGNANCY

1. *Prematurity*

In prematurity, Aubry and Nesbitt (1970) found normal excretion of HCG, and could not detect a trend of prelabor increase or decrease.

In premature parturition umbilical arterial and venous HCG concentrations were above those found in normal term pregnancies (Berle and Schultze-Mosgau, 1967).

2. *Prolonged Pregnancy*

In prolonged pregnancy no changes in the excretion of HCG were detected (Daniëlsson, 1965).

G. SUMMARY

Immunological methods have transformed the field of HCG assay. Biological assays and immunological assays may give rather different results. Immunological techniques measure a spectrum of "gonadotropins" different from that detected by biological methods. The trend of values obtained by biological tests is usually the same as that obtained by immunoassay. In pathological pregnancy variations of HCG concentrations reflect changing production rates rather than altered renal excretion. A fetal metabolism of HCG occurs. In general there are wide inter- and intrapersonal fluctuations of HCG.

The use of serum HCG and urinary HCG excretion is of prognostic value in early threatened abortion, but not in late abortion. Increased HCG excretion is not necessarily associated with hydatidiform mole pregnancy. Determination of urinary B:I ratio can be a useful additional diagnostic step. Serum HCG is nearly always elevated in molar pregnancy. Serum HCG and/or urinary HCG titers are of paramount importance in the detection of choriocarcinoma following a mole and in the clinical evaluation of patients submitted to chemotherapy. Intracranial or spinal cord metastases can be detected by HCG determinations in cerebrospinal fluid.

Considerable amounts of HCG are excreted for several weeks after termination of abdominal pregnancy with the placenta left *in situ*. There is a slowly declining production of HCG under these circumstances.

Female fetuses are associated with higher HCG levels than male fetuses, which may suggest that the fetus exerts some control over placental HCG synthesis. In multiple pregnancy, urinary HCG excretion has been reported to be above or at the upper limit of normal values. Serum HCG is abnormally high or in the normal range.

In hypertension without superimposed preeclampsia, the HCG excretion is in the normal range. The HCG excretion values do not change prior to or at the moment of intrauterine fetal death. The balance of evidence suggests that the mean values of serum and urinary HCG are mostly higher in severe toxemia than in normal pregnancy. This is correlated with a higher placental concentration of HCG. Routine HCG assays are of no value in the clinical management of toxemia of pregnancy. In cases of severe Rh isoimmunization, the serum and urinary HCG values are increased, presumably because of the increased HCG production by the large and hydropic placenta. In terms of fetal viability HCG determinations are of no value. In pregnancy complicated with diabetes there is no relationship between HCG levels in the body fluids and the outcome of pregnancy.

In prematurity and postmaturity the excretion of HCG is in the normal range.

III. Human Placental Lactogen (HPL)

A. Introduction

1. Presence in Serum, Urine, and Umbilical Cord and Half-Life

Josimovich and MacLaren (1962) partially purified a polypeptide, found in large amounts in placental tissue, human placental lactogen (HPL), called lactogen because of its lactogenic activity in the pigeon crop and in pseudopregnant rabbit assays and its possible role in breast enlargement and the initiation of lactation (Section III, A, 2). They demonstrated its presence in the peripheral circulation during pregnancy. For an excellent review concerning the chemical nature (extraction and purification; purity; biochemical, and physicochemical properties), biological properties, and site of synthesis (the placenta, very probably the cytoplasm of the syntrophoblastic layer of the chorionic villi), the reader is referred to Brody (1969a) and Saxena (1971). From day 35 onward serum HPL is detectable, increasing until term. The half-life is 20–30 minutes (Kaplan and Grumbach, 1965a; Frantz et al., 1965; Samaan et al., 1966; Saxena et al., 1968; Kaplan et al., 1968). The 24-hour excretion increases until term (Kaplan and Grumbach, 1965a). Relatively small quantities of HPL are detectable in umbilical cord blood, indicating only a minor transplacental transfer of this protein (Kaplan and Grumbach, 1965a,b; Samaan et al., 1966).

2. Possible Physiopathological Role of HPL

El Tomi et al. (1971) blocked the HPL action in rabbits by active immunization. Ovulation and implantation rates were not reduced. However, none of the pregnant HPL-immunized rabbits showed a normal course of pregnancy. Partial or complete fetal resorption was observed. The few young that were born alive all died within 36 hours after delivery since the mother failed to nurse them. The mammary glands of these mothers were underdeveloped compared to the puerperal controls. The ovaries showed a reduced weight as well as an impaired enzyme activity. These experiments suggest an important physiological role for HPL in the maintenance of pregnancy and initiation of lactation. Mouse mammary tissue stimulation by HPL (Turkington and Topper, 1966) and the observation of gynecomastia in a male with a HPL-secreting choriocarcinoma of the testis (Frantz et al., 1965; Josimovich et al., 1969) also indicate that this hormone may play an important role in breast enlargement and the initiation of lactation. Moreover, HPL might play an important role in the regulation of carbohydrate metabolism in pregnancy (Section III, C, 3).

3. Range of Normal Values and Clinical Usefulness, Especially in Late Pregnancy

The short half-life of HPL (Section III, A, 1) and its autonomous trophoblastic production (Spellacy et al., 1967) would suggest serum HPL assays to be of great value in the assessment of placental function in early as well as late pregnancy. However, there exists a wide range of normal values (e.g., Singer, 1970), particularly during the second half of pregnancy. The unexplained large variability in the in vitro rate of synthesis of HPL in apparently normal placentas following normal pregnancies (Suwa and Friesen, 1969) may be of interest in this context. The wide range of normal values should be stressed, since serial sampling over several days or weeks may be necessary for HPL determinations to represent a reasonable prognostic index. Transient drops in HPL values may have no significance, particularly after week 38 of gestation. In view of the autonomy of the placenta, measurement of serum HPL cannot be expected to be of value when fetal distress is secondary to primary fetal abnormality. However, this is seldom the case.

Spellacy and Teoh (1969) and Spellacy et al. (1971) have analyzed more than 4000 samples of serum during pregnancy from 200 normal women and from 350 women who had medical complications which are known to cause fetal death—erythroblastosis fetalis, diabetes mellitus, and hypertension (BP > 140/90). Values less than 4 μg/ml serum after

30 weeks reflected a risk for the fetus. This abnormally low zone was termed the fetal danger or F-D zone. Saxena *et al.* (1969) proposed that a 50% fall during late pregnancy indicates the need for prompt induction of labor or for cesarean section, since it suggests an extensive placental dysfunction. This proposal has been challenged on the basis of the data presented by Spellacy (1969). Saxena *et al.* (1969) have subsequently clarified their interpretation (Selenkow, 1969), and they do not recommend interruption of the pregnancy. The use of HPL estimation as a placental function test might be promising (Spellacy and Teoh, 1969; Spellacy *et al.*, 1970), but considerably more work needs to be done before interruption can be recommended on the basis of HPL levels alone.

B. Abortion, Hydatidiform Mole Pregnancy, and Choriocarcinoma

1. *Abortion*

In normal pregnancy and in 5 women with threatened abortion who ultimately went to term, Genazzani *et al.* (1969) found steadily rising plasma levels of HPL; in contrast, in 8 pregnancies which ended in spontaneous abortion, plasma levels were either barely detectable or rapidly decreased until abortion. Saxena *et al.* (1969) found that the decrease in plasma HPL levels preceded abortion by periods ranging from 5 to 10 days. Also Singer (1970) and Singer *et al.* (1970) found a correlation between decreased HPL levels and the outcome of pregnancy in patients with threatened abortion.

It can be concluded that the determination of serum HPL seems to be of prognostic significance in threatened abortion. However, the number of reported cases is still limited.

2. *Hydatidiform Mole Pregnancy and Choriocarcinoma*

Tumor extracts from patients with hydatidiform moles and choriocarcinoma were shown to have HPL or HPL-like activity (Currie *et al.*, 1966; Ehnholm *et al.*, 1967). However, whereas HCG is elevated (Section II, B, 2), serum HPL is subnormal in the range of that of early pregnancy (Frantz *et al.*, 1965; Samaan *el al.*, 1966; Yen *et al.*, 1967; Ehnholm *et al.*, 1967; Saxena *et al.*, 1968; Goldstein, 1971). Based on an extensive study of 121 patients, the level of HPL was found to be inversely proportional to the degree of malignancy (Goldstein, 1971). Saxena *et al.* (1968) found normal HPL values in 4 patients incorrectly suspected of having molar pregnancy, and clearly lower levels than in normal pregnancy in 51 patients with choriocarcinoma and molar pregnancy. According to Saxena *et al.* (1968), the finding of a serum HPL level one-tenth or less the expected normal value, in conjunction with a normal or elevated urinary HCG level after 8 weeks of pregnancy is virtually pathognomonic of molar pregnancy. The prompt reduction and disappearance of HPL in parallel with serum HCG activity following the removal of a molar pregnancy or during chemotherapy for tropho- blastic disease (Ehnholm *et al.*, 1967) confirms trophoblastic tissue as its source. As might be expected, in view of the relatively smaller amounts present, measurement of HPL activity is not as sensitive an indicator of remission as is the level of serum or urinary HCG (Saxena *et al.*, 1968).

C. HYPERTENSION, RH ISOIMMUNIZATION, AND CARBOHYDRATE METABOLISM

1. *Hypertension*

In mild toxemia without fetal underdevelopment or fetal distress a normal production of HPL has been reported by several authors (Saxena *et al.*, 1969; Samaan *et al.*, 1969, 1971). In the extensive study of Spellacy *et al.* (1971), 8% of the 432 serum samples from 163 patients with mild toxemia were found in the fetal-danger (F-D) zone (Section III, A, C), as compared with 1% in normal pregnancies. In severe toxemia (224 samples in 76 women) this percentage was increased to 18%. In all the 13 cases with fetal death HPL values were found in the F-D zone for several days to weeks prior to the death, whereas no death occurred in the severely toxemic women with normal HPL values. Samaan *et al.* (1971) reported 3 patients with severe toxemia and fetal death: all 3 showed low HPL values. Josimovich *et al.* (1970) found lowered HPL values in 41% of their patients with severe hypertension. They did not report the clinical outcome in these patients. In contrast, Singer *et al.* (1970) found high HPL levels in about half of the patients with pre- eclamptic toxemia.

The balance of evidence suggests that possibly by measuring HPL in toxicosis a group can be separated in which fetal distress is to be ex- pected in a much higher frequency than in patients with normal HPL values.

2. *Rh Isoimmunization*

In patients with rhesus incompatibility, normal to slightly elevated HPL values were found by Samaan *et al.* (1969), Josimovich *et al.* (1970), Singer *et al.* (1970), and Spellacy *et al.* (1971). Spellacy *et al.* (1971) as well as Samaan *et al.* (1969) did not observe any correlation with the fetal outcome. In the 15 cases with fetal death occurring in the 57 patients reported by Spellacy *et al.* (1971), normal HPL values were found in all samples. This is in contrast with the data reviewed in Section III, C, 1, where, in fetal death in cases of severe toxemia, HPL was found in the F-D zone for several days to weeks prior to death. Thus, in Rh isoimmunization there is no correlation of HPL with fetal outcome.

3. *Carbohydrate Metabolism*

No unanimity of opinion exists concerning the changes in HPL secretion in pregnant women with diabetes mellitus. In patients delivering normal babies, normal values have been reported by Beck *et al.* (1965), Gusdon (1969), Josimovich *et al.* (1970), Samaan *et al.* (1971), and Spellacy *et al.* (1971). Significant increases were found by Saxena *et al.* (1969), Zuckermann *et al.* (1970), Singer *et al.* (1970), and M. Cohen *et al.* (1970). In diabetic patients with fetal distress (retarded fetal growth or fetal death), lower values were observed in 3 cases (Saxena *et al.,* 1969), and Samaan *et al.* (1971) found subnormal or declining values in 5 of 8 patients. In contrast to these reports, Spellacy *et al.* (1971) found normal HPL levels in 4 of the 5 fetal deaths in diabetic patients; however, the pregnancy of the patient with subnormal values was also complicated by hypertension. These data seem to suggest that serum HPL is not of prognostic value as regards imminent fetal death in diabetes and Rh isoimmunization, in contrast to intrauterine fetal death due to toxemia (Section III, C, 1). Samaan *et al.* (1969) and Spellacy and Teoh (1969) found HPL levels of no prognostic significance in diabetic patients.

Large doses of HPL in normal subjects (Grumbach *et al.,* 1966; Beck and Daughaday, 1967; Samaan *et al.,* 1968) can induce some metabolic changes of pregnancy, such as elevated circulating free fatty acid levels and decreased peripheral glucose uptake. HPL administration to stable diabetics increases glucosuria and fasting blood glucose levels (Dominguez *et al.,* 1965; Samaan *et al.,* 1968). Thus, HPL might be responsible for the well known disturbance of equilibrium of diabetes in pregnancy. However, the evidence that increased circulating free fatty acid levels, decreased peripheral glucose uptake, and difficulties in regulating diabetic pregnancy are due to HPL is circumstantial and awaits further experimentation.

D. FETAL WEIGHT AND RETARDED FETAL GROWTH

Serum concentrations below the normal range have been found in retarded intrauterine growth by Saxena *et al.* (1969) (5 patients),

M. Cohen *et al.* (1970), and Zuckermann *et al.* (1970). However, Josimovich *et al.* (1970) could not find a correlation between fetal outcome and randomly obtained placental lactogen levels in the serum of patients with small-for-date babies.

No correlation was found between term serum HPL or amniotic fluid HPL and placental weight in normal pregnancy (Spellacy *et al.*, 1966; J. J. Sciarra *et al.*, 1968; Singer, 1970; Cramer *et al.*, 1971). Saxena *et al.* (1969) are the only group reporting a high degree of correlation between serum-HPL and placental weight. However, these authors divided their subjects into three different categories: diabetics, women with normal pregnancies, and patients with placental insufficiency; this could perhaps explain their identification of correlations not found by other workers.

Thus in retarded fetal growth, serum HPL is sometimes low. In normal pregnancy, serum HPL and placental weight are not correlated, whereas in pathological pregnancy they are correlated. Thus, lowered serum HPL might be a manifestation of lowered placental weight.

E. MISCELLANEOUS

Normal or elevated levels were observed in twin pregnancy (Grumbach *et al.*, 1968; Saxena *et al.*, 1969; Singer *et al.*, 1970; M. Cohen *et al.*, 1970; Zuckermann *et al.*, 1970).

In cases with fetal death due to nonplacental causes, normal, or near-normal values were found (Saxena *et al.*, 1969; Singer, 1970).

In 4 patients with prolonged pregnancy a gradual fall in serum HPL values occurred (Saxena *et al.*, 1969).

F. SUMMARY

In normal and in pathological human pregnancy, the placental trophoblast produces HPL. There is minimal transfer from the mother to the fetus. The half-life of circulating HPL is 20–30 minutes. Based on animal experiments and circumstantial evidence, HPL might also play an important role in the human species in the maintenance of pregnancy in breast enlargement, initiation of lactation, and carbohydrate metabolism in pregnancy. Despite its short half-life and its autonomous trophoblastic production, there is a wide range of serum HPL values in normal and pathological pregnancies, limiting the practical clinical usefulness of HPL determinations.

Serum HPL seems to be of prognostic significance in threatened abortion. HPL is present in tissue of hydatidiform mole and choriocarcinoma. Serum HPL is low in these conditions, and in conjunction with normal or elevated urinary HCG this finding is pathognomonic of molar pregnancy. Serum HCG determination is superior to serum HPL as an indicator of remission during chemotherapy.

In mild toxemia HPL is normal, whereas in severe toxemia serum HPL levels are generally reported to be subnormal. Due to the large variability, the clinical usefulness, if any, of such assays is very limited. In Rh isoimmunization, serum HPL and fetal outcome are not correlated. Circumstantial evidence points to the fact that HPL might play a role in the exacerbation of diabetes in pregnancy. The clinical usefulness of HPL determinations in diabetes and pregnancy is also very limited.

In retarded fetal growth serum HPL may sometimes be low, possibly as a manifestation of lowered placental weight. In twin pregnancy, due to the large placental mass, serum HPL may be elevated, whereas normal serum HPL has been reported in fetal death due to nonplacental causes.

IV. ESTROGENS

A. EXCRETION

1. Total "Estrogens" versus "Estriol"

Many methods (J. B. Brown, 1955; Eberlein et al., 1958; Ittrich, 1960a,b; Beling, 1963; Frandsen and Stakemann, 1963a; Greene and Touchstone, 1963; S. Cohen, 1966; Schindler and Herrmann, 1966; Jaffe and Levitz, 1967; Oakey et al., 1967; Strickler et al., 1967; Scommegna and Chattoraj, 1967, 1968; Acevedo et al., 1968; Rourke et al., 1968; Scommegna, 1969; Cummings et al., 1969; Heron, 1969; Dito and Shelly, 1969; Nilson, 1970; de la Torre et al., 1970) have been published for measuring estriol and "total estrogens" in the urine during pregnancy. The range of normal values reported by different laboratories can vary greatly. In general, estriol excretion has been found to increase progressively from levels of 1.0–2.0 mg in 24 hours at 8–12 weeks gestation to 12.0–50.0 mg in 24 hours at term. The reliability criteria for all these methods are different. Although estriol is almost certainly the main single component of the total estrogens in pregnancy, the quantitative relationships have not always been particularly clear. Confusion has sometimes resulted from the term "total estrogens" to denote the "classical" compounds: estrone, estradiol-17β, and estriol. It is now known that several other phenolic steroid metabolites may contribute significantly to total urinary estrogens (see, e.g., the review by Diczfalusy and Troen, 1961). However, estriol is excreted in huge quantities in human pregnancy urine as compared with other estrogens. Also, the rise in estriol excretion during pregnancy is quantitatively much more marked than, for example, that of estrone and estradiol. Hobkirk *et al.* (1970) showed that estriol accounted for an average of 74% of the principal Kober-positive steroids in the urine of 13 women during uncomplicated pregnancies. This proportion is independent of the stage of pregnancy from 20 weeks until term. The average ratio of estriol to ring D α-ketols (mainly 16-hydroxyestrone and 16 ketoestradiol-17β) is about 5:1 over the same period. In 17 pregnant women with diabetes, urinary estriol averaged 63% of the "total steroids" during a similar period, and the average ratio of estriol to ring D α-ketols was 3:1.

The quantitative importance of these ketolic steroids may introduce a problem in deciding whether to measure estriol or "total estrogens" when evaluating fetal viability in complicated pregnancies. The elucidation of this quantitative importance necessitates further studies. It is beyond the scope of this review to discuss all hitherto known methods for estrogen excretion and their reliability. The reader is referred to Klopper (1969). The choice of the method of assay depends on reliability criteria, rapidity and on clinical correlation. Beling (1963) observed that the monosulfate conjugates of estrone, estradiol, and estriol were eluted in peak II aliquots according to the method involving gel filtration (Beling, 1963) along with estriol 16-glucuronide. E. R. Smith and Kellie (1967) have shown this major peak II estrogen to be estriol 16-glucuronide. Beling has suggested that peak II estrogens are a more precise reflection of the fetal status than the total estrogen. Into this framework fit, for example, the observations of Carpenter (1970) in studying the rising post-transfusion estrogen excretion in rhesus incompatibility. He found that after initial depression the rise of Beling's peak II estrogens was indicative of a fetus with long-term survival.

The measurement of steroids that are produced only by the fetus and that are not further metabolized in the placenta or the maternal organism would be expected to give a more accurate indication of the fetal state. It has been suggested (WHO Scientific Group, 1971) that at least three steroids may fulfill these requirements. The first of these is estetrol, a compound having an additional hydroxyl group at the 15α-position of estriol, and formed predominantly in the fetus. About 80% of the estetrol originates from fetal precursors (Heikkilä and Luukkainen, 1971), and it has been claimed to be a specific product of the fetal liver (Adlercreutz and Luukkainen, 1970; Zucconi *et al.*, 1967; Hagen *et al.*, 1965). Another steroid which appears to be exclusively a product of fetal metabolism is 11-dehydro-17α-estradiol. The third compound that has been firmly established as a purely fetal steroid is 15-hydroxyprogesterone. However, concerning these last two steroids, only very limited information is available on quantitative measurements during normal pregnancy and none at all in abnormal pregnancy. The question arises whether—except for very exceptional situations—it makes much sense to measure purely fetal steroids, because in pathological pregnancy the dissociation between placental and fetal pathology is very rare (e.g., anencephalic monsters, or the situation in which a real knot in the umbilical cord interferes with the fetal circulation).

In addition to urinary estriol assays, plasma estriol can be measured (e.g., Ratanasopa et al., 1967). Increase or decrease of plasma and urinary estriol levels in pregnancy correlate well. Introduction of protein-binding techniques and, particularly, the related technique of radio-immunoassay of steroids would open new perspectives. However, the future value of plasma assays will depend entirely on the magnitude of the variability of normal levels. Precise definition of the physiological factors, such as diurnal variations, activity, or posture, that may influence plasma steroid levels wil be a prerequisite for the application of such assays in obstetric disease.

Berman et al. (1968) found amniotic fluid estriol less than 100 μg per liter indicative of fetal jeopardy. Amniotic fluid volume did not correlate with the amniotic fluid estriol concentration, but the latter correlated fairly closely with maternal urinary estriol.

2. Dynamic Tests

Hausknecht (1967) reported that adrenal suppression in 2 pregnant women resulted in no change in the urinary excretion of estriol; however, Simmer et al. (1966) and Warren and Cheatum (1967) have shown that a marked drop in estriol excretion occurs after administration of dexamethasone to women in the second and third trimesters of gestation. In order to elucidate the regulatory mechanisms involved in estriol production in pregnancy, Scommegna et al. (1968) administered to women in the second and third trimesters of normal and pathological pregnancies ACTH intravenously, metyrapone orally, and dexamethasone orally. DHAS was infused intravenously in relatively large doses in a similar group of patients. Urinary estriol was measured before and after these treatments. After ACTH, DHAS, and metyrapone administration, only a small rise was observed in urinary estriol excretion in normal and in pathological pregnancies. However, a sharp decrease occurred after dexamethasone-induced adrenal suppression. These findings were interpreted by Scommegna et al. (1968) as an indication that in normal pregnancy the enzymatic systems involved in estriol synthesis are almost completely saturated by the available precursors, and that in pathological pregnancies the decreased estriol excretion might be related to diminished enzymatic activity more than to a decrease in the availability of precursors. In contrast, Hausknecht and Mandelbaum (1969) found that in normal pregnancy intra-amniotic instillation of 200 mg of DHAS brings about a pronounced rise in urinary estriol excretion, which suggests that the various enzyme systems in the fetus and placenta under normal conditions are not fully saturated at term.

An explanation of the discrepancy between the findings of Scommegna et al. (1968) and of Hausknecht and Mandelbaum (1969) might be the route of administration of DHAS, but further observations are needed to clarify this subject. Arguments will be presented that also a decrease in the availability of precursors plays an important role in some kinds of pathological pregnancies, e.g., anencephalic monsters (Section IV, D, 1), and preeclamptic toxemia (Section IV, E, 1). For an appraisal of the factors responsible for the progressive increase in estrogen production in human pregnancy, the reader is referred to the review by Oakey (1970).

The balance of evidence seems to indicate that in addition to a possibly diminished enzymatic activity there is certainly also a decreased availability of precursors in certain kinds of pathological pregnancy.

3. Variations in the Day-to-Day Excretion of Estrogens

Values obtained will vary according to methodology. Even if technical errors of measurement are excluded and if collection of urine is not incomplete, urinary estrogen output shows wide fluctuations from day to day and from one individual to another (e.g., Frandsen, 1963; Booth et al., 1964). There can be as much as 30–50% variation in daily estriol output (e.g., Greene, 1970). It is commonly agreed that a single test is worthless. Once the laboratory's normal range is known, depending on the method of assay used, variability may partly be eliminated by performing serial estrogen determinations in one patient.

a. Errors of Measurement. Errors that may play a part in the day-to-day variations of estrogens excreted can be, for example, acid hydrolysis applied to urine in pregnancy complicated by varying amounts of glycosuria, resulting in false results (E. S. Taylor et al., 1963; Greene and Touchstone, 1963). According to Luukkainen and Adlercreutz (1967), the method of J. B. Brown et al. (1957) would overestimate estrogens. Several drugs cause errors of measurements. Mackay et al. (1967) and Eraz and Hausknecht (1969) report abnormally low urinary estrogen levels in pregnancy in patients receiving the urinary antiseptic drug methenamine mandelate, the breakdown product, formaldehyde, being responsible for the interference observed. However, the drug does not interfere with plasma estriol determinations (Eraz and Hausknecht, 1969). Meprobamate, methenamine mandelate, and phenazopyridine HCl directly interfere with the chemical analysis according to the short method reported by Ittrich (1960a,b). Hydrochlorothiazide can, by impairment of proximal tubular reabsorption, promote increased estrogen excretion (Timonen et al., 1965). ACTH and corticosteroids may cause variations of urinary estriol by elevating or suppressing maternal and/ or fetal production of DHAS and/or 16α-hydroxy-DHAS (MacDonald and Siiteri, 1965; Houtzager and Van Leusden, 1971). Also competitive inhibition by prednisone of placental conversion of 16α-hydroxy-DHAS into estriol has been established by Dony et al. (1971).

b. Renal Factors. These factors also play an important role in determining the amount of estrogens excreted (E. S. Taylor et al., 1965; Yousem et al., 1966; Pion, 1967; MacNaughton, 1967). Many observers (e.g., Courey et al., 1970) have noted the apparent increase in urinary estriol levels when patients are put at bed rest, and renal function has been demonstrated to be extremely sensitive to changes in the patient's position also during pregnancy (Dickey et al., 1966; Vedra and Horska, 1969). According to Dickey et al. (1966), estrogen excretion in patients ambulant or at bed rest closely paralleled changes in creatinine excretion, reflecting alterations in renal plasma flow and glomerular filtration. C. H. Brown et al. (1964) have presented evidence for tubular secretion of estriol, demonstrating that the mean clearance of estriol may reach 200% of the mean clearance of creatinine measured at the same time. This would appear to be a varying phenomenon related to plasma concentration of estriol with a tubular secretory maximum hypothesized at high plasma concentrations. These findings seem to be in contradiction with those reported in Section IV, A, 3, c, and warrant further experimentation. Estriol clearance was found by Talbert and Easterling (1967) to be reduced in hypertensive pregnant patients, but DHAS in cord serum was lowered, suggesting that reduced production of fetal precursors was more responsible for lowered urinary estriol than depressed maternal renal function. Increased mobilization of peripheral fluid (Timonen et al., 1965) during initial bed rest might increase urinary estriol excretion. Massive hydration leading to a 200% increase in urinary output could sometimes induce increased estrogen excretion: Courey et al. (1969) found a significant relationship between urine output and total estriol excreted. Furthermore, potential changes in urinary estriol excretion may be the result of liver or intestinal disease by interference with enterohepatic steroid metabolism (Breborowicz et al., 1965).

c. Estriol:Creatinine in Pregnancy Urine. The excretion rates of estriol and creatinine in normal pregnancy bear a constant relationship throughout the 24-hour period (Kahmann *et al.*, 1968, 1969a,b; Mackay *et al.*, 1968; Welshman *et al.*, 1969; Cummings *et al.*, 1969; Kahmann, 1970a,b). Estriol/creatinine per 24 hours is much more constant than estriol 16-glucuronide excretion per 2 hours (Kahmann *et al.*, 1968; 1969a,b). The same applies to 24-hour specimens from the same patient in Beling's method for serial estriol determination. In a case of repeated partial placental abruption, diminished excretion of estriol-6-glucuronide concomitant with a rather constant creatinine excretion for 24 hours appeared not to be due to renal failure, but to disturbance of estriol-16-glucuronide production within the fetoplacental unit (Kahmann, 1970a,b). Such evidence of variations of estriol synthesis in pathological pregnancy caused within the fetoplacental unit deserves further experimentation.

4. *Corticosteroids and Estrogen Excretion*

Estrogen excretion was reported to be normal (Jailer and Knowlton, 1950), but more usually very much reduced (e.g., Baulieu *et al.*, 1956; Hammerstein and Nevinny-Stickel, 1965; Badarau, 1966; Wallace and Michie, 1966; MacLeod *et al.*, 1967; Michie, 1967; J. B. Brown *et al.*, 1967, 1968; Scommegna *et al.*, 1968; Driscoll, 1969; J. Morrison and Kilpatrick, 1969; Dony *et al.*, 1971) during administration of corticosteroids in human pregnancy. The effect on estriol excretion is probably dose dependent (Dony *et al.*, 1971), whereas placental function as assessed by pregnanediol excretion is normal in otherwise uncomplicated pregnancies.

Estrone, estradiol, and estriol are reduced. Fetal synthetic routes should be involved to account for the amounts of estriol. Fetal adrenal steroid formation could well be suppressed. However, THE and THF excretion in infants born of mothers receiving corticosteroids during pregnancy was normal (Kulin *et al.*, 1966). Since Dony *et al.* (1971) found competitive inhibition by prednisone of estriol formation from 16α-hydroxy DHA in preparations of human placenta *in vitro*, suppression of placental enzymatic systems could play a role.

B. ABORTION, HYDATIDIFORM MOLE PREGNANCY, AND CHORIOCARCINOMA

1. *Abortion*

Lowered estriol excretion preceding expulsion of the product of conception or before the abortion manifested itself was reported by Borth (1960), Booth *et al.* (1965), Frandsen and Stakemann (1966), Klopper and MacNaughton (1965), and J. B. Brown *et al.* (1970a,b). The same applies to estrone excretion (Timonen and Tervilä, 1968). Also in missed abortion, estriol excretion is low (Bengtsson and Forsgren, 1966). However, Wei *et al.* (1968) did not find that estriol values could predict the outcome of pregnancy in threatened abortion. If abortion was merely threatened (Frandsen and Stakemann, 1966) or due to an incompetent cervix (Booth *et al.*, 1965), estriol output was generally within the normal range.

In contrast with the findings of Allan and Dodds (1935) and the temporary postoperative fall in estriol excretion after bilateral oophorectomy in early pregnancy reported by Mancuso (1962), most authors agree that urinary estriol is not changed after bilateral oophorectomy in early pregnancy (Amati, 1928; Waldstein, 1929; Szarka, 1930; Guldberg, 1936; Diczfalusy and Borell, 1961; Rebbe and Alling Møller, 1966). Thus, lowered estriol excretion in abortion is caused by changes within the fetoplacental unit.

2. Hydatidiform Mole Pregnancy

a. Excretion, Production Rate and Tissue Content of Estrogens. An increased excretion of estrogens in molar pregnancy has been reported by a number of investigators: Payne (1941), Hinglais and Hinglais (1949), Lajos and Szontagh (1950), M. Keller (1953), Erb *et al.* (1961), and Bonanno *et al.* (1963). Frandsen and Stakemann (1964b) found greater excretion of estriol by women with hydatidiform moles than in nonpregnant women, but less than in normal pregnancy. Excretion of estrone, estradiol, and estriol in molar pregnancy can even be equal to that of normal pregnancies of a comparable duration (Kock *et al.*, 1965; MacNaughton, 1965; J. B. Brown *et al.*, 1970a,b). In some cases there was an immediate fall in estrogen excretion after evacuation, in others the values remained elevated for several weeks (J. B. Brown *et al.*, 1970a,b). Low estriol excretion values were found by Wei *et al.* (1968). Since the ratio of estriol to estrone plus estradiol is mostly similar to that of nonpregnant women, the source of estriol was suggested to be the often hyperstimulated ovaries, and not the molar tissue. Siiteri and MacDonald (1966) studied 6 women with hydatidiform mole. The production rate of estradiol during weeks 12 to 19 of molar pregnancy ranged from 2 to 11 mg per day. The amount of estradiol produced in four of these patients was comparable to that found during the third trimester of human pregnancy. Chamberlain *et al.* (1968) found that estriol was virtually absent from mole tissue, which is lower than in normal placental tissue of equivalent age as reported by Diczfalusy *et al.* (1961); estrone and estradiol were present in mole tissue within the limits found in normal placentae (25–200 μg/kg in each case).

b. Formation of Estrone, Estradiol, and Estriol. It has been shown that during normal pregnancy a 16-hydroxylated neutral metabolite (Bolté *et al.*, 1964a,b,c) possibly formed dehydroepiandrosterone sulfate circulating in the fetus (Ryan, 1959) and/or a 16-hydroxylated phenolic intermediate formed by the fetus from placental estrone (Ryan, 1959) can be converted into estriol by the midgestational and term human placenta. Siiteri and MacDonald (1963, 1966) have emphasized the importance of DHAS [present in higher concentrations in fetal than in maternal blood (e.g., Simmer *et al.*, 1964)] as an estrogen precursor. Interruption of the fetoplacental connection resulted in a sudden drop in the excretion of estrogens by the mother, whereas artificial perfusion of the placenta *in situ* with maternal blood maintained the excretion at preoperative levels (Cassmer, 1959), possibly by supplying estrogen precursor steroids to the placenta. The decrease in the excretion of estriol was particularly pronounced in these experiments. Thus, whereas in the nonpregnant individual urinary estriol is derived primarily from the catabolism of estrone and estradiol (Fishman *et al.*, 1962; Gurpide *et al.*, 1962), most urinary estriol in normal pregnancy is derived from sources other than the catabolism of estrone and estradiol in the maternal compartment. The experimental situation of Cassmer (1959) exists as a natural experiment: in hydatidiform mole pregnancy, there is no circulation in the chorionic villi and the fetus is absent. The absence of the fetal compartment of the fetoplacental unit does not explain the considerable amounts of estrogens, especially of estriol, which may be excreted in molar pregnancy. Thus, steroidogenesis in hydatidiform moles is of special interest. A large number of *in vitro* incubation studies with moles providing information regarding the formation and metabolism of a number of estrogens with tissue and homogenates have been reported and described in detail (Van Leusden and Villee, 1966, 1967; Houtzager *et al.*, 1967, 1970; Van Leusden *et al.*, 1967; Houtzager, 1968, 1970; Van Leusden and Siemerink, 1969; Van Leusden, 1970a,b, 1971). In initial experiments (Van Leusden and Villee, 1966) using [7α-^{3}H] pregnenolone and [4-^{14}C]DHA incubated in the presence of molar tissue and homogenates, the synthesis of any labeled estriol during the incubations was excluded by crystallization. On the other hand, in these same experiments [^{14}C]estrone and [^{14}C]estradiol were isolated in a radiochemically homogeneous form. In incubation experiments with DL-[5-^{3}H]mevalonate, incorporation of radioactive material into sterols, cholesterol, estrone, estradiol, and estriol was excluded. Thus, in the molar compartment pregnenolone is not metabolized into estrone, estradiol, and estriol. However, major quantities of DHA as well as DHAS are converted into estrone and estradiol.

In other incubation experiments with [1,2-^{3}H]testosterone and [4-^{14}C] androstenedione, the synthesis of estriol during the incubations was excluded by crystallization (Houtzager et al., 1970). Incubations with testosterone resulted in the formation of estrone and estradiol. Kinetic studies with [4-^{14}C]androstenedione and [7α-^{3}H]testosterone indicated that androstenedione is a more effective precursor of estrone and estradiol than is testosterone. Equilibrium of estrone $\rightleftharpoons$ estradiol was reached much earlier than of androstenedione $\rightleftharpoons$ testosterone. In the incubations involving shorter periods conversion of testosterone into estradiol was twice that into estrone, indicating that a direct pathway, testosterone $\rightarrow$ estradiol, prevailed in such incubations. Appropriate corrections for endogenous production of androstenedione, testosterone, estrone, and estradiol synthesized in molar tissue during *in vitro* incubations were calculated from monitoring experiments modified according to the method of Cameron and Griffiths (1968) and reported in detail (Houtzager et al., 1970). Estrone is the most important steroid produced *in vitro*. Recently Coutts and MacNaughton (1971) have also found conversion of DHA into estrone and estradiol by molar tissue. The data concerning the formation of estrogens by hydratidiform moles agree well with the conversion of C_{19} steroids to estrogens found in preparations of placentas of normal pregnancies (Ryan, 1959). The observations (Van Leusden, 1971) that pregnenolone was not converted into estrone, estradiol, or estriol and that no estriol was formed from androstenedione, testosterone, estrone, or estradiol are of interest in view of the fact that the same preparations of molar tissue converted DHA very effectively into estrone and estradiol. DL-[5^{3}H]mevalonic acid was not incorporated into sterols, squalene, or cholesterol. This and the finding that pregnenolone is not converted into estrogens seem to indicate that estrogens are not produced *de novo* in hydatidiform moles. Since DHAS was incorporated into estrone and estradiol as well as DHA, molar tissue, like normal placenta, is rich in sulfatase activity. Thus the molar compartment could utilize DHAS for estrogen production *in vivo*. DHAS served as a precursor *in vivo* of a large proportion of the estrogen produced by a patient with a hydatidiform mole, as was proved by Siiteri and MacDonald (1963, 1966).

These results of *in vitro* incubations are in agreement with findings *in vivo* that after administration of labeled 17β-estradiol to patients with hydatidiform moles the specific activity of the estriol excreted was only 13–32% less than that of the estrone or estradiol (MacDonald and Siiteri, 1964). In contrast, only 10% of the estriol in late pregnancy arises from the catabolism of estrone and estradiol in the maternal compartment (Fishman et al., 1962). Urinary estriol in patients with vesicular moles is derived primarily from the catabolism of estrone and estradiol in the maternal compartment. Maternal DHA(S) can serve as an effective precursor of estrone and estradiol in hydratidiform moles. DHA(S) may be of maternal adrenal origin, since administration of 9α-fluoro-16α-methylprednisolone to a patient with a mole resulted in a decrease of the urinary excretion of estrone, estradiol, and estriol of 77, 79, and 85%, respectively (Houtzager and Van Leusden, 1969).

3. Choriocarcinoma

a. *Excretion.* Akasu *et al.* (1969) reported low urinary estrogen excretion. However, an increase in the excretion of estrogens has been found by Payne (1941) and Frandsen and Stakemann (1964b).

b. *Biosynthesis of Estrogens in Choriocarcinoma.* Barlow *et al.* (1967), found in only 4 out of 12 women with malignant trophoblastic disease *in vivo* conversion of DHAS into estrogens, and conclude that this conversion is characteristic only for benign trophoblast. However, like preparations of hydatidiform moles and of normal placentas, a case of choriocarcinoma showed formation of progesterone from pregnenolone and aromatization of DHA into estrone and estradiol *in vitro* (Section V, E, 3). In contrast to molar and normal placental tissue, choriocarcinoma showed side-chain cleavage *in vitro* (Van Leusden, 1970c, 1971). Since chorionepithelioma apparently possesses more enzymatic properties, these *in vitro* observations do not seem to support the theory that chorio-carcinoma would result from hydatidiform mole. A simpler explanation would be that chorionepithelioma arises before differentiation of the fertilized ovum into cells of the trophoblast (exhibiting 3β-dehydrogenase activity, but no side-chain cleavage) and cells resulting in the fetus *strictu sensu.* The mole (and of course the normal placenta) would then arise after this differentiation. However, since recent studies by Telegdy *et al.* (1970) have shown that the human midgestational placenta does possess an (albeit very limited) ability to synthesize 17β-estradiol from cholesterol, this theory on the origin of choriocarcinoma should be viewed with caution and should be subjected to further experimentation.

C. ABDOMINAL PREGNANCY

When, after termination of abdominal pregnancy by cesarean section, the placenta is left *in situ,* in contrast with pregnanediol excretion (Section V, F), excretion of estrone, estradiol, and predominantly of estriol is lowered, resulting in a sharp decrease in the ratio estriol: estrone + estradiol (Hamersma and Schopman, 1967; Van Wering, 1969). These data illustrate the important fetal contribution to estriol formation. However, in a similar case with a 4-month pregnancy (Maguin *et al.,* 1967) estrogen excretion remained at the same level. As shown by Kim *et al.* (1971) and Borth *et al.* (1971) from plasma estrone and estradiol disappearance rates, the estrogens still excreted (Michie et al., 1966; Hamersma and Schopman, 1967; Friedman et al., 1969) reflect slowly declining production.

D. CONGENITAL DEFECTS, FETAL SEX, AND MULTIPLE PREGNANCY

1. Anencephalic Monsters

Low excretion of estriol (Frandsen and Stakemann, 1961, 1964a; Nakayama et al., 1967), in contrast with normal pregnanediol excretion, has been established in anencephalic pregnancy. There is a correlation between fetal adrenal development and maternal estriol excretion (Frandsen and Stakemann, 1964a). Cord estriol is 12.5–25%, whereas estrone and estradiol are 50%, of the normal values (Nakayama et al., 1967), and in contrast to normal pregnancy, very low amounts of $\Delta^5,3\beta$-hydroxysteroids (Eberlein, 1965) are present in fetal blood of these monsters. Maternal plasma estrogen values (Nakayama et al., 1967) also are low in this condition. Placental preparations of anencephalic fetuses aromatize DHA as well as normal placentas (Nakayama et al., 1967; Van Leusden, 1972c). Low estriol concentration (Schindler and Ratanasopa, 1968; Aleem et al., 1969a,b) and low or nondetectable 16-keto adrenostenediol and 16α-hydroxy DHA, but normal DHA and pregnanediol values (Schindler and Ratanasopa, 1968) have been reported in the amniotic fluid in anencephalic pregnancy. Unconjugated 17-hydroxycorticosteroids are high, and 17-oxosteroid and 17-hydroxy-corticosteroid concentrations are low (Abramovich, 1969) in this condition in the amniotic fluid as compared with normal pregnancy. However, when the polyhydramnios of anencephalic pregnancies is taken into account, the amount of steroid in the fluid surrounding such a fetus is as great as, or greater than, that surrounding a normal fetus.

These data on steroid determinations, correlated with the well documented morphological underdevelopment of the fetal adrenal cortex, especially the fetal zone, in anenchephalic pregnancy (Meyer, 1912; Angevine, 1938; Nakayama et al., 1967), point to a deficient fetal adrenocortical steroid precursor production for placental estrogen synthesis and subsequent estrogen excretion. This is confirmed by the studies of MacDonald and Siiteri (1965) and Siiteri and MacDonald (1966), and is harmony with the studies of Frandsen and Stakemann (1961, 1963a,b), who postulated that the fetal adrenals produce a substance which serves as a precursor for estrogen biosynthesis in the placenta. Dynamic tests by instillation of DHAS into the amniotic cavity (Michie, 1966) have been employed in anencephalic monsters and resulted in an increase of the excretion of estrone, estradiol, and predominantly of estriol. Since estetrol has been claimed (Section IV, A, 1) to be a specific product of the fetal liver, whereas estriol would be relatively more specific to the fetal adrenals, a study of estetrol excretion in anencephalic pregnancy would be of interest.

Since ACTH administration to newborn babies inhibits postnatal involution of the fetal zone (Daenen, 1965) and in anencephalic monsters causes differentiation of the atrophic fetal adrenal glands, especially the fetal zone (Lanman, 1962; Johannisson, 1968), ACTH seems to play an important role in the differentiation of the fetal adrenal glands. These data and the fact that anencephalic monsters nearly always show adrenal atrophy are in agreement with the hypothesis that ACTH does not pass from the mother to the fetus. In animal experiments, in which fetal rats were decapitated and left in their intrauterine environment (Jost et al., 1962) and after hypophysectomy (Kitchell and Wells, 1952), the fetal adrenals became atrophic.

The paradoxical findings of Migeon et al. (1956) that during ACTH administration the fetal plasma 17-hydroxycorticosteroid concentration is increased, can be explained by passage of increased maternal 17-hydroxycorticosteroids to the fetus.

In normal pregnancy, but not in pregnancies with intrauterine fetal death ACTH administration gives rise to increased estriol excretion (Dässler, 1966; Maeyama et al., 1969). Although these findings could suggest passage of ACTH from the mother to the fetus, the explanation could as well be maternal adrenocortical stimulation, resulting in increased conversion of maternal adrenocortical estrogen precursors into estrogens by healthy, but not by pathological placentas in cases of intrauterine fetal death. In contrast herewith, Maeyama et al. (1969) reported low urinary estriol even after ACTH administration in anencephalic pregnancy, whereas one case in whom the adrenal gland had a thin but distinct fetal area, showed an increase of estriol excretion after ACTH administration. Under their experimental conditions the most simple explanation of these findings would be passage of ACTH from the mother to the fetus. Jeffery et al. (1970) found that increasing ACTH concentration in the maternal compartment did not cause regular rises in estrogen excretion in anencephalic pregnancies. The lack of fetal adrenal 3β-hydroxysteroid dehydrogenase in normal pregnancy (Diczfalusy, 1964; Goldman et al., 1966) results in high concentrations of Δ^5, 3β-hydroxycorticosteroids in normal umbilical cord blood (Eberlein, 1965). The low cortisol concentrations in umbilical cord blood (Eberlein, 1965) would come from the maternal circulation (Migeon et al., 1956) and could inhibit fetal ACTH production. This would result in large fetal adrenals, especially fetal zones, found under normal conditions (Tähkä,

1951; Jackson, 1960). Already in the first month postpartum the fetal zone has undergone rapid involution (Moeri, 1951; Lanman, 1953).

Further investigations are necessary to study the factors regulating the passage of 17-hydroxycorticosteroids from the mother to the fetus. Thus maternal ACTH by influencing fetal 17-hydroxycorticosteroid concentration could control fetal ACTH and fetal adrenocortical activity. It is assumed that the deficient hypothalamohypophyseal system of anencephalic monsters would lead to a lack of fetal adrenocortical growth. However, there is as yet no strict proof that ACTH is absent or low in umbilical blood of anencephalic monsters. Moreover, further investigations are needed on the possible passage of ACTH from the mother to the fetus.

2. Prenatal Diagnosis of Adrenogenital Syndrome

Amniotic fluid 17-ketosteroid (Merkatz et al., 1969) and pregnanetriol concentration at term (Jeffcoate et al., 1965; Merkatz et al., 1969; Nichols, 1969; Nichols and Gibson, 1969; New, 1970) is suggestively elevated in fetuses with congenital adrenogenital syndrome. The presence of the disease could not be predicted during early or mid-pregnancy.

One could argue that, just as fetal adrenocortical hypoplasia entails a very low estrogen excretion, adrenocortical hyperplasia in the fetus is likely to cause increased excretion of estrogens. In accordance with this, Cathro et al. (1969a,b) found very high values for estriol excretion in a case of a mother pregnant with a virilized girl with congenital adrenocortical hyperplasia. Nichols (1970) reported a case with increased pregnanetriol concentration in the amniotic fluid, which decreased after injection of hydrocortisone to the fetus. However, injection of 25 mg of hydrocortisone into the fetus on 4 occasions in a week did not change the (normal) maternal excretion of estriol, and Nichols and Gibson (1969) reported a case of an affected child with normal maternal estriol excretion before delivery and increased pregnanetriol concentration of amniotic fluid.

3. Fetal Sex

The concentration of estrogens is not different in the first voided urine of male or female newborns (Dickey, 1969; Dickey and Robertson, 1969), and there are no reports correlating fetal sex with maternal estriol excretion.

4. Multiple Pregnancy

Except for the report of Wei et al. (1968), who found normal estriol excretion in subjects bearing twins and triplets, most authors (Borth *et al.*, 1959; Kellar *et al.*, 1959; B. Zondek and Pfeiffer, 1959; Frandsen and Stakemann, 1960; Beischer *et al.*, 1968a,b,c; Khoo and MacKay, 1970) find increased excretion of estrogens in multiple pregnancy as compared with normal pregnancy.

E. HYPERTENSION, RH ISOIMMUNIZATION, AND
    CARBOHYDRATE METABOLISM

1. *Hypertension*

In hypertension and pregnancy without superimposed toxemia and normal fetal viability, the excretion of estriol is in the normal range (Klopper, 1966). The same was found by Aubry and Nesbitt (1970). However, when the patients are divided into severe (BP > 180/110) and mild (BP 140–180/90–110) hypertension, the mean estriol excretion in the former group is lower, especially beyond week 26 of pregnancy, possibly due to a lower mean fetal weight in the severe hypertensive group.

In preeclamptic toxemia estriol excretion is below the normal range (see below; e.g., also, Oakey *et al.*, 1967) but the scatter may be large to within the normal range. Occasionally (Würtele, 1962; Beling, 1967) there may be a normal estriol excretion. Other investigators note only a wider scatter than normal (Kellar *et al.*, 1959) or no reduction in estriol excretion even in severe toxemia (Timonen and Hirvonen, 1964). Since arguments are lacking that estriol excretion is lowered preceding the onset of toxemia (J. B. Brown, 1960; Jayle *et al.*, 1965), lowered estriol excretion is the result, not the cause, of toxemia. Severity of toxemia (as measured by blood pressure, albuminuria, and fetal growth retardation) is correlated with lowering of estriol excretion (E. S. Taylor *et al.*, 1958; Lenters, 1958; Klopper, 1965; Duhring and Greene, 1966; Tenhaeff and Karajiannis, 1968). In proteinuria alone (Reid *et al.*, 1968), estriol excretion is usually normal. The lowering of estriol excretion has been found to be correlated with microscopic placental alterations by Lenters (1958), but not by Breborowicz *et al.* (1965), reduction of uterine blood flow (E. S. Taylor *et al.*, 1958), and decreased placental (e.g., Würtele, 1963; Breborowicz *et al.*, 1965) and fetal weight (Section IV, F, 1 and 2). Renal clearance (low estriol clearance) may be disturbed (Talbert and Easterling, 1967) in toxemia. Plasma estriol (Ratanasopa *et al.*, 1967), erythrocyte estrogen concentration (Lachowicz, 1969), and amniotic fluid estriol levels in the period 37–40 weeks (Aleem *et al.*, 1969a,b) are lowered in severe preeclampsia. *In vitro* conversion of 19-hydroxyadrostenedione, androstenedione, and testosterone into estrogens by preparations of toxemic placentas is lowered as compared with normal placentas (Laumas *et al.*, 1968). Moreover, the concentration of fetal steroid precursors for placental estrogen synthesis may be lowered since Talbert and Easterling (1967) reported lowered levels of DHAS in cord plasma, compared to normal.

The balance of evidence would indicate that the cause of the decreased estriol excretion in toxemia must be sought in the placenta as well as in the fetus, thus in the whole fetoplacental unit; in addition to diminished enzymatic activity there is a decreased availability of precursor steroids (see also Section IV, A, 2).

The practical usefulness of monitoring estriol excretion in toxemia of pregnancy for the handling of individual cases is very limited (Booth et al., 1964; Müller and Nielsen, 1967), despite the optimistic feelings of some authors (e.g., MacLeod et al., 1967). This is due to the wide scatter. A fall in estriol output may only be used as one of the symptoms in the whole clinical picture. On the other hand, it has been well established (Aubry and Nesbitt, 1970) that a terminal dramatic fall in estriol levels occurs often only just prior to the death of the fetus. The report (Heikkilä and Luukkainen, 1971) that in some cases of toxemia the amount of estetrol excreted is more reliable for monitoring the intrauterine fetal condition than that of estriol deserves further study (see also Section IV, A, 1).

2. Rh Isoimmunization

Normal to high-normal values of estriol excretion have been found in Rh isoimmunization (Banerjea, 1962; E. S. Taylor et al., 1963; Frandsen, 1965; Klopper and Stephenson, 1966; Lundvall and Stakemann, 1969; Heys et al., 1969; Samaan et al., 1969). Except for Mandelbaum and Evans (1969) and Mandelbaum et al. (1970), most investigators (e.g., Frandsen, 1965; Klopper and Stephenson, 1966) regard maternal estriol excretion as not related to the fetal status, and observe a decrease only after intrauterine fetal death. Schindler et al. (1967) found very low estriol values only within 24 hours of fetal death. A similar lack of correlation has been established between plasma estriol and the degree of fetal damage (Schindler et al., 1967; Ratanasopa et al., 1967), and Lachowicz (1969) even found a marked increase of erythrocyte estrogen concentration in Rh isoimmunization. In contrast to estriol, urinary estetrol excretion was found to bear a linear correlation to the cord blood hemoglobin concentration (Heikkilä and Luukkainen, 1971). Fetal liver damage in Rh incompatability would result in a specific lowering of urinary estetrol. (Section IV, A, 1).

After the well established initial depression of estriol excretion following intrauterine transfusion (Bjerre et al., 1968; Dickey et al., 1968; Carpenter, 1970), which also occurs after introduction of the intraperitoneal catheter without transfusion of red cells (Dickey et al., 1968), the determination of urinary estriol excretion seems to be useful as a guide for the assessment of the fetal condition (Bjerre *et al.*, 1968; Carpenter, 1970; Mandelbaum *et al.*, 1970).

Low or nondetectable amniotic fluid estriol (Schindler and Herrmann, 1966; Schindler and Ratanasopa, 1968; Aleem *et al.*, 1969a,b), 16-keto-androstenediol and 16α-hydroxy DHA (Schindler and Ratanasopa, 1968) contents have been found in cases of severe Rh isoimmunization. In contrast, amniotic fluid DHA and pregnanediol concentrations do not appear to be significantly influenced under these circumstances unless intrauterine fetal death had already occurred (Schindler and Ratanasopa, 1968). The contents of estriol and bilirubin in the amniotic fluid are correlated (Breborowicz *et al.*, 1969) and the estriol concentration of the amniotic fluid reflects the condition of the fetus better than maternal plasma or urinary estriol values (Schindler *et al.*, 1967). Amniotic fluid estriol determination has been suggested as a further diagnostic step, in addition to the Liley procedure (Schindler *et al.*, 1967). Since in intrauterine transfusion blood spillage does not interfere with amniotic fluid estriol determination (as it will with spectral analysis), estriol determinations in this condition seem to be of great value.

Estriol glucuronoside and estriol sulfate are excreted into the amniotic fluid, the greater portion being the glucuroniside (Troen *et al.*, 1961). The ratio estriol glucuronoside: estriol sulfate is increased by a selective gradient imposed by the membranes, the transfer of estriol glucuronoside through the membranes occurring only at a slow rate (Mikhail *et al.*, 1963a,b; Katz *et al.*, 1965; Goebelsmann *et al.*, 1966; Levitz, 1966). Estriol glucuronoside is largely excreted into the amniotic fluid via fetal urine (Goebelsmann *et al.*, 1966). The concentration of estriol glucurono-side in amniotic fluid reflects to a large extent the enzymatic activity involved in glucuronidic acid transfer in the fetus. Fetal liver damage in Rh isoimmunization thus would result in lowered amniotic fluid estriol.

3. Carbohydrate Metabolism

In diabetes and pregnancy, estriol excretion has been reported higher than the normal range (Ten Berge *et al.*, 1957; Samaan *et al.*, 1969), but mostly in the lower limit of the normal range (Rubin *et al.*, 1946; Hobkirk *et al.*, 1960; Hobkirk and Nilson, 1962; Coyle and Brown, 1963; Greene *et al.*, 1965; E. S. Taylor *et al.*, 1965; Wyss and Meyer, 1966; Beling, 1967). Larger than normal scatter of values was reported by Magendantz *et al.* (1968), and Heys *et al.* (1969) reported inconclusive findings on estriol excretion in diabetic pregnancy. Lauritzen and Lehmann (1971) found excretion values within the normal range. Thus in diabetes and pregnancy estriol excretion may be in the lower limit of the normal range, in the normal range, or higher than the normal range. No correlation of grade of diabetes to estriol excretion was found by Frandsen et al. (1962), Wyss and Meyer (1966), and Wyss (1968). However, a correlation of urinary estriol excretion with the severity of diabetes was established by Southren et al. (1968). Anderson et al. (1969) found depressed estriol excretion only in class C and D diabetics (classes according to White, 1949). Also Beling (1967) established lower values in more severe diabetes. A correlation between fetal weight (Section IV, F, 1) and estriol excretion has been well established. The often large fetus and bulky placenta in diabetic pregnancy could thus cause a rather high excretion of estriol. The large babies do not seem to be caused by fetal growth hormone excess in diabetic pregnancy (Cole et al., 1970). In diabetic pregnancy complicated by hypertension, estriol excretion is below the normal range (Aubry and Nesbitt, 1970). Estetrol excretion seems to give a more reliable clue to the state of the fetus than estriol in those patients in whom toxemia is superimposed (Heikkilä and Luukkainen, 1971).

Plasma estriol in diabetic pregnancy is in the lower normal range (Roy and Kerr, 1964; Wodrig and Göretzlehner, 1964) or low (Ratanasopa et al., 1967).

The concentrations of umbilical arterial DHAS and 16-OH-DHAS are normal in diabetic pregnancy if not complicated by toxemia (Lauritzen and Lehmann, 1971). The clearance of DHAS, which is mostly a uteroplacental clearance, is not reduced in the diabetic patient, except when the diabetes is complicated by toxemia. However, Lauritzen and Lehmann (1971) and Van Leusden (1972c) found reduction of the aromatization of DHA into estrone in diabetic placentas in vitro. These authors stated that since estrogen and DHA values in plasma and urine are mostly normal some unknown factor must compensate for the placental defect. This factor might well be the hypertrophy of the placenta in diabetic pregnancy.

Amniotic fluid estriol has been reported to be low or undetectable (Schindler and Ratanasopa, 1968); 16-ketoandrostenediol and 16α-hydroxy DHA are low or undetectable (Schindler and Ratanasopa, 1968), whereas DHA and pregnanediol are in the normal range.

Clinical judgment in diabetic pregnancy is difficult since classification and treatment of diabetes and pregnancy differ from clinic to clinic. Schwarz et al. (1969) considered in 8 of 113 gestational diabetics preterm delivery necessary because of falling estriol excretion. Echt and Cohen (1970) did not encounter perinatal fetal death as long as estriol excretion remained above 12.0 mg per 24 hours within 48 hours of labor.

However, it is wise to keep in mind that every diabetic patient may show a precipitous fall in urinary estriol, frequently associated with intrauterine death (Talbert et al., 1969; Aubry and Nesbitt, 1970). Thus, normal estriol excretion in diabetic pregnancy may give a false sense of security. Clinical judgment based on low or falling estriol excretion may be used as an additional argument in clinical management. Repeated determinations of amniotic fluid estriol concentration might prove to be of great help in the future.

F. Fetal Weight, Retarded Fetal Growth, Fetal
   Acidosis, and Intrauterine Death

1. *Fetal Weight and Retarded Fetal Growth*

In following patients with retarded fetal growth, serial assays are of crucial importance. In retarded fetal growth (these fetuses nearly always have a low placental weight) in the absence of recognizable maternal disease, such as preeclampsia or chronic hypertension, the estriol excretion is low (Yousem et al., 1966; Wallace and Michie, 1966; Bell et al., 1967; Oakey et al., 1967; Michie, 1966; Reid et al., 1968; Iyengar, 1968; Beischer et al., 1968a,b,c; Heys et al., 1969; Greene et al., 1969; Elliott, 1970). The general impression is that in addition to estriol, estrone and estradiol excretion are lowered as well. If growth retardation is a result of obstetrical maternal disease, predominantly preeclamptic toxemia, estrogen excretion is lowered as well (Bell et al., 1967; Neill and Macafee, 1968; Aubry and Nesbitt, 1970). Normal estriol output is only exceptionally associated with low birth weight (Frandsen and Stakemann, 1963a; Klopper, 1966). Except for Klopper and Billewicz (1963), who found no such relationship in normal pregnancy, all other investigators (Frandsen and Stakemann, 1960; Greene and Touchstone, 1963; Coyle and Brown, 1963; Beling, 1963, 1967; Frandsen, 1963; Yousem et al., 1966; Aoba, 1966; Neill and Macafee, 1968; Beischer et al., 1968a,b,c; Goecke, 1969; Easterling and Talbert, 1970; Aubry and Nesbitt, 1970) have reported that in normal pregnancy fetal weight is correlated with estriol excretion. Dickey (1969) and Dickey and Robertson (1969) have measured the estrogen concentration and the ratio estrogen:creatinine in the first voided urine of 147 newborn infants. Estrogen concentration and the ratio were found to be related to birth weight.

Amniotic fluid estriol concentration is correlated with fetal weight (Aleem et al., 1969a,b). Goecke (1969) established a positive correlation between estriol excretion and placental surface. Conversion of infused DHAS into total estrogens (Lauritzen, 1969) is lowered in placental insufficiency and is absent if the fetus is dead. If Diamox is given to pregnant women with abnormally low estriol excretion, an increase of urinary estriol would indicate a favorable fetal condition, whereas in retarded fetal growth urinary estriol does not change (Aoba, 1966). The excretion of DHA in infants whose mothers had decreased estriol is not altered, whereas both 16α-hydroxy DHA and 16 ketoandrostenediol are markedly reduced.

Thus, arguments are accumulating that the various enzyme systems in the fetus *and* placenta exhibit a low activity in retarded fetal growth. Scommegna *et al.* (1968) found that in pathological pregnancies the decreased estriol excretion might be related to diminished enzymatic activity more than to a decrease in the availability of precursors (see also Section IV, A, 2). In contrast, Hausknecht and Mandelbaum (1969) found that in normal pregnancy the intra-amniotic instillation of 200 mg DHA brings about a pronounced rise in urinary estriol excretion. This would indicate that the various enzyme systems in the fetus and placenta under normal conditions are not fully saturated at term, and that there is certainly also a decreased availability of steroid precursors (see also Section IV, A, 2). From the data presented it cannot be denied that there is certainly also a decreased availability of steroid precursors in retarded fetal growth.

Wallace and Michie (1966) reported serious neurological problems in 5 of 14 infants with low birth weight and abnormally low maternal estriol excretion throughout gestation. However, as established by Greene *et al.* (1969), low estriol excretion before delivery is compatible with normal development and intelligence of the infant.

From the practical point of view serial assays of estriol can be of help as additional evidence to establish growth retardation. However, when estriol is low, growth retardation is so obvious that estriol determinations are of little additional value (Booth *et al.*, 1965). The decision whether or not labor should be induced depends on the whole clinical picture. This is illustrated by the findings of Martin and Hahnel (1964), who found no difference between estriol output of mothers with growth-retarded babies who succumbed and those who survived.

2. Fetal Acidosis and Intrauterine Death

a. Fetal Acidosis. A number of studies have demonstrated a relationship between fetal acidosis and the condition of the fetus at birth (e.g., Saling, 1965; Beard *et al.*, 1966). In this connection the study of Fliegner *et al.* (1969) is of interest. These authors measured urinary estriol excretion and fetal acid-base status in 80 patients with high-risk pregnancies. Estriol excretion was below normal limits in 24 patients

(30%), and in this group the incidence of pH values less than 7.20 was 41%, which was significantly different from that in patients with normal estriol values. Thus, the detection of low urinary estriol excretion by screening of all high-risk pregnancies would enable more accurate selection of those patients who require fetal blood pH measurement.

b. *Intrauterine Death.* It is fairly well established that when estriol excretion values are consistently below 2.0–4.0 mg per 24 hours after week 33, fetal death is imminent, if it has not already occurred (Greene, 1970). If termination of pregnancy is being considered in a case with such low values, fetal X-ray examination for gross anomalies is essential, to exclude, e.g., anencephaly. Regardless of the cause of fetal death, estriol excretion drops to very low levels, the amounts depending on the methods used by the authors (B. Zondek, 1954; B. Zondek and Goldberg, 1957; Frandsen and Stakemann, 1960; Banerjea, 1962; Coyle *et al.*, 1962; Beling, 1963; Greene and Touchstone, 1963; Wray and Russel, 1964; Greene *et al.*, 1965; Jayle *et al.*, 1965; Strand, 1966; Nilsson and Bengtsson, 1968; Heys *et al.*, 1968; Wei *et al.*, 1968; Nelson, 1969; Aubry and Nesbitt, 1970; Echt and Cohen, 1970). Welshman *et al.* (1969) found no cases of stillbirth with normal values. However, there are exceptions: Booth *et al.* (1965), MacLeod *et al.* (1967), and Oakey *et al.* (1967) have also found normal urinary estriol values even after the death of the fetus. Plasma estriol has been reported low in fetal death (Ratanasopa *et al.*, 1967) Starting from the observation that there exists a positive correlation between estriol excretion and placental surface, Goecke (1969) asked himself after what period placental removal is followed by a fall of estriol excretion. In a collection period of 3–6 hours postpartum, the mean estriol excretion was 50% of the antepartum period. From these data Goecke (1969) concluded that the earliest fall of estrogen excretion is in a period starting 3 hours after the placenta has been affected deleteriously.

A circumstance restricting the use of estriol excretion values might be the fact that antepartum as well as postpartum there is a positive correlation between the excretion of estriol and plasma volume (Goecke, 1969). According to this author, this might explain the fact that after intrauterine fetal death the excretion of urinary estriol is sometimes within the normal range. On the other hand, when a placenta is functionally handicapped to the extent of about one-third of its volume, there is not necessarily a significant fall of urinary estriol.

Thus in intrauterine fetal death estriol excretion is very low, with rare exceptions. Also plasma estriol is low. Fetal acidosis and low estriol excretion are correlated. Many authors (Lenters, 1958; B. Zondek and Pfeiffer, 1959; Ten Berge, 1961; Furuhjelm, 1962; Würtele, 1962; Greene and Touchstone, 1963; MacLeod *et al.*, 1967; Heys *et al.*, 1968, 1969; Magendantz *et al.*, 1968; Klopper, 1969; Echt and Cohen, 1970) have defined more or less fixed levels of estriol excretion that would indicate that fetal death is going to occur. These values differ from method to method, and are of rather limited value. The amount of lowering of estriol excretion per unit of time preceding intrauterine death (thus a dynamic criterion) has not been accurately defined as yet, and will depend on the cause of the intrauterine accident. From the practical point of view estriol determinations may help to diagnose intrauterine death.

G. Anemia

Urinary estriol values below normal were found after 30 weeks' gestation in 25% of 133 patients with hemoglobin levels below 10 gm/100 ml (Beischer *et al.*, 1968a,b). It was found that in the low estriol group 6.6% of patients had β-thalassemia minor whereas the incidence was only 2.1% in the normal estriol group. Thus anemia should be classified with other conditions described as being associated with low estriol values.

H. Antepartum Hemorrhage

Beischer *et al.* (1967) found normal estriol excretion in patients with placenta previa, but low values in patients with other causes of bleeding. Kahmann (1970a,b) found reversible lowering of estriol excretion in repeated partial placental abruptions. Dickey and Robertson (1969) and Dickey (1969) compared E:C ratios in patients with various pregnancy complications and newborn diseases and in normal cases by analysis of covariance, thereby removing the effect of weight. The E:C ratio of infants born following pregnancies complicated by maternal hemorrhage was significantly below the average found for normal infants. Patients with antepartum hemorrhage can be divided into two main categories on the basis of estriol excretion. First, those with placenta previa and some of those classified after delivery as having bleeding of unknown origin, in whom the bleeding does not affect placental function. The second category includes the remainder of patients in whom bleeding causes placental damage, temporary or permanent.

I. Prematurity, Onset of Labor, and Postmaturity

1. *Prematurity*

Diminished estriol excretion in prematurity has been reported by E. S. Taylor *et al.* (1965); Heys *et al.* (1968), in a group of 403 pregnancies with increased fetal risk found 38 premature deliveries following subnormal estriol excretion. In patients with repeated premature births (delivered 2 or more low birth weight infants, >1500 < 2500 grams, in the past) estriol excretion was found by Aubry and Nesbitt (1970) to be depressed to the low normal range as early as week 24 of pregnancy. In all these instances the lowering of estriol excretion might be related to the fact that the mean birth weight is lower in these patients than in the control group. However, Aubry and Nesbitt (1970) did not find recognizable dysmaturity in their group. No sharp decreases in estriol excretion were noted prior to the onset of premature labor.

It is clear that if prematurity is defined in terms of low birth weight, estriol excretion is low as compared with the group with normal birth weight (Section IV, F, 1). However, if prematurity is defined in terms of duration of pregnancy, estriol excretion is not necessarily lowered.

2. Onset of Labor

Liggins *et al.* (1966, 1967) have shown that in the ewe pregnancy could be prolonged by destruction of the fetal adrenals, pituitary, or hypothalamus. Liggins (1968, 1969) induced premature delivery in the ewe by infusing ACTH, cortisol, or dexamethasone into the intact sheep fetus *in utero,* whereas deoxycorticosterone and corticosterone did not induce premature delivery.

In the human it is well known that in cases of anencephalic monsters without polyhydramnios very often there may be considerable postmaturity. A duration of 53 weeks of pregnancy has been reported (e.g., Papiernik-Berkhauer and Hamelin, 1968). In anencephalic monsters the fetal adrenal cortex is nearly always absent or underdeveloped (Section IV, D, 1). Turnbull and Anderson (1969) established a greatly increased fetal adrenal weight in many infants delivered as a result of "unexplained" premature labor after week 20 compared to those of similar gestational age delivered because of a specific complication of pregnancy.

Urinary excretion of estriol and estrone at week 34 of pregnancy showed that in patients with a high level of uterine activity and early onset of labor estriol excretion was high and estrone was low. The lower the urinary estriol or the higher the estrone at that stage, the more prolonged was the pregnancy. Pregnanediol excretion was not related to the gestational length at the onset of labor (Turnbull *et al.,* 1967).

The above-mentioned data strongly suggest that there might be a fetal mechanism acting as a signal for the onset of labor, involving the fetal hypophysis hypothalamus and adrenals. Estriol synthesis within the fetoplacental unit might be involved, as a cause or a result. However, the onset of parturition in the ewe is not necessarily identical with that in the human. Moreover, the sound clinical evidence that at term a dead fetus *in utero* is mostly delivered spontaneously proves that the absence of a functional hypophyseal–hypothalamic–adrenal axis is certainly not the only cause for the onset of labor.

3. *Prolonged Pregnancy and Postmaturity Syndrome*

The expected data of delivery is usually calculated from the date of the last period, according to the rule of Nägele. If pregnancy continues after the calculated date, a state of postmaturity is assumed to be present, but there is no unanimous agreement on the exact definition of this condition. In general, prolonged pregnancy can be defined as a pregnancy that is more than 14 days past term (term = 280 days after the first day of the last menstrual period), provided the menstrual cycle is regular, and the time of quickening agrees with the calculation. Many American authors feel that postmaturity is unimportant, whereas most European obstetricians are of the opinion that postmaturity involves an increased risk for the baby. In a careful study of postmaturity, Strand (1956) concluded that perinatal mortality increases with increasing length of gestation, especially in nulliparae. Lindell (1956) found that in multiparae the perinatal mortality was unchanged (approximately 1%) for gestation of 40–44 weeks' duration, whereas in nulliparae the mortality increased to 6.3% for gestations of over 42 weeks' duration.

Pseudo-prolonged pregnancy due to retarded ovulation remains always a possibility, but it has been well established that part of the prolonged pregnancy fetuses have a postmaturity syndrome (reduced liquor amnii, meconium staining, desquamation of skin), a condition associated with a high perinatal mortality. Prolonged pregnancy may lead to placental senescence in the absence of maternal disease.

Thus prolonged pregnancy is a mixture of pseudo-prolonged pregnancy and of fetuses with postmaturity syndrome. K. Smith *et al.* (1966), Lundvall and Stakemann (1966), and Beischer *et al.* (1968a,b, 1969) found that prolonged pregnancy may be associated with normal and high estriol excretion without fetal jeopardy, but also with low or falling estriol output. Holtorff *et al.* (1968) have determined total estrogen excretion per 24 hours according to Ittrich in 20 cases with prolonged pregnancy in which the children had a typical postmaturity syndrome (Clifford I–III). The data were compared with those for a control group of 46 women whose children had no postmaturity syndrome. They found that in individual cases, even with serial determinations, intrauterine danger in prolonged pregnancy is extremely difficult to recognize. Jenkins *et al.* (1970) found that the progressive rise in estrogen excretion seen in the preterm period is not continued after the expected date of confinement. There is a leveling off to a plateau in mean estrogen excretion.

Amnioscopic observations and/or fluid analysis after transabdominal puncture have become of much more importance in the clinical management of prolonged pregnancy than serial determinations of estriol. However, a continuous rise in estriol excretion might be an additional argument not to induce labor as long as the amniotic fluid does not become meconium-stained.

J. SUMMARY

Of the estrogens, estriol is excreted in disproportionately large quantities in the course of human gestation. Estriol excretion is certainly altered in pathological pregnancy. A more accurate indication of the fetal state in human pathological pregnancy might be expected from determinations of estetrol, arising to the extent of 80% from fetal precursors, and of 11-dehydro-17α-estradiol and 15-hydroxyprogesterone, which are purely fetal steroids. Dynamic tests (infusing intravenously or intra-amniotically maternal or fetal precursor steroids such as DHAS, and measuring their urinary metabolites) have tentatively suggested that in normal pregnancy the enzymatic systems involved in estriol synthesis are almost completely saturated by the available precursors. In pathological pregnancies, decreased estriol excretion might be related to diminished enzymatic activity in addition to a decrease in the availability of precursors. Even if technical errors of measurement are excluded and if collection of urine is not incomplete, urinary estrogen output shows wide variations from day to day and from one individual to another. A single test is worthless. Errors of measurement and renal factors are discussed. Determination of estriol:creatinine might reduce variations and thus increase the clinical usefulness of such assays.

In abortion the lowered estriol excretion is caused by changes within the fetoplacental unit. In hydatidiform mole pregnancy the excretion of estrogens is lower than in normal pregnancy of comparable duration. Maternal DHAS, presumably of adrenal origin, can serve as an effective precursor of estrone and estradiol, but not of estriol. In this condition, estriol arises from the catabolism of estrone-estradiol in the maternal compartment. In choriocarcinoma, in contrast to hydatidiform moles, *in vitro* studies indicate an ability to perform steroid side-chain cleavage; these observations are in agreement with the hypothesis that chorion-epithelioma would arise before differentiation of the fertilized ovum into trophoblast and fetal cells *strictu sensu* takes place, thus that choriocarcinoma would not arise from hydatidiform mole.

In abdominal pregnancy, excretion of estrogens, predominantly estriol, decreases very rapidly after cesarean section with the placenta left *in situ,* illustrating the important fetal contribution to maternal urinary estriol.

In anencephalic monsters, estriol excretion is low, related to the under-development of the fetal adrenal cortex. ACTH would not seem to pass from the mother to the fetus. However, ACTH determinations in the fetus, especially in anencephalic monsters are lacking. In fetuses with congenital adrenogenital syndrome amniotic fluid pregnanetriol and 17-ketosteroid concentrations are suggestively elevated at term. Fetal sex is not related to estriol excretion and in multiple pregnancy estriol excretion is increased as compared with normal pregnancy.

In preeclamptic toxemia estriol excretion is lowered, and arguments are presented that the cause of decreased estriol excretion must be sought in the placenta as well as in the fetus, due to a generalized disturbance of estrogen metabolism. In Rh isoimmunization, excretion of estriol is in the high normal range, and there is no correlation with the degree of fetal damage. Estetrol excretion might become of much greater value, and as amniotic fluid estriol determinations correlate better with fetal state than estriol excretion, further studies on amniotic fluid estriol in Rh isoimmunization might be promising.

In diabetes and pregnancy estriol excretion may be higher than normal. Data concerning correlation with the grade of diabetes are conflicting, possibly due to meticulous insulin titration of patients with diabetes and pregnancy. Placental aromatization *in vitro* is inhibited, but normal estrogen excretion may then still be present due to the compensatory total capacity of the large and bulky placenta.

Estrogen excretion is correlated with fetal weight with such over-whelming evidence that it is tempting to speculate that in all kinds of pathological pregnancy resulting in reduced fetoplacental mass estrogen excretion is lowered, regardless of the cause (e.g., toxemia, idiopathic growth retardation). If, on the other hand, the fetoplacental mass is increased (the large baby and placenta in diabetes and Rh isoim-munization), estriol excretion may be high, even such that a deteriorating clinical condition of the fetus is masked. In cases of intrauterine fetal death estrogen excretion is extremely low. There are studies indicating a correlation between fetal acidosis and lowered estriol excretion. How-ever, the amount of decrease of estriol excreted per unit of time preced-ing fetal death has not been accurately defined.

In anemia and pregnancy, estriol excretion may be low, sometimes also in antepartum hemorrhage, but a placenta which is functionally handi-capped for about one-third of its volume is not necessarily associated with a significant fall of urinary estriol.

In prematurity, estriol excretion may be low; this is probably related to a decreased fetal weight as compared with controls. Animal experiments and observations in anencephalic monsters strongly suggest the existence of a fetal mechanism acting as a signal for the onset of labor involving the fetal hypophysis–hypothalamus and adrenals. Estriol synthesis within the fetoplacental unit might be involved as a cause or as a result. In prolonged pregnancy there are indications that the progressive rise in estrogen excretion seen in the preterm period is not continued after the expected date of confinement. A continuous rise of estriol excretion might be an additional argument not to induce labor as long as the amniotic fluid does not become meconium stained.

If one compartment of the fetoplacental unit is lacking (e.g., anencephalic monsters) or is experimentally or naturally put out of circuit, formation of estriol more than that of estrone and estradiol is the most vulnerable within the fetoplacental unit. From these observations and from the experiments of Diczfalusy and his school, insight into the localization of disturbances within the fetoplacental unit resulting in changing estriol excretion has increased tremendously. Isolated disturbances within the fetoplacental unit bring about specific changes of estriol excretion. However, the reverse situation, changed estriol excretion pointing to specific disturbances within the fetoplacental unit, hardly ever exists, since isolated lesions, such as in anencephalic monsters, are extremely rare. From the clinical point of view, lowering of estriol excretion is mostly caused by generalized disturbances in the fetus and in the placenta. This and the large inter- and intraindividual variability of estriol excretion limit the practical usefulness of the measurement of estriol excretion in toxemia, Rh isoimmunization, diabetes and pregnancy, retarded fetal growth, intrauterine death, anemia, antepartum hemorrhage, prematurity, and prolonged pregnancy, as far as the management of individual cases is concerned. Serial determinations may contribute to a more reliable assessment of the whole clinical picture.

V. Progesterone

A. Excretion

1. *Pregnanediol, Pregnanetriol, and Pregnanolone*

Simultaneous estimations of total estrogens, pregnanetriol, pregnanediol, and pregnanolone in the same urine sample were carried out by Acevedo et al. (1968). These authors established the pattern of excretion of these compounds in a total of 170 normal and abnormal pregnancies in various stages of gestation. They considered 107 patients as normal, and the results from this group gave the basis for criteria of normalcy. The lower limit of normalcy was arbitrarily drawn in such a way that at least 98% of the values found are inside the area of excretion. Their results obtained with normals showed a parallelism between pregnanetriol and total estrogen excretion, on one hand, and of pregnanolone and pregnanediol, on the other. The results in terms of range of pregnanetriol excretion are quite different from those of Fotherby et al. (1965) and of Harkness and Love (1966). The difference may very well be due to methodology. The results of Fotherby et al. (1965) showed a lack of correlation between pregnanediol and pregnanetriol excretions. It is suggested that the fetal compartment of the fetoplacental unit is the main source of urinary pregnanetriol in pregnancy, but a fraction of the urinary steroid is also due to the maternal compartment.

2. Progesterone and Urinary Pregnanediol

A number of authors (Sommerville and Marrian, 1950; Zander, 1954; Klopper and Michie, 1956; Pearlman, 1957) determined the conversion of progesterone into urinary pregnanediol in nonpregnant patients. Within 5 days 0–25% of progesterone administered appears in the urine as pregnanediol. In pregnant women the conversion was determined by Venning and Browne (1940), Davis and Fugo (1947), Sommerville and Marrian (1950), Guterman (1953), Klopper and Michie (1956), Pearlman (1957), Plotz et al. (1963), and Henssen (1969). The same or a somewhat higher percentage of conversion was found in pregnant women than in nonpregnant individuals.

The percentage of conversion seems to depend on the stage of gestation and changes in pathological pregnancy. Fotherby (1970) investigated patients between weeks 8 and 14 of pregnancy who were scheduled for termination of pregnancy. They were given [^{14}C]progesterone intravenously and urine was collected for 5 days; 9.2% of the administered progesterone was recovered as pregnanediol; a minimum of 6% of the administered dose of progesterone was metabolized to 6-oxygenated steroids. Henssen (1969) established a mean percentage of 15 for the conversion of progesterone into pregnanediol. In normal pregnancy a lowering of the percentage of conversion from 20.8 to 18.5% was established from week 30 until week 36, after which a sharp decrease to 12.0% was observed until week 39. Pregnancies with low birth weight with or without hypertension showed a lower mean percentage of conversion from week 30 until week 36 as compared with normal pregnancies. MacNaughton and Greig (1965) reported a lower percentage of conversion in patients with disturbed pregnancy than in normal pregnancy.

The determination of the percentage of conversion during pregnancy is hampered by the fact that the quantity of urinary pregnanediol after administration of progesterone must be corrected for the amount of endogenously produced progesterone. This is difficult in pregnant women because of the relatively large coefficient of variation between the values in successive 24-hour urines from the same subject (Section V, A, 3), limiting the reliability of the secretion rate of progesterone (PSR) (Section V, C) calculated from the percentage of conversion. Another difficulty in the interpretation of changing pregnanediol excretion is the possibility of a change in fecal excretion, which may go as high as 30% of the progesterone administered (Davis et al., 1960). Limited amounts also are excreted through the skin (Wiest et al., 1955; Davis and Plotz, 1958; Sandberg and Slaunwhite, 1958; Zander, 1959; Klopper and Mac-Naughton, 1959; Chang et al., 1960). Cassmer (1959), after ligation of the umbilical cord, and Klopper and Stephenson (1966), after intra-amniotic administration of hypertonic saline in therapeutic abortion, noted a lowering of about 20% in urinary pregnanediol. Thus some contribution by the fetal compartment to urinary pregnanediol certainly cannot be excluded.

3. Day-to-Day Variation in Pregnanediol Excretion

There are large variations in urinary pregnanediol levels from day to day in normal pregnancy (Coyle et al., 1956; Shearman, 1959; Kanka-anrinta, 1963; Klopper and Billewicz, 1963). Klopper (1964) found the average coefficient of variation between successive 24 hour urine samples from the same subject to be 24%. In pathological pregnancy, such as severe preeclamptic toxemia, the coefficient of variation was even higher than in normal pregnancy (Kankaanrinta, 1963) (Section V, H, 1).

B. MATERNAL AND FETAL ADRENALS

1. Maternal Adrenal Cortex and Progesterone in Pregnancy

The concentration of pregnenolone sulfate of 10 μg per 100 ml of plasma from an adrenalectomized woman in week 11 of pregnancy, whereas 6 weeks after delivery pregnenolone sulfate could not be demonstrated in the plasma (Conrad et al., 1967), suggested that during pregnancy pregnenolone sulfate could originate in the fetoplacental unit.

From this evidence the suggestion arises that the maternal adrenal cortex is not responsible for fundamental endocrinological changes in human pregnancy. However, a possible exception might be aldosterone (Solomon et al., 1964). Increased progesterone secretion by the adrenal cortex does not seem to occur at all in view of the observations in pregnant women with Addison's disease having a normal excretion of pregnane-diol; also, after subtotal adrenalectomy normal excretion of pregnanediol has been well established (Samuels *et al.*, 1943; Knowlton *et al.*, 1949; Baulieu *et al.*, 1956; Tivenius, 1959; Venning *et al.*, 1959; Dellepiane and Andreoli, 1961; Hammerstein and Nevinny-Stickel, 1965; Harkness *et al.*, 1966). It seems that maternal secretion of adrenal progesterone and pregnenolone sulfate during pregnancy is the same as in the nonpregnant individual; from the data observed in adrenalectomized women it appears that the fetoplacental unit contributes to a similar secretion of pregnenolone sulfate and progesterone as in normal pregnant women.

2. *Fetal Adrenals and Progesterone Formation in Pregnancy*

A limited contribution from the fetus as such to urinary pregnanediol cannot be excluded (Cassmer, 1959; Klopper and Stephenson, 1966). However, in intrauterine death due to a nonplacental cause (Kloosterman and Huis in 't Veld, 1961) and in anencephalic monsters (Frandsen and Stakemann, 1961), the pregnanediol excretion is in the normal range. Also Lurie *et al.* (1966) found an unchanged maternal plasma progesterone concentration after intrauterine fetal death. Since after termination of abdominal pregnancy with the placenta left *in situ* the pregnanediol excretion remains elevated (Section V, F), a substantial fetal adrenal contribution to urinary pregnanediol can be excluded. Conrad *et al.* (1967) established a higher plasma pregnenolone sulfate concentration in the umbilical arteries as compared with that in the umbilical vein. Their data could be explained by the assumption that the placenta secretes pregnenolone as well as progesterone. It has been well established that the placenta has substantial sulfatase activity, whereas the fetus conjugates steroids with sulfuric acid on a large scale (Mikhail *et al.*, 1963a,b; Diczfalusy, 1964; Bolté *et al.*, 1964a,b,c; Schwers *et al.*, 1965a,b), however, it was claimed that the fetus in week 20 of gestation cannot metabolize pregnenolone sulfate to other steroids. One could assume a fetoplacental circle in this respect: the placenta secretes pregnenolone to the fetus, where pregnenolone is sulfurylated. Pregnenolone sulfate is carried back to the placenta, where one part of it is desulfated whereas another part would escape into the fetal and maternal circulation. This assumption would also explain the increased concentration of pregnenolone sulfate found in pregnant adrenalectomized women. In view of the *in vitro* experiments of G. Morrison *et al.* (1965), who established conversion of cholesterol into pregnenolone by the placenta, and the *in vivo* experiments of Jaffe *et al.* (1965), Jaffe (1967), Jaffe and Ledger (1966) and Telegdy *et al.* (1970), who established pregnenolone formation in the placental perfusate as well as in the placenta after perfusion with cholesterol, this hypothesis does not seem unlikely.

C. PROGESTERONE SECRETION RATE IN PATHOLOGICAL PREGNANCY

The limitations of the calculation of the secretion rate of progesterone (PSR) have been discussed (Section V, A, 2). The possible influence of additional compartments (fetus, placenta, amniotic fluid) with their selective permeabilities may make calculation of PSR in pregnancy extremely complex.

The possible passage of progesterone from the mother to the fetus in PSR determinations in human pregnancy might be of importance.

Castren *et al.* (1962) determined the permeability of the human placenta to [4-¹⁴C]progesterone in mid-pregnancy, and Haskins and Soiva (1960) did so in term pregnancy. Their data suggest that labeled progesterone disappears from the maternal blood very quickly and spreads through the tissues. Part of it passes at a slower rate to the fetus, where a further spread takes place through the fetal plasma and tissues.

From the experiments of Plotz and Davis (1957), it appears that the quantity of progesterone passing is certainly <1%, from which one might conclude that when normal (300–400 mg per day) progesterone secretion exists in the last trimester of pregnancy, the passage of progesterone from the maternal organism to the fetus would be in the order of magnitude of less than 3–4 mg per day.

Secretion of Progesterone by the Placenta to the Fetus

The investigators who assessed PSR during pregnancy all used Pearlman's method. No investigator takes the "consumption" by the fetus into account. Such a "consumption" is not unlikely to occur, as the concentration of progesterone in the umbilical vein and arteries is 37 and 14 µg per 100 ml, respectively (Runnebaum and Zander, 1962); Greig *et al.* (1962) and Harbert *et al.* (1964) also established a higher concentration of progesterone in the umbilical vein than in the arteries. Taking the data of Runnebaum and Zander (1962), the difference in concentration between umbilical arterial and venous blood is 23 µg/100 ml. Assuming (Hytten and Leitch, 1964) a fetal placental circulation of 250 ml of blood per minute, the net "consumption" of progesterone by the fetus would be in the order of magnitude of 80 mg per day. This progesterone is converted into other steroids by the fetus. In making this calculation a number of assumptions were made, which may or may not be valid. However, it is clear that when Pearlman's method is used for the assessment of the PSR in the third trimester of pregnancy, the extrafetal compartment has to be taken into account. Gurpide *et al.* (1962) and

Henssen (1969) proposed the introduction of a correction factor in the formula of Pearlman. The correct value of this factor has not been defined, but if a correction factor is not used, the values found for the PSR could well be in the order of magnitude of 80 mg per day too low because of consumption by the fetus. Further experimentation is needed to clarify this point.

D. The Progesterone Block Theory

1. Introduction

As early as 1929 Allen and Corner found that progesterone prevents the expulsion of fetuses in the rabbit after castration. According to the theory of the local action of placental progesterone postulated by Csapo (1956, 1966, 1969a,b), progesterone is secreted by the placenta and reaches the overlying myometrium directly in a high concentration before being transported into the systemic circulation. Furthermore, it is suggested that the distribution of the hormone in the myometrium is not uniform and that the highest concentrations occur near the placenta, producing a nonuniform block. Therefore, the myometrial concentrations are higher than can be achieved by systemic administration of progesterone, since this hydrophobic steroid is only slightly soluble in blood. Since the site of progesterone production in early pregnancy is the corpus luteum, a change in the nature of the block from uniform to nonuniform is predicted to occur when progesterone synthesis shifts to the placenta (Csapo, 1969a,b). There is nowadays controversy concerning the applicability of the progesterone block theory to the human.

2. Early Pregnancy

From the data presented in Section V, E, 1, it may be concluded that ovariectomy in early pregnancy certainly does not always result in abortion, even if accompanied by a steep fall in pregnanediol excretion. Thus the existence of a progesterone block in the human may be questioned. Progesterone therapy in threatened abortion (Section V, E, 1, d) does not seem to be of much value. Csapo (1969a) and Csapo et al. (1969) demonstrated that hypertonic saline treatment induced a gradual and statistically significant progesterone withdrawal, correlated with increasing uterine pressure during abortion induced by hypertonic saline solution. However, correlation does not necessarily indicate a causal relationship. Klopper et al. (1966) reported a steep fall in estriol output immediately after the saline was injected, because the fetus dies within a short time. Pregnanediol excretion, however, was maintained at about

80% of the presaline level until the placenta was expelled, when it fell very rapidly.

3. Late Pregnancy

Progesterone has been shown to inhibit uterine activity in species that depend upon the presence of the ovaries throughout pregnancy. However, in species such as the human, in which the ovaries may be removed without interrupting pregnancy (Section V, E, 1, *a*), no evidence of inhibition of uterine activity has been shown. Large doses of progesterone were without significant effect upon the uterine activity at term in women (Pose and Fielitz, 1959; Csapo *et al.*, 1966). Progesterone fails to prolong pregnancy (Zarrow *et al.*, 1963; Schofield, 1964) and is not a myometrial blocking agent in the guinea pig (Porter, 1969). In the ewe progesterone does not prolong pregnancy (Bengtsson and Schofield, 1963). Kerr *et al.* (1966) could not provide any evidence to suggest that declining placental progesterone production initiated laborlike contractions. Sommerville (1969) found considerable variation in the results of 4-hour analyses of plasma progesterone, but no consistent circadian rhythm. He found that the plasma concentration in peripheral venous blood did not fall significantly prior to spontaneous labor in women. However, Csapo *et al.* (1971) found that plasma progesterone reached peak values at different times during the last 4 weeks of gestation in individual patients, but subsequently a slight decrease occurred with the onset of clinical labor.

It may be concluded that the applicability of the progesterone-block theory to early and in late pregnancy in the human species is still a controversial subject.

E. ABORTION, HYDATIDIFORM MOLE PREGNANCY, AND CHORIOCARCINOMA

1. Abortion

a. Pregnanediol Excretion after Ovariectomy. A temporary fall of pregnanediol excretion after ovariectomy has been reported by H. W. Jones and Weil (1938) in a pregnancy of 58 days, Seegar and Delfs (1940), Trolle (1955a,b), and Tulsky and Koff (1957) (49 days' pregnancy). In two of 14 patients 35 and 41 days pregnant, pregnanediol excretion became low and abortion resulted (Tulsky and Koff, 1957). No interference with pregnanediol excretion by ovariectomy was observed by Browne *et al.* (1937) or Tulsky and Koff (1957) in patients 49 or more days pregnant, by Diczfalusy and Borrell (1961) in a 78 days pregnancy, or by Mancuso (1962). Thus ovariectomy in early pregnancy, even before day 49, does not necessarily result in abortion. Also, a temporary fall of pregnanediol excretion after ovariectomy is not necessarily accompanied by abortion. It appears that hormone production by the ovary is certainly not always essential for the maintenance of human pregnancy.

b. *Progesterone Production in Early Pregnancy. Role of the corpus luteum versus the fetoplacental unit.* Since plasma progesterone rises after the tenth week, whereas 17α-hydroxyprogesterone declines at about 10 weeks (Yoshimi *et al.,* 1969; Holmdahl *et al.,* 1971), it was suggested that the functional life-span of the corpus luteum, which very probably synthesizes 17α-hydroxyprogesterone, is completed at about 10 weeks.

Therapeutic abortion before week 9 was accompanied by slowly declining plasma progesterone levels, suggesting that the corpus luteum was producing substantial amounts of progesterone (Holmdahl *et al.,* 1971). In contrast, abortion between weeks 12 and 16 resulted in a more rapid decline, showing the placenta at that time to be the main organ for progesterone production. Lebech (1971) established in early pregnancy (6–12 weeks of gestation), 24–48 hours after therapeutic abortion, progesterone plasma concentrations in the range of 5–20% of the initial values. After removal of the corpus luteum in weeks 8 and 9 of gestation, a rapid decline of plasma progesterone to about 50% of the initial values was observed in all patients during the first 24 hours. After abortion there was a rapid further decline. According to Lebech (1971), in weeks 8 and 9 of pregnancy about half of the progesterone is produced by the corpus luteum and half by the placenta. More studies are needed to evaluate the relative contribution of the corpus luteum and the fetoplacental unit to progesterone production in early pregnancy.

c. *Progesterone and Pregnanediol in Abortion and in Threatened Abortion.* Urinary levels of the metabolite pregnanediol are frequently taken as an index of (placental) progesterone production, but not more than about 20% of the hormone is excreted as urinary pregnanediol (Section V, A, 2). This limitation to considering pregnanediol excretion as an index of progesterone production should be realized.

Normal excretion of pregnanediol has been reported if abortion was only threatened, whereas pregnanediol excretion was found to be lowered if abortion was actually the final result (Guterman, 1946; de Watteville, 1951; Furuhjelm, 1953; Alder and Krieger, 1957; Rawlings, 1965; Jayle, 1967; Acevedo *et al.,* 1968, 1969; J. B. Brown *et al.,* 1970a,b). Vaginal smears suggesting an insufficient progesterone effect may be associated with a poor prognosis in habitual abortion (Langer and Hockstaedt, 1959; Hughes *et al.,* 1964). However, Robson and Gornall (1955), Baker *et al.* (1955), MacNaughton and Michie (1960), and Langmade *et al.*

(1961) consider pregnanediol excretion in threatened abortion to be of no prognostic value. Russell *et al.* (1957, 1960) measured pregnanediol excretion in 68 women threatening to abort, of whom 41 finally delivered viable infants. There were no significant differences between the 27 patients who did abort and the 41 who did not.

The balance of evidence seems to indicate often, but not always, a correlation between low pregnanediol excretion and poor outcome; however, normal pregnanediol excretion is not always correlated with a favorable outcome. Correlation of low pregnanediol excretion and poor prognosis thus does not seem to point to a causal relationship. According to Klopper and MacNaughton (1965), the pregnanediol output shows little change until the fetoplacental unit is irretrievably damaged.

d. Progesterone and Synthetic Oral Progestogens in Abortion. In those cases in which progesterone deficiency is a secondary effect of fetoplacental damage, not its cause, there is little point in treating impending abortion by the administration of progesterone—the more so since the applicability of the progesterone-block theory to the human is questionable (Section V, D, 2). More commonly the reason for abortion is a defect of the germ plasm (blighted ova, showing only trophoblastic tissue without organized fetal structures; chromosomal aberrations), but there might be occasional instances where progesterone deficiency is the basic cause of an abortion. In at least 19% of spontaneous abortions (see, e.g., WHO Scientific Group, 1966), chromosomal aberrations can be found in the pregnancy products.

It has been claimed that progestogens are effective in the treatment of threatened and recurrent abortion when progesterone deficiency can be demonstrated (Randall *et al.*, 1955; Banks *et al.*, 1964; Jacobson, 1965; MacRae, 1965; Thierstein, 1965). It should be realized that intravenous infusion would be difficult to prepare and would probably have to be continuous to attain blood levels of the hormone within the range normally present in early pregnancy (Taubert and Haskins, 1963; Fuchs *et al.*, 1963). Other investigators (Hansen *et al.*, 1963; Shearman and Garrett, 1963; Goldzieher, 1964; L. Nilsson, 1964; Møller and Fuchs, 1965; Klopper and MacNaughton, 1965; Fuchs and Olsen, 1966), in double-blind clinical trials, have failed to confirm the value of progesterone treatment. Burton and Wachtel (1967) made a trial of the cyclopentyl-3-enol ether of progesterone (Enol Luteovis) and did not find that the ability of this compound (in the dosage used) to convert a "poor" or "fair" smear to "good" improves the ultimate prognosis in apparently progesterone-deficient patients. In the controlled studies on the use of progestogens in women who were habitual aborters and who showed evidence of low endogenous progesterone levels (Sherman and

Garrett, 1963; Goldzieher, 1964), the overall abortion rate was about 20%. The favorable prognosis for women who have had repeated abortions, even where there is low pregnanediol excretion, may (Goldzieher, 1964) also explain why a great variety of gynecological, endocrine, or psychotherapeutic treatments have all achieved the same level of therapeutic "benefit": a salvage rate of approximately 80%.

A point to take into consideration in reviewing reports concerning progestogens in threatened abortion is that a woman who had already aborted two or three times was until recently supposed to be very liable to do so in subsequent pregnancies, and after four abortions she would have a nearly 100% chance of aborting in the fifth pregnancy. However, although women who have had several abortions are very liable to abort in subsequent pregnancies, the risk does not increase with the number of previous abortions. Many of our beliefs about the efficacy of a particular therapeutic regime for abortion were based upon an erroneously high expectation of abortion in the untreated patient. The incidence of a further abortion in women who have had three or more previous abortions (Speert, 1954; Warburton and Fraser, 1959; Goldzieher, 1964; Eastman and Hellman, 1966) is very much lower than the calculated predictions of over 70% (Malpas, 1938; Eastman, 1946), which assume that the population is static and that all the women who have miscarried will continue to conceive. The result of treating habitual abortion should be weighed against a control abortion rate of around 23% (Goldzieher, 1964).

There is not much knowledge concerning the possible metabolic fate of a number of synthetic progestogens administered in early pregnancy. Incubation studies with placental minces and homogenates in the presence of labeled retroprogesterone, dydrogesterone, and progesterone indicate 17α-hydroxylating activity (Van Leusden, 1970a,b). However, the $9\beta,10\alpha$ configuration inhibits 17α-hydroxylation as well as 20α-hydroxylation of retroprogesterone and dydrogesterone. The bulk of progesterone, retroprogesterone, and dydrogesterone appeared not to be metabolized under these experimental conditions. These studies would indicate that if progesterone, retroprogesterone, and dydrogesterone reach the placenta they may exert their biological activity as such. The question what the biological activity of progesterone or of synthetic oral progestogens is, still remains to be answered. Of interest are the observations by Sharp and Wood (1966) showing that dydrogesterone increases the expansile properties of the nonpregnant human uterus.

Summarizing, ovariectomy in early pregnancy, even before day 49, does not necessarily result in abortion; abortion does not necessarily result after ovariectomy even if there is a fall of pregnanediol excretion.

There are indications that the functional life-span of the corpus luteum of pregnancy is completed at about 10 weeks. More studies are needed to evaluate the contribution of the corpus luteum and of the feto-placental unit to progesterone formation in the different stages of early human gestation. There is often, but certainly not always, a correlation between low pregnanediol excretion and poor outcome in threatened abortion. However, as normal pregnanediol excretion is not always correlated with a favorable outcome, correlation of low pregnanediol excretion and poor prognosis does not point to a causal relationship. More commonly the reason for abortion is a defect of the germ plasm, but there might be occasional instances where progesterone deficiency is the basic cause of an abortion. In this light it can be understood that double-blind clinical trials have failed to confirm the value of progesterone treatment in threatened abortion. The metabolic fate of synthetic progestogens in human trophoblast is incompletely known.

2. Hydatidiform. Mole Pregnancy

a. Excretion or Tissue Content of Progesterone, Pregnanediol, and Pregnanetriol. Increased excretion of pregnanediol has been established in molar pregnancy by Payne (1941), Hinglais and Hinglais (1949), Lajos and Szontagh (1950), Erb et al. (1961), and Frandsen and Stakemann (1964b,c). Coutts et al. (1968), Van Leusden and Siemerink (1969), and Acevedo et al. (1970) have reported an increased excretion of pregnanetriol by patients with hydatidiform mole. MacNaughton (1965) found that pregnanediol excretion was frequently but not invariably low. J. B. Brown et al. (1970a,b) found low and normal pregnanediol excretion in hydatidiform mole pregnancy. After evacuation of the mole in 4 patients there was an immediate fall in pregnanediol excretion; in the other 6, the values remained elevated for periods of up to 7 weeks.

Chamberlain et al. (1968) compared the steroids of normal placentas and of three hydatidiform moles. They found lower concentrations of progesterone in the moles than in full-term placentas. They also had lower levels than those reported for normal placentas of equivalent age; these authors give 3000–6000 μg/kg wet weight for 3-month placentas.

It has been shown that conversion of progesterone into pregnanediol in hydatidiform mole is less than in normal pregnancy (MacNaughton and Greig, 1965) (see also Section V, A, 2). In such a study the ratio urinary pregnanediol:pregnanetriol was approximately 2:1 (Coutts et al., 1969), as compared with 20:1 in normal pregnancy (Harkness and Love, 1966). Stitch et al. (1966) found pregnanetriol excretion to remain high in a case of hydatidiform mole after evacuation of the uterus. This would suggest pregnanetriol to be of ovarian origin.

b. Formation of Progesterone, 17α-Hydroxypregnenolone and 17α-Hydroxyprogesterone. Experiments with labeled acetate failed to show incorporation into pregnenolone and progesterone in molar vesicles (Van Leusden and Siemerink, 1969; Van Leusden, 1971). Thus the biosynthesis of 17α-hydroxypregnenolone, 17α-hydroxyprogesterone, and progesterone was investigated in vesicles of hydatidiform moles incubated with [7α-³H]pregnenolone. From a series of incubation experiments with molar trophoblast in the presence of [7α-³H]pregnenolone, radiochemically homogeneous progesterone was isolated (Van Leusden and Siemerink, 1969; Van Leusden, 1971). 17α-Hydroxyprogesterone was obtained in a radiochemically homogeneous form in a number of experiments using [7α-³H]pregnenolone as a precursor. The radiometabolite was incubated with 20β-hydroxysteroid dehydrogenase, subsequently acetylated, and retained the same specific activity. The percentage conversion was 2%. Other experiments with molar throphoblast indicated formation of radiochemically homogeneous [³H]17α-hydroxypregnenolone from [7α-³H]pregnenolone. The radiometabolite retained the same specific activity upon acetylation. The percentage conversion from pregnenolone was 5%.

Coutts *et al.* (1969) and MacNaughton *et al.* (1970) reported that tissue of a mole incubated in the presence of labeled pregnenolone *in vitro* synthesized 17α-hydroxypregnenolone, progesterone, 16α-hydroxyprogesterone, and 16β-hydroxyprogesterone, but no 17α-hydroxyprogesterone. However, from theca lutein cyst fluid 17α-hydroxyprogesterone was recovered. These findings would suggest urinary pregnanetriol to be of ovarian origin. However, a possibly limited contribution to maternal urinary pregnanetriol from 17α-hydroxyprogesterone synthesized in the mole cannot be excluded (Van Leusden, 1971).

In summary, it can be said that failure of incorporation of acetate into pregnenolone and progesterone, and the absence of conversion of mevalonate into steroids, squalene and cholesterol (Van Leusden, 1971), strongly suggest that pregnenolone, 17α-hydroxypregnenolone, and progesterone are not produced *de novo* in the moles. The experimental data provide evidence that 17α-hydroxyprogesterone and progesterone produced in the molar trophoblast *in situ* may contribute to the sometimes considerable amounts of pregnanetriol and pregnanediol excreted by patients with a mole. The quantitative importance of the contribution of ovarian 17α-hydroxyprogesterone to maternal urinary pregnanetriol deserves further experimentation.

3. Choriocarcinoma

In choriocarcinoma an increase of the excretion of pregnanediol has been found by Payne (1941) and Frandsen and Stakemann (1964b).

Huang *et al.* (1969) reported that a pure trophoblastic cell line of human choriocarcinoma grown in tissue culture on incubation with [7α-³H]pregnenolone synthesized progesterone *in vitro*. Tritiated pregnenolone and carbon-labeled DHA incubated with fresh choriocarcinoma yielded radiochemically homogeneous [³H]progesterone, [³H-¹⁴C]androstenedione, [³H-¹⁴C]testosterone, [³H-¹⁴C]estrone, and [³H-¹⁴C]-estradiol (Van Leusden, 1971). Thus, conversion of C_{21} into C_{19} steroids can occur in chorionepithelioma in contrast to molar trophoblast. These findings do not seem to support the hypothesis that choriocarcinoma would arise from molar trophoblast, and they suggest further studies.

It is clear that progesterone produced in choriocarcinoma may contribute to the pregnanediol excreted by patients with chorionepithelioma.

F. ABDOMINAL PREGNANCY

Considerable amounts of pregnanediol are excreted in the urine for several weeks after the termination of an abdominal pregnancy with the placenta left *in situ* (Allen, 1953; Hamersma and Schopman, 1967; Michie *et al.*, 1966; Friedman *et al.*, 1969). Kim *et al.* (1971) determined plasma progesterone after termination with the placenta left *in situ*. Progesterone levels decreased only slightly (-4% per day) from day 1 to day 8 and even less (-2% per day) from day 9 to day 28. The decline from pregnancy levels lasted 9–10 weeks. These findings reflect slowly declining production rather than metabolic clearance of progesterone.

G. CONGENITAL DEFECTS OF THE FETUS AND MULTIPLE PREGNANCY

1. Anencephalic Monsters

Frandsen and Stakemann (1961, 1964a) have observed normal excretion of pregnanediol in pregnancies with anencephalic monsters, in contrast with low excretion of estrogens (Section IV, D).

2. Experimental Ligation of and Naturally Occurring Real Knot in the Umbilical Cord

A considerable contribution of the fetal adrenals to the secretion of progesterone and of pregnenolone or its sulfate seems unlikely in view of the observations of Cassmer (1959) after ligation of the umbilical cord around week 20 of pregnancy. He found a slightly changed excretion of pregnanediol. Kloosterman and Huis in 't Veld (1961) after intrauterine death due to a real knot in the umbilical cord (thus due to a nonplacental cause) found hardly any change of pregnanediol excretion.

3. Multiple Pregnancy

With twins, triplets, and quadruplets the blood progesterone level goes up and up, depending on the number of fetuses (Short, 1969). Progesterone secretion rate in twin pregnancy has been reported to be in the normal range (Pearlman, 1957) or far above the normal range (Bengtsson and Ejarque, 1964).

H. HYPERTENSION, RH ISOIMMUNIZATION, AND CARBOHYDRATE METABOLISM

1. Hypertension

Pregnanediol excretion in preeclamptic toxemia has been reported below the normal range by, e.g., G. Smith and Smith (1948), de Watteville (1951), and Borth (1954), but scatter and overlap with the normal range may be considerable (Kankaanrinta, 1963; Strand, 1966). This overlap exists *a fortiori* in nonsevere toxemia as compared with normal pregnancy.

Aubry and Nesbitt (1970) in "chronic hypertension in pregnancy" (defined as 140/90 or greater either prior to the pregnancy or prior to week 24 of the pregnancy under study) divided this group into severe (BP > 180/110) versus mild (BP 140–180/90–110) hypertension. If the outcome was normal they observed a trend to lower excretion of pregnanediol in the severe hypertensive group, but this was not so striking as in the case of estriol excretion. Three subjects with intrauterine fetal death had values below the normal range just prior to fetal death. Three hypertensive diabetics with intrauterine fetal death had values within the normal range. Impending fetal death (Coyle *et al.*, 1962) is certainly not always preceded by lowered pregnanediol excretion. No correlation with fetal prognosis was found by Trolle (1955a,b) and Van der Molen and Hart (1961). Acevedo *et al.* (1968) assume that the simultaneous determination of urinary pregnanolone and pregnanediol represents an index of the progestational activity of the placenta (or the corpus luteum of pregnancy in the early stages of gestation). Total estrogens and pregnanetriol would constitute an index of the status of the fetal compartment of the fetoplacental unit provided adrenal differentiation has taken place. Based on a small number of patients they thus found suggestive evidence that the alteration in the fetal compartment is secondary to placental impairment in toxemia of pregnancy. In severe toxemia, pregnanediol excretion may become on the whole about 50% of the normal value (Kankaanrinta, 1963); however, this author also reported that the large variation coefficient of pregnanediol excretion in normal pregnancy is even larger in severe toxemia (coefficient of variation 32%). PSR (Solomon *et al.*, 1964) in nonsevere toxemia is somewhat higher than the mean values established for normal pregnancy of the same duration. Values of PSR in severe toxemia were nearly all lower than in normal pregnancy of the same duration. In hypertension with normal birth weight and in retarded fetal growth with or without hypertension, PSR and placental weight were not correlated, whereas PSR and fetal weight were correlated (Henssen, 1969). Because of the wide scatter, it can be concluded that the practical usefulness of determination of pregnanediol excretion in toxemia of pregnancy is very limited.

2. *Rh Isoimmunization*

The mean urinary pregnanediol excretion in Rh isoimmunization is in the normal range (Klopper and Stephenson, 1966; Samaan *et al.*, 1969). Thus the measurement of pregnanediol excretion offers no help in the management of isosensitized patients. In severe Rh isoimmunization, Schindler and Ratanosopa (1968) found a normal amniotic fluid preg-nanediol concentration unless fetal death had occurred. This is in sharp contrast to the estriol concentration, which was found to be very low or undetectable (Section IV, E, 2).

3. *Carbohydrate Metabolism*

Urinary pregnanediol excretion in the normal range (Southren *et al.*, 1968) or in the upper range of the normal nondiabetic pattern (Samaan *et al.*, 1969; Aubry and Nesbitt, 1970) has been found in pregnant diabetics with a normal outcome of pregnancy. A greater mean placental weight among the diabetic group may be responsible at least in part for the upper normal range values reported by Aubry and Nesbitt (1970). These authors found no warning of impending fetal death in pregnanediol excretion in diabetes and pregnancy. Schindler and Ratanasopa (1968) found normal pregnanediol concentrations in am-niotic fluid in diabetic pregnancy, whereas estriol was low or undetectable. High birth weight and high placental weight in this group of patients are correlated with increased PSR as compared with normal pregnancies of the same duration (Henssen, 1969).

I. FETAL WEIGHT, RETARDED FETAL GROWTH, AND INTRAUTERINE FETAL DEATH

1. *Fetal Weight and Retarded Fetal Growth*

In following patients with retarded fetal growth, serial assays are of crucial importance.

a. In normal pregnancy some investigators have found no correlation of pregnanediol excretion and fetal and placental weight (Kankaanrinta, 1963; Henssen, 1969), whereas Shearman (1959), Van der Molen and Hart (1963), and Brush et al. (1966) found a positive correlation between fetal weight and pregnanediol excretion. Thus, in contrast to estriol in normal pregnancy, there is no unanimity concerning the existence of a correlation of pregnanediol and fetal weight.

b. In retarded fetal growth in the absence of recognizable maternal disease, such as preeclampsia or chronic hypertension, pregnanediol excretion is low (e.g., Henssen, 1969; Brush et al., 1970). Aubry and Nesbitt (1970) observed a tendency to lower values in this group of patients, but to a less striking extent than in the case of estriol; the spread of the values was greater, but the mean excretion showed a tendency to fall in the lower control range beyond 28 weeks.

c. If growth retardation is a result of obstetrical maternal disease, predominantly preeclamptic toxemia, pregnanediol excretion is reported to be correlated with fetal and placental weight (Russell et al., 1957, 1960; Shearman, 1959; Kankaanrinta, 1963; Strand, 1966; Henssen, 1969), except by Dässler (1967). In "uteroplacental insufficiency" (with or without hypertension) pregnanediol levels are reported generally within or just below the normal range (Bell et al., 1967).

PSR in retarded fetal growth, regardless of its cause, is lowered after week 33 as compared with normal pregnancy (Henssen, 1969); PSR and fetal weight are correlated.

Brush et al. (1970) found in incubations carried out with labeled pregnenolone measuring placental progesterone synthesis that the decline in placental progesterone production in patients with retarded fetal growth is due to a decrease in the total mass of functional placental tissue rather than to qualitative changes in the metabolism of pregnenolone.

Thus, pregnanediol excretion is correlated with fetal weight and lowered in retarded fetal growth, whatever the cause of the growth retardation. Owing to the large variability, predictions of fetal size by means of a single urinary pregnanediol determination as a screening test show an appreciable error (Brush et al., 1970). Serial determinations might be of additional help to establish growth retardation. However, large intra-individual variations greatly limit the practical use of such determinations.

2. Intrauterine Death

In view of Cassmer's experiments (1959) after experimental ligation of the umbilical cord, and of the observations of Kloosterman and Huis in 't Veld (1961) after a real knot in the umbilical cord, it is clear that a fall in pregnanediol excretion can hardly be expected to occur very soon after fetal death due to nonplacental causes. Lurie *et al.* (1966) showed that plasma progesterone did not decrease, even in the case of fetal death, until after delivery of the placenta. Thus a normal excretion of pregnanediol does not exclude intrauterine fetal death due to a non-placental cause. However it should be realized that fetal death is mostly the final result of placental insufficiency, correlated with lowered placental and fetal weight and lowered excretion of pregnanediol (Section V, I, 1). PSR revealed low values in intrauterine fetal death with an anencephalic monster (4 weeks dead, 28 weeks pregnancy), toxicosis (2 days dead, 35 weeks pregnancy), 2 unknown causes (28 and 30 weeks, 3 and 2 weeks dead), and one case of "habitual abortion" (16 weeks, 1 week dead) (Solomon *et al.*, 1964). In contrast, one case with fetal death due to Rh isoimmunization (23 weeks, 3 weeks dead) and one case with unknown cause (30 weeks, 2 days dead) had normal PSR.

J. PREMATURITY, ONSET OF LABOR, AND POSTMATURITY

1. *Prematurity*

Lowered excretion of pregnanolone and pregnanediol in the presence of normal excretion of pregnanetriol and total estrogens was described by Acevedo *et al.* (1968) in 3 of 4 patients with prematurity. Aubry and Nesbitt (1970) observed a wider range of values for pregnanediol excretion than for estriol in the same subjects. One third of the values fell below the normal control range. No pattern of prelabor decrease was noted.

2. *Onset of Labor*

A fall of pregnanediol excretion is not found prior to spontaneous labor. In contrast to the observations of Kerr *et al.* (1966) and Sommerville (1969), Csapo *et al.* (1971) found a slight decrease of plasma progesterone with the onset of clinical labor.

Short (1969) (Section V, G, 3) reported that in women with twins, triplets, and quadruplets the blood progesterone level goes up and up, depending on the number of fetuses. Yet the gestation length tends to be shorter and shorter. Short (1969) suggests that the total mass of adrenal tissue might dictate the length of gestation, and that the total fetal volume may not be as important as Turnbull and Anderson (1969) believe.

3. *Postmaturity*

The curve of pregnanediol excretion flattens off in the last 2 weeks of pregnancy and continues to decline after term (Strand, 1966).

K. SUMMARY

There seems to be a parallelism between pregnanetriol and total estrogen excretion on the one hand, and pregnanolone and pregnanediol on the other hand, in normal and pathological pregnancy. The fetal compartment of the fetoplacental unit is the main source of urinary pregnanetriol. The percentage of conversion progesterone into pregnanediol in pregnancy is the same or somewhat higher than in the nonpregnant state. The percentage of conversion probably depends on the stage of gestation, and changes in pathological pregnancy. Because of the coefficient of variation between successive 24-hour urine samples from the same subject, the correction of the quantity of urinary pregnanediol for the amount of endogenously produced progesterone is difficult. The varying amount of fecal (and skin?) excretion of metabolites of progesterone may interfere. Some contribution of the fetal compartment to urinary pregnanediol cannot be excluded.

Maternal adrenal progesterone and pregnenolone secretion during pregnancy is the same as in the nonpregnant individual. Whereas a contribution from the fetal compartment to urinary pregnanediol cannot be excluded, there does not seem to be a major contribution by the fetal adrenal to urinary pregnanediol.

The PSR in pathological pregnancy is complex because of additional compartments (fetus, placenta, amniotic fluid) with selective permeability. Passage of progesterone from the maternal compartment to the fetus would seem to be in the order of magnitude of less than 3–4 mg per day. Based on the fact that the progesterone concentration in the umbilical vein is much higher than in the umbilical arteries, it could be calculated that the fetus would convert approximately 80 mg of progesterone per day into other steroids. In using Pearlman's method for the assessment of PSR during pregnancy the "consumption" by the fetus is not taken into account.

The applicability of the progesterone-block theory to the human species is controversial. Ovariectomy in early pregnancy even before day 49 does not necessarily result in abortion, and abortion does not necessarily result after ovariectomy even if there is a fall in pregnanediol excretion.

In term human pregnancy, large doses of progesterone are without any significant effect on uterine activity. Some authors report a slight decrease of plasma progesterone with the onset of clinical labor. There are indications that the functional life-span of the corpus luteum of pregnancy is completed at about 10 weeks. More studies are needed to evaluate the contribution of the corpus luteum and of the fetoplacental unit to progesterone formation at the different stages of early human gestation. There is often, but certainly not always, a correlation between low pregnanediol excretion and poor outcome in threatened abortion. However, as normal pregnanediol excretion is not always correlated with a favorable outcome, correlation of low pregnanediol excretion and poor prognosis does not point to a causal relationship. Thus it can be understood that double-blind clinical trials have failed to confirm the value of "progesterone" treatment in threatened abortion. The metabolic fate of synthetic progestogens is often unknown.

In hydatidiform mole pregnancy excretion of pregnanediol and of pregnanetriol may be increased. Incubation experiments with molar trophoblast failed to show incorporation of acetate into pregnenolone and progesterone. Also, the absence of conversion of mevalonate into sterols, squalene, and cholesterol strongly suggests that pregnenolone, 17α-hydroxypregnenolone and progesterone are not produced *de novo* from acetate in the moles. 17α-Hydroxyprogesterone and progesterone produced in the molar trophoblast *in situ* from pregnenolone and possibly from cholesterol may contribute to the sometimes considerable amounts of pregnanetriol and pregnanediol excreted by patients with mole. The quantitative contribution of ovarian 17α-hydroxyprogesterone to maternal urinary pregnanetriol deserves further experimentation. Choriocarcinoma grown in tissue culture or as such can convert pregnenolone into progesterone *in vitro*, and this progesterone may contribute to the pregnanediol excreted by patients with chorionepithelioma.

Considerable amounts of pregnanediol are excreted following the termination of an abdominal pregnancy with the placenta left *in situ*. These findings reflect slowly declining production.

In anencephalic monsters pregnanediol excretion is in the normal range, in contrast to estriol excretion. Experimental or naturally occurring ligation of the umbilical cord causes hardly any change in pregnanediol excretion in contrast to estrogen excretion. Multiple pregnancy is associated with higher blood progesterone than is normal pregnancy. PSR is in the normal or above normal range.

In toxemia of pregnancy the alterations in the fetal compartment are secondary to placental impairment. Pregnanediol excretion may be below or within the normal range. Owing to the wide intra-individual scatter it can be understood that the practical usefulness of the measurement of pregnanediol excretion in toxemia of pregnancy is very limited.

PSR in severe toxemia is lowered as compared to that in normal pregnancy. The urinary excretion and amniotic fluid concentration of pregnanediol in Rh isoimmunization are in the normal range.

Urinary pregnanediol in the normal or in the upper normal range and normal amniotic fluid pregnanediol concentration have been observed in pregnant diabetics. Pregnanediol excretion gives no warning of impending fetal death. The PSR is increased, correlated with high birth weight and high placental weight in this group of patients.

In retarded fetal growth in the absence or in the presence of recognizable maternal disease, pregnanediol excretion is reported to be low (with a large coefficient of variation of successive 24-hour urine samples), and to be correlated with fetal and placental weights. The decline of placental progesterone production as followed by pregnanediol excretion seems to be due to a decrease in the total mass of functional placental tissue rather than to qualitative changes in the metabolism of pregnenolone. Serial determinations of pregnanediol might be of additional help in establishing growth retardation. However, large intra-individual variations limit their practical use. PSR in intrauterine fetal death is often, but not always, low.

In intrauterine fetal death due to nonplacental causes, pregnanediol excretion does not show any rapid changes. Mostly, however, fetal death is due to placental insufficiency, correlated with low placental and fetal weight and lowered excretion of pregnanediol.

In prematurity, urinary pregnanolone and pregnanediol excretion may be low. Pregnanediol excretion is not lowered prior to spontaneous labor. Some, but not all, investigators have reported a slight decrease of plasma progesterone with the onset of clinical labor. After term the curve of pregnanediol excretion, flattening off in the last 2 weeks of pregnancy, continues to decline.

VI. Concluding Remarks

From the evidence presented in this review, it may be concluded that there are definite hormonal changes in pathological pregnancy. Excretion, plasma, placental tissue and amniotic fluid content, umbilical arterial and venous blood concentrations, and the secretion rates of several hormones are altered in pathological pregnancy. In addition, the data obtained from dynamic tests, experiments of nature, such as hydatidiform mole pregnancy and anencephalic monsters, and incubation experiments point to changing production, metabolism, and excretion of hormones in pathological pregnancy. However, much of this work does not have immediate clinical implication. The practical usefulness of determinations of HCG, HPL, estrogens, and pregnanediol is limited by inter- and intra-individual variability. The causes of this variability should be studied, because in this way control mechanisms might be elucidated.

Despite its variability, HCG determinations by measuring trophoblastic growth are of considerable prognostic value in threatened abortion and are useful to diagnose hydatidiform mole pregnancy. Moreover, HCG determinations have become indispensable in measuring chemotherapeutic effects in the treatment of choriocarcinoma.

Information concerning HPL has been rather limited. Similarly to HCG, HPL is of prognostic significance in threatened abortion. However, the paradoxical behavior of HPL and HCG in trophoblastic tumors is intriguing and requires elucidation.

If one compartment of the fetoplacental unit is lacking or is experimentally or naturally put out of function, formation of estriol is more vulnerable than formation of estrone and estradiol within the fetoplacental unit. Isolated disturbances within the fetoplacental unit bring about specific changes of estriol excretion. However, the reverse, changed estriol excretion pointing to specific disturbances within the fetoplacental unit, hardly ever occurs. Lowered estriol excretion is mostly caused by generalized disturbances in the fetus and the placenta. There is hardly ever dissociation of pathology of the fetus and the placenta. This and the large inter- and intra-individual variability of estriol excretion limit the practical usefulness of estriol determinations.

Even continuous low excretion of estrogens and pregnanediol in late pregnancy should be regarded critically; such values do not always necessitate the termination of pregnancy. Excretion of pregnanediol can be regarded as a placental function test, and is fundamental: a too low excretion of pregnanediol indicates that estrogen excretion also is lowered.

From the evidence presented, it becomes clear that in all kinds of pathological pregnancy resulting in reduced fetoplacental mass, the excretion of estrogens and of pregnanediol is lowered, whereas if the fetoplacental mass is increased, estrogen and pregnanediol excretion may be high, even to such an extent that a deteriorating clinical condition of the fetus may be masked. It is concluded that serial hormone determinations in pathological pregnancy are of additional help in the clinical management of individual cases. However, clinical judgment should never be based on hormone determinations alone.

Acknowledgments

The author wishes to express his gratitude to Professor Egon Diczfalusy for the time and effort he has taken to review the manuscript and to Professor L. A. M. Stolte for critical remarks.

Part of the expense of investigations reported was defrayed by Stichting voor Fundamenteel Geneeskundig Onderzoek (Fungo), den Haag.

REFERENCES

Abdul Enein, M. A., and Sharman, A. (1967). *J. Obstet. Gynaecol. Brit. Commonw.* **74**, 583.

Abramovich, D. R. (1969). *Med. J. Austr.* **2**, 408.

Acevedo, H. F., Strickler, H. S., Gilmore, J., Vela, B. A., Campbell, M. T., and Arras, B. J. (1968). *Amer. J. Obstet. Gynecol.* **102**, 867.

Acevedo, H. F., Vela, B. A., Campbell, E. A., Strickler, H. S., Gilmore, J., Moraca, J. I., and Arras, B. J. (1969). *Amer. J. Obstet. Gynecol.* **104**, 964.

Acevedo, H. F., Vela, B. A., Campbell, E. A., Gilmore, J., Strickler, H. S., Merkow, L. P., Hayeslip, D. W., Maydak, J. J., and Ferraro, R. J. (1970). *Obstet. Gynecol.* **35**, 857.

Adlercreutz, H., and Luukkainen, T. (1970). *Ann. Clin. Res.* **2**, 365.

Akasu, F., Kuwabara, S., Iwakami, T., and Sumitani, J. (1969). *Endocrinol. Jap.* **16**, 205.

Alder, R. M., and Krieger, V. I. (1957). *Med. J. Aust.* **2**, 122.

Aleem, F. A., Neill, D. W., and Pinkerton, J. H. M. (1969a). *Steroids* **13**, 651.

Aleem, F. A., Pinkerton, J. H., and Neill, D. W. (1969b). *J. Obstet. Gynaecol. Brit. Commonw.* **76**, 200.

Allan, H., and Dodds, E. C. (1935). *Biochem. J.* **29**, 285.

Allen, W. M. (1953). In discussion of A. B. Hunt and W. M. McConahey, *Amer. J. Obstet. Gynecol.* **66**, 970.

Allen, W. M., and Corner, G. W. (1929). *Amer. J. Physiol.* **88**, 340.

Amati, G. (1928). *Zentralbl. Gynaekol.* **52**, 2639.

Anderson, A. B. M., Laurence, K. M., and Turnbull, A. C. (1969). *J. Obstet. Gynaecol. Brit. Commonw.* **76**, 196.

Angevine, D. M. (1938). *Arch. Pathol.* **26**, 507.

Aoba, H. (1966). *Tohoku J. Exp. Med.* **89**, 121.

Aubry, R. H., and Nesbitt, F. (1970). *Amer. J. Obstet. Gynecol.* **107**, 48.

Badarau, L. (1966). *Amer. J. Obstet. Gynecol.* **96**, 323.

Bagshawe, K. D., Golding, P. R., and Orr, A. H. (1969). *Brit. Med. J.* **3**, 733.

Baker, W. S., Bancroft, C. E., Lyda, E. W., and Lehman, J. J. (1955). *Amer. J. Obstet. Gynecol.* **69**, 405.

Banerjea, S. K. (1962). *J. Obstet. Gynaecol. Brit. Commonw.* **69**, 963.

Banks, A. L., Rutherford, R. N., and Coburn, W. A. (1964). *Fert. Steril.* **15**, 94.

Barlow, J. J., Goldstein, D. P., and Reid, D. E. (1967). *J. Clin. Endocrinol. Metab.* **27**, 1028.

Baulieu, E. E., Bricaire, H., and Jayle, M. F. (1956). *J. Clin. Endocrinol. Metab.* **16**, 690.

Baumgarten, K. (1966). *Wien. Klin. Wochenschr.* **78**, 141.

Beard, R. W., Morris, E. D., and Clayton, S. G. (1966). *J. Obstet. Gynaecol. Brit. Commonw.* **73**, 562.

Beck, P., and Daughaday, W. H. (1967). *J. Clin. Invest.* **46**, 103.

Beck, P., Parker, M. L., and Daughaday, W. H. (1965). *Clin. Res.* **13**, 318.

Behrman, S. J., and Niemann, P. (1955a). *Fert. Steril.* **6**, 263.

Behrman, S. J., and Niemann, P. (1955b). *Fert. Steril.* **6**, 415.

Beischer, N. A., Brown, J. B., MacLeod, S. C., and Smith, M. A. (1967). *J. Obstet. Gynaecol. Brit. Commonw.* **74**, 51.

Beischer, N. A., Townsend, L., Holsman, M., Brown, J. B., and Smith, M. A. (1968a). *Amer. J. Obstet. Gynecol.* **102**, 819.

Beischer, N. A., Bhargava, V. L., Brown, J. B., and Smith, M. A. (1968b). *J. Obstet. Gynaecol. Brit. Commonw.* **75**, 1024.

Beischer, N. A., Brown, J. B., and Smith, M. A. (1968c). *J. Obstet. Gynaecol. Brit. Commonw.* **75**, 622.

Beischer, N. A., Brown, J. B., Smith, M. A., and Townsend, L. (1969). *Amer. J. Obstet. Gynecol.* **103**, 483.

Beischer, N. A., Bettinger, H. F., Fortune, D. W., and Pepperell, R. (1970). *J. Obstet. Gynaecol. Brit. Commonw.* **77**, 263.

Beling, C. G. (1963). *Acta Endocrinol. (Copenhagen), Suppl.* **79**, 1.

Beling, C. G. (1967). *Advan. Obstet. Gynecol.* **1**, 88–102.

Bell, E. T., Loraine, J. A., McEwan, H. P., and Charles, D. (1967). *Amer. J. Obstet. Gynecol.* **97**, 562.

Bengtsson, L. P., and Ejarque, P. M. (1964). *Acta Obstet. Gynecol. Scand.* **43**, 49.

Bengtsson, L. P., and Forsgren, B. (1966). *Acta Obstet. Gynecol. Scand.* **45**, 155.

Bengtsson, L. P., and Schofield, B. M. (1963). *J. Reprod. Fert.* **5**, 423.

Berle, P. (1969). *Acta Endocrinol. (Copenhagen)* **61**, 369.

Berle, P., and Schultze-Mosgau, H. (1967). *Zentralbl. Gynaekol.* **89**, 771.

Berle, P., and Schultze-Mosgau, H. (1968). *Acta Endocrinol. (Copenhagen)* **58**, 339.

Berman, A. M., Kalchman, G. G., Chattoraj, S. C., Scommegna, A., and Petropoulou, M. (1968). *Amer. J. Obstet. Gynecol.* **100**, 15.

Bjerre, S., Gold, C. C., Wilson, R., and Doran, T. A. (1968). *Amer. J. Obstet. Gynecol.* **102**, 275.

Bolté, E., Mancuso, S., Eriksson, G., Wiqvist, N., and Diczfalusy, E. (1964a). *Acta Endocrinol. (Copenhagen)* **45**, 535.

Bolté, E., Mancuso, S., Eriksson, G., Wiqvist, N., and Diczfalusy, E. (1964b). *Acta Endocrinol. (Copenhagen)* **45**, 560.

Bolté, E., Mancuso, S., Eriksson, G., Wiqvist, N., and Diczfalusy, E. (1964c). *Acta Endocrinol. (Copenhagen)* **45**, 576.

Bonanno, P., Patti, A. A., Frawley, T. F., and Stein, A. A. (1963). *Amer. J. Obstet. Gynecol.* **87**, 210.

Booth, R. T., Stern, M., Wood, C., Sharples, M. J., and Pinkerton, J. H. (1964). *J. Obstet. Gynaecol. Brit. Commonw.* **71**, 266.

Booth, R. T., Stern, M. I., Wood, C., Sharples, M. J., and Pinkerton, J. H. (1965). *J. Obstet. Gynaecol. Brit. Commonw.* **72**, 229.

Borth, R. (1954). *Gynecol. Obstet.* **53**, 27.

Borth, R. (1960). *In* "Symposion on Prenatal Care," p. 57. Noordhof, Groningen.

Borth, R., Lunenfeld, B., Stamm, O., and de Watteville, H. (1959). *Acta Obstet. Gynecol. Scand.* **38**, 417.

Borth, R., Kim, M. H., McCleary, P., Woolever, C. A., and Young, P. C. M. (1971). *Acta Endocrinol. (Copenhagen), Suppl.* **155**, 133.

Bradbury, J. T., and Goplerud, C. P. (1963). *Obstet. Gynecol.* **21**, 330.

Breborowicz, H., Krzywinska, F., and Pisarski, T. (1965). *Amer. J. Obstet. Gynecol.* **91**, 1107.

Breborowicz, H., Baraniecka, K., Biniszkiewicz, W., and Breborowicz, A. (1969). *Endokrynol. Pol.* **20**, 109.

Brewer, J. J., Gerbie, A. B., Dolkart, R. E., Skom, J. H., Nagle, R. G., and Torok, E. E. (1964). *Amer. J. Obstet. Gynecol.* **90**, 566.

Brody, S. (1969a). *In* "Foetus and Placenta" (A. Klopper and E. Diczfalusy, eds.), pp. 299–412, Blackwell, Oxford.

Brody, S. (1969b). *Acta Endocrinol. (Copenhagen), Suppl.* **142**, 113.

Brody, S., and Carlström, G. (1960). *Lancet* **2**, 99.

Brody, S., and Carlström, G. (1962a). *J. Clin. Endocrinol. Metab.* **22**, 564.

Brody, S., and Carlström, G. (1962b). *Acta Endocrinol. (Copenhagen), Suppl.* **67**, 19.
Brody, S., and Carlström, G. (1962c). *Ciba Found. Colloq. Endocrinol.* [*Proc.*] **14**, 329.
Brody, S., and Carlström, G. (1965a). *Acta Obstet. Gynecol. Scand.* **44**, 32.
Brody, S., and Carlström, G. (1965b). *J. Clin. Endocrinol. Metab.* **25**, 792.
Brown, C. H., Saffan, B. D., Howard, C., and Preedy, J. R. (1964). *J. Clin. Invest.* **43**, 295.
Brown, J. B. (1955). *Biochem. J.* **60**, 185.
Brown, J. B. (1960). *Advan. Clin. Chem.* **3**, 157.
Brown, J. B., Bulbrook, R. D., and Greenwood, F. C. (1957). *J. Clin. Endocrinol. Metab.* **16**, 49.
Brown, J. B., MacLeod, S. C., Beischer, N. A., and Smith, M. A. (1967). *Aust. N. Z. J. Obstet. Gynaecol.* **7**, 25.
Brown, J. B., Beischer, N. A., and Smith, M. A. (1968). *J. Obstet. Gynaecol. Brit. Commonw.* **75**, 819.
Brown, J. B., Beischer, N. A., Campbell, D. G., Evans, J. H., and Townsend, L. (1970a). *Proc. Roy. Soc. Med.* **63**, 1092.
Brown, J. B., Evans, J. H., Beischer, N. A., Campbell, D. G., and Fortune, D. W. (1970b). *J. Obstet. Gynaecol. Brit. Commonw.* **77**, 690.
Browne, J. S. L., Henry, J. S., and Venning, E. H. (1937). *J. Clin. Invest.* **16**, 678.
Brush, M. G., Taylor, R. W., and Maxwell, R. (1966). *J. Obstet. Gynaecol. Brit. Commonw.* **73**, 954.
Brush, M. G., Maxwell, R., Scherer, J., Taylor, R. W., and Tye, G. (1970). *Proc. Roy. Soc. Med.* **63**, 1098.
Burton, E. R., and Wachtel, E. G. (1967). *J. Obstet. Gynaecol. Brit. Commonw.* **74**, 533.
Cameron, E. H. D., and Griffiths, K. (1968). *J. Endocrinol.* **41**, 327.
Campbell, D. G., Brown, J. B., Fortune, D. W., Pepperell, R., and Beischer, N. A. (1970). *J. Obstet. Gynaecol. Brit. Commonw.* **77**, 410.
Carlsson, M. G. (1964). *Acta Endocrinol. (Copenhagen)* **46**, 142.
Carpenter, C. W. (1970). *Amer. J. Obstet. Gynecol.* **107**, 69.
Cassmer, O. (1959). *Acta Endocrinol. (Copenhagen), Suppl.* **45**, 1.
Castrén, O., Hirvonen, L., Närvänen, S., and Soiva, K. (1962). *Acta Endocrinol. (Copenhagen)* **39**, 506.
Cathro, D. M., Bertrand, J., and Coyle, M. G. (1969a). *Lancet* **1**, 732.
Cathro, D. M., Bertrand, J., and Coyle, M. G. (1969b). *Lancet* **1**, 1099.
Chamberlain, J., Morris, N. F., and Smith, N. C. (1968). *J. Endocrinol.* **41**, 289.
Chang, E., Slaunwhite, W. R., and Sandberg, A. A. (1960). *J. Clin. Endocrinol. Metab.* **20**, 1568.
Cohen, M., Haour, F., Bertrand, J., and Dumont, M. (1970). *Gynecol. Obstet.* **69**, 197.
Cohen, S. (1966). *J. Clin. Endocrinol. Metab.* **26**, 994.
Cole, H. S., Bilder, J. H., Camerini-Davalos, R. A., and Grimaldi, R. D. (1970). *Pediatrics* **45**, 394.
Connon, A. F. (1966). *Austr. N. Z. J. Obstet. Gynaecol.* **6**, 248.
Conrad, S. H., Pion, R. J., and Kitchin, J. D. (1967). *J. Clin. Endocrinol. Metab.* **27**, 114.
Courey, N. G., Stull, R. L., Fisher, B. N., Stull, C. G., and Lundstrom, P. (1969). *Obstet. Gynecol.* **34**, 523.

Courey, N. G., Stull, R. L., Fisher, B., Stull, C. G., and Lundstrom, P. (1970). *Obstet. Gynecol.* **35**, 178.

Coutts, J. R. T., and MacNaughton, M. C. (1971). *Acta Endocrinol. (Copenhagen), Suppl.* **155**, 136.

Coutts, J. R. T., MacNaughton, M. C., and Ross, P. E. (1968). *J. Endocrinol.* **43**, XXVII.

Coutts, J. R. T., MacNaughton, M. C., Ross, P. E., and Walker, J. (1969). *J. Endocrinol.* **44**, 335.

Coyle, M. G., and Brown, J. B. (1963). *J. Obstet. Gynaecol. Brit. Commonw.* **70**, 225.

Coyle, M. G., Mitchell, F. L., and Russell, C. S. (1956). *J. Obstet. Gynaecol. Brit. Emp.* **63**, 560.

Coyle, M. G., Greig, M., and Walker, J. (1962). *Lancet* **2**, 275.

Cramer, D. W., Beck, P., and Makowski, E. L. (1971). *Amer. J. Obstet. Gynecol.* **109**, 649.

Csapo, A. (1956). *Amer. J. Anat.* **98**, 273.

Csapo, A. (1966). *Bibl. Gynaecol.* **42**, 93.

Csapo, A. (1969a). *Ciba Found. Study Group* [Pap.] **34**, 13–55.

Csapo, A. (1969b). *Postgrad. Med. J.* **45**, 57.

Csapo, A., de Sousa-Filho, M. B., de Souza, J. C., and de Sousa, O. (1966). *Fert. Steril.* **17**, 621.

Csapo, A., Knobil, E., Sommerville, I. F., van der Molen, H. J., and Wiest, W. G. (1969). As cited by Csapo (1969a).

Csapo, A., Knobil, E., van der Molen, H. J., and Wiest, W. G. (1971). *Amer. J. Obstet. Gynecol.* **110**, 630.

Cummings, R. V., Rourke, J. E., and Shelley, T. F. (1969). *Amer. J. Obstet. Gynecol.* **104**, 1047.

Currie, A. R., Beck, J. S., Ellis, S. T., and Read, C. H. (1966). *J. Pathol. Bacteriol.* **92**, 395.

Daenen, M. (1965). *Bull. Soc. Roy. Belge Gynecol. Obstet.* **35**, 385.

Daniëlsson, M. (1965). *Amer. J. Obstet. Gynecol.* **91**, 895.

Dässler, C. G. (1966). *Acta Endocrinol. (Copenhagen)* **53**, 401.

Dässler, C. G. (1967). *Acta Endocrinol. (Copenhagen)* **56**, 333.

Davis, M. E., and Fugo, N. W. (1947). *Proc. Soc. Exp. Biol. Med.* **65**, 283.

Davis, M. E., and Plotz, E. J. (1958). *Amer. J. Obstet. Gynecol.* **76**, 939.

Davis, M. E., Plotz, E. J., Lupu, C. I., and Ejarque, P. M. (1960). *Fert. Steril.* **11**, 18.

dela Torre, B., Johannisson, E., and Diczfalusy, E. (1970). *Acta Obstet. Gynecol. Scand.* **49**, 165.

Delfs, E. (1957). *Obstet. Gynecol.* **9**, 1.

Delfs, E. (1959). *Ann. N. Y. Acad. Sci.* **80**, 125.

Delfs, E., and Jones, G. E. S. (1948). *Obstet. Gynecol. Surv.* **3**, 680.

Dellepiane, G., and Andreoli, C. (1961). *Gynecol. Prat.* **12**, 231.

de Watteville, H. (1951). *J. Clin. Endocrinol. Metab.* **11**, 251.

Dickey, R. P. (1969). *Amer. J. Obstet. Gynecol.* **104**, 68.

Dickey, R. P., and Robertson, A. F. (1969). *Amer. J. Obstet. Gynecol.* **104**, 551.

Dickey, R. P., Cortes, W. T., Besch, P. K., and Ullery, J. C. (1966). *Amer. J. Obstet. Gynecol.* **96**, 127.

Dickey, R. P., Besch, P. K., and Ullery, J. C. (1968). *Amer. J. Obstet. Gynecol.* **102**, 222.

Diczfalusy, E. (1964). *Fed. Proc., Fed. Amer. Soc. Exp. Biol.* **23**, 791.

Diczfalusy, E., and Borell, U. (1961). *J. Clin. Endocrinol. Metab.* **21**, 119.

Diczfalusy, E., and Mancuso, S. (1969). *In* "Foetus and Placenta" (A. Klopper and E. Diczfalusy, eds.), pp. 191–249. Blackwell, Oxford.

Diczfalusy, E., and Troen, P. (1961). *Vitam. Horm. (New York)* **19**, 229.

Diczfalusy, E., Nilsson, L., and Westman, A. (1958). *Acta Endocrinol. (Copenhagen)* **28**, 137.

Diczfalusy, E., Cassmer, O., Alonso, C., and de Miguel, M. (1961). *Recent Progr. Horm. Res.* **17**, 147.

Dito, W. R., and Shelly, J. (1969). *Amer. J. Clin. Pathol.* **51**, 177.

Dominguez, J. M., Cottini, E. P., and Fabregat, A. N. (1965). *Excerpta Med. Found. Int. Congr. Ser.* **99**, 72.

Dony, J., Siemerink, M., and Van Leusden, H. A. (1971). *Acta Endocrinol. (Copenhagen), Suppl.* **155**, 131.

Driscoll, A. M. (1969). *Brit. Med. J.* **1**, 556.

Duhring, J. L., and Greene, J. W. (1966). *Clin. Obstet. Gynecol.* **9**, 935.

Easterling, W. E., and Talbert, L. M. (1970). *Amer. J. Obstet. Gynecol.* **107**, 417.

Eastman, N. J. (1946). *In* "Progress in Gynecology" (J. V. Meigs and S. H. Sturgis, eds.), p. 262. Grune & Stratton, New York.

Eastman, N. J., and Hellman, L. M. (1966). "William's Obstetrics," 13th ed., p. 518. Appleton, New York.

Eberlein, W. R. (1965). *J. Clin. Endocrinol.* **25**, 1101.

Eberlein, W. R., Bongiovanni, A. M., and Francis, C. M. (1958). *J. Clin. Endocrinol. Metab.* **18**, 1274.

Echt, C. R., and Cohen, L. (1970). *Amer. J. Obstet. Gynecol.* **107**, 947.

Ehnholm, C., Seppälä, M., Tallberg, T., and Widholm, O. (1967). *Ann. Med. Exp. Biol. Fenn.* **45**, 318.

Ehrhardt, K. (1931). *Med. Klin. (Munich)* **27**, 426.

Eik-Nes, K. B., and Hall, P. F. (1965). *Vitam. Horm. (New York)* **23**, 153.

Elliott, P. M. (1970). *Austr. N. Z. J. Obstet. Gynaecol.* **10**, 18.

El Tomi, A. E. F., Crystle, C. D., and Stevens, V. C. (1971). *Amer. J. Obstet. Gynecol.* **109**, 74.

Eraz, J., and Hausknecht, R. (1969). *Amer. J. Obstet. Gynecol.* **104**, 924.

Erb, H., Keller, M., Hauser, G. A., and Wenner, R. (1961). *Gynaecologia* **152**, 317.

Fishman, J., Brown, J. B., Hellman, L., Zumoff, B., and Gallagher, T. F. (1962). *J. Biol. Chem.* **237**, 1489.

Fliegner, J. R. H., Renou, P., Wood, C., Beischer, N. A., and Brown, J. B. (1969). *Amer. J. Obstet. Gynecol.* **105**, 252.

Fotherby, K. (1970). *Proc. Roy. Soc. Med.* **63**, 1091.

Fotherby, K., James, F., and Kamyab, S. (1965). *J. Endocrinol.* **33**, 133.

Frandsen, V. A. (1963). "The Excretion of Oestriol in Normal Human Pregnancy." Munksgaard, Copenhagen.

Frandsen, V. A. (1965). *In* "Estrogen Assays in Clinical Medicine" (C. A. Paulsen, ed.), pp. 234–238. Univ. of Washington Press, Seattle.

Frandsen, V. A., and Stakemann, G. (1960). *Dan. Med. Bull.* **7**, 95.

Frandsen, V. A., and Stakemann, G. (1961). *Acta Endocrinol. (Copenhagen)* **38**, 383.

Frandsen, V. A., and Stakemann, G. (1963a). *Acta Endocrinol. (Copenhagen)* **44**, 183.

Frandsen, V. A., and Stakemann, G. (1963b). *Acta Endocrinol. (Copenhagen)* **43**, 184.

Frandsen, V. A., and Stakemann, G. (1964a). *Acta Endocrinol. (Copenhagen)* **47**, 265.

Frandsen, V. A., and Stakemann, G. (1964b). *Acta Endocrinol. (Copenhagen)*, *Suppl.* **90**, 81.

Frandsen, V. A., and Stakemann, G. (1964c). *Acta Endocrinol. (Copenhagen)*, *Suppl.* **90**, 45.

Frandsen, V. A., and Stakemann, G. (1966). *Acta Endocrinol. (Copenhagen)* **53**, 93.

Frandsen, V. A., Pedersen, J., and Stakemann, G. (1962). *Acta Endocrinol. (Copenhagen)* **40**, 40.

Frantz, A. G., Rabkin, M. T., and Friesen, H. (1965). *J. Clin. Endocrinol. Metab.* **25**, 1136.

Friedman, S., Gans, B., Eckerling, B., Goldman, J., Kaufman, H., and Rumny, M. (1969). *J. Obstet. Gynaecol. Brit. Commonw.* **73**, 554.

Fuchs, F. (1962). *Acta Obstet. Gynecol. Scand.* **41**, Suppl. 1, 7.

Fuchs, F., and Olsen, P. (1966). *Ugeskrift Laeger* **128**, 1461.

Fuchs, F., Fuchs, A. R., and Short, R. V. (1963). *J. Endocrinol.* **27**, 333.

Furuhjelm, M. (1953). *Acta Endocrinol. (Copenhagen)* **14**, 353.

Furuhjelm, M. (1962). *Acta Obstet. Gynecol. Scand.* **41**, 370.

Gastineau, C. F., Albert, A., and Randall, L. M. (1949). *J. Clin. Endocrinol. Metab.* **9**, 615.

Genazzani, A. R., Aubert, M. L., Casoli, M., Fioretti, P., and Felber, J. P. (1969). *Lancet* **1**, 1385.

Goebelsman, U., Wiqvist, N., Diczfalusy, E., Levitz, M., Condon, G. P., and Dancis, J. (1966). *Acta Endocrinol. (Copenhagen)* **52**, 550.

Goecke, C. (1969). *Wien. Med. Wochenschr.* **119**, 805.

Goldman, A. S., Yakovac, W. C., and Bongiovanni, A. M. (1966). *J. Clin. Endocrinol. Metab.* **26**, 14.

Goldstein, D. P. (1971). *Amer. J. Obstet. Gynecol.* **110**, 583.

Goldstein, D. P., and Reid, D. E. (1967). *Clin. Obstet. Gynecol.* **10**, 313.

Goldzieher, J. W. (1964). *J. Amer. Med. Ass.* **188**, 651.

Greene, J. W. (1970). *Postgrad. Med.* **47**, 213.

Greene, J. W., and Touchstone, J. C. (1963). *Amer. J. Obstet. Gynecol.* **85**, 1.

Greene, J. W., Smith, K., Kyle, C. G., Touchstone, J. C., and Duhring, J. L. (1965). *Amer. J. Obstet. Gynecol.* **91**, 684.

Greene, J. W., Beargie, R. A., Clark, B. K., and Smith, K. (1969). *Amer. J. Obstet. Gynecol.* **105**, 730.

Greig, M. G., Coyle, M. G., Cooper, W., and Walker, J. (1962). *J. Obstet. Gynaecol. Brit. Commonw.* **69**, 772.

Grumbach, M. M., Kaplan, S. L., Abrams, C. L., Bell, J. J., and Conte, F. A. (1966). *J. Clin. Endocrinol. Metab.* **26**, 478.

Grumbach, M. M., Kaplan, S. L., Sciarra, J., and Burr, I. M. (1968). *Ann. N. Y. Acad. Sci.* **148**, 501.

Guldberg, E. (1936). *Acta Obstet. Gynecol. Scand.* **15**, 345.

Gurpide, E., Angers, M., Van de Wiele, R. L., and Lieberman, S. (1962). *J. Clin. Endocrinol. Metab.* **22**, 935.

Gusdon, J. P. (1969). *Obstet. Gynecol.* **33**, 397.

Guterman, H. S. (1946). *J. Amer. Med. Ass.* **131**, 378.

Guterman, H. S. (1953). *Recent Progr. Horm. Res.* **8**, 293.

Hagen, A. A., Barr, M., and Diczfalusy, E. (1965). *Acta Endocrinol. (Copenhagen)* **49**, 207.

Hamburger, C. (1944). *Acta Obstet. Gynecol. Scand.* **24**, 45.

Hamburger, C. (1958). *Ciba Found. Colloq. Endocrinol.* [*Proc.*] **12**, 190.

Hamersma, K., and Schopman, W. (1967). *Ned. Tijdschr. Verlosk. Gynäecol.* **67**, 26.

Hammerstein, J., and Nevinny-Stickel, J. (1965). *Acta Endocrinol. (Copenhagen)* **48**, 375.

Hansen, H., Nilsson, L., and Zettergren, L. (1963). *Acta Obstet. Gynecol. Scand.* **42**, 117.

Harbert, G. M., McGaughey, H. S., Scoggin, W. A., and Thorton, W. N. (1964). *Obstet. Gynecol.* **23**, 314.

Harkness, R. A., and Love, D. N. (1966). *Acta Endocrinol. (Copenhagen)* **51**, 526.

Harkness, R. A., Menini, E., Charles, D., Kenny, F. M., and Rombaut, R. (1966). *Acta Endocrinol. (Copenhagen)* **52**, 409.

Haskins, A. L. (1967). *Amer. J. Obstet. Gynecol.* **97**, 777.

Haskins, A. L., and Sherman, A. I. (1952). *J. Clin. Endocrinol. Metab.* **12**, 385.

Haskins, A. L., and Soiva, K. U. (1960). *Amer. J. Obstet. Gynecol.* **79**, 674.

Hausknecht, R. U. (1967). *Amer. J. Obstet. Gynecol.* **97**, 1085.

Hausknecht, R. U., and Mandelbaum, N. (1969). *Amer. J. Obstet. Gynecol.* **104**, 433.

Heikkilä, J., and Luukkainen, T. (1971). *Amer. J. Obstet. Gynecol.* **110**, 509.

Helbing. W., Radzuweit, H., and Mlytz, H. (1969). *Deut. Gesundheitsw.* **24**, 969.

Hellema, M. J. C. (1965). *Ned. Tijdschr. Geneesk.* **109**, 163.

Hellema, M. J. C. (1971). *J. Endocrinol.* **49**, 393.

Henssen, S. G. F. (1969). Ph.D. Thesis, Nÿmegen. Crouzen, Maastricht.

Hepp, H. (1967). *Geburtsh. Frauenheilk.* **27**, 990.

Hepp, H., Fettig, O., and Hoshi, J. (1968). *Muenchen. Med. Wochenschr.* **110**, 2128.

Heron, H. J. (1969). *N. Z. Med. J.* **69**, 20.

Hertz, R., Bergenstal, D. M., Lipsett, M. B., Price, E. B., and Hilbish, T. F. (1958). *J. Amer. Med. Ass.* **168**, 845.

Heys, R. F., Scott, J. S., Oakey, R. E., and Stitch, S. R. (1968). *Lancet* **1**, 328.

Heys, R. F., Scott, J. S., Oakey, R. E., and Stitch, S. R. (1969). *Obstet. Gynecol.* **33**, 390.

Hinglais, H., and Hinglais, M. (1949). *C. R. Soc. Biol.* **143**, 61.

Hobkirk, R., and Nilson, M. (1962). *J. Clin. Endocrinol. Metab.* **22**, 142.

Hobkirk, R., Blahey, P. R., Alfheim, A., Raeside, J. I., and Joron, G. E. (1960). *J. Clin. Endocrinol. Metab.* **20**, 805.

Hobkirk, R., Anuman-Rajadhon, Y., Nilsen, M., and Blahey, P. R. (1970). *Clin. Chem.* **16**, 235.

Hobson, B. M. (1955). *J. Obstet. Gynaecol. Brit. Emp.* **62**, 354.

Hobson, B. M. (1958). *J. Obstet. Gynaecol. Brit. Emp.* **65**, 253.

Hobson, B. M., and Wide, L. (1964). *Acta Endocrinol. (Copenhagen)* **46**, 623.

Holmdahl, T. H., Johansson, E. D. B., and Wide, L. (1971). *Acta Endocrinol. (Copenhagen)* **67**, 353.

Holtorff, J., Nitzsche, P., and Schollberg, K. (1968). *Zentralbl. Gynaekol.* **90**, 289.

Hon, E. H., and Morris, J. (1955). *Surg., Gynecol. Obstet.* **101**, 59.

Hon, E. H., and Morris, J. (1956). *J. Clin. Endocrinol. Metab.* **16**, 1354.

Houtzager, H. L. (1968). Ph.D. Thesis, Centrale Drukkerij, Nijmegen.

Houtzager, H. L. (1970). *Ned. Tijdschr. Geneesk.* **114,** 532.

Houtzager, H. L., and Van Leusden, H. A. (1969). *Ned. Tijdschr. Geneesk.* **113,** 1272.

Houtzager, H. L., and Van Leusden, H. A. (1971). *Ned. Tijdschr. Geneesk.* **115,** 65.

Houtzager, H. L., Van Leusden, H. A., and Mastboom, J. L. (1967). *Acta Physiol. Pharmacol. Neer.* **14,** 512.

Houtzager, H. L., Van Leusden, H. A., and Siemerink, M. (1970). *Acta Endocrinol. (Copenhagen)* **46,** 17.

Huang, W. Y., Patillo, R. A., Delfs, E., and Mattingly, R. F. (1969). *Steroids* **14,** 755.

Hughes, H. E., Loraine, J. A., and Bell, E. T. (1964). *Amer. J. Obstet. Gynecol.* **90,** 1297.

Hytten, F. E., and Leitch, I. (1964). "The Physiology of Human Pregnancy," p. 195. Blackwell, Oxford.

Ittrich, G. (1960a). *Zentralbl. Gynaekol.* **82,** 429.

Ittrich, G. (1960b). *Acta Endocrinol. (Copenhagen)* **35,** 34.

Iyengar, L. (1968). *Amer. J. Obstet. Gynecol.* **102,** 834.

Jackson, C. M. (1960). *Amer. J. Anat.* **9,** 119.

Jacobson, B. D. (1965). *Fert. Steril.* **16,** 604.

Jaffe, R. B. (1967). *Proc. Int. Congr. Horm. Steroids, 2nd, 1966* Int. Congr. Ser. No. 132, p. 547.

Jaffe, R. B., and Ledger, W. J. (1966). *Steroids* **8,** 61.

Jaffe, R. B., and Levitz, M. (1967). *Amer. J. Obstet. Gynecol.* **90,** 992.

Jaffe, R. B., Eriksson, G., and Diczfalusy, E. (1965). *Excerpta Med. Found. Int. Congr. Ser.* **99,** No. 403.

Jailer, J. W., and Knowlton, A. I. (1950). *J. Clin. Invest.* **29,** 1430.

Jayle, M. F. (1967). *Rev. Fr. Endocrinol. Clin.* **8,** 467.

Jayle, M. F., Scholler, R., Veyrin-Forrer, F., and Mege, F. (1965). *Eur. Rev. Endocrinol., Suppl.* **1,** 77.

Jeffcoate, I. N. A., Fliegner, J. R. H., Russell, S. H., Davis, J. C., and Wade, A. P. (1965). *Lancet* **2,** 553.

Jeffery, J., Swapp, G. H., and Wilson, G. R. (1970). *Proc. Roy. Soc. Med.* **63,** 1088.

Jenkins, D. M., Farquhar, J. B., and Oakey, R. E. (1970). *Proc. Roy. Soc. Med.* **63,** 1096.

Johannisson, E. (1968). *Acta Endocrinol. (Copenhagen), Suppl.* **130,** 1.

Johnson, F. D., Jacobs, E. M., and Silliphant, W. M. (1968). *Calif. Med.* **108,** 1.

Jones, G. E. S., Gey, G. O., and Gey, M. K. (1943). *Bull. Johns Hopkins Hosp.* **72,** 26.

Jones, G. E. S., Delfs, E., and Stran, H. M. (1944). *Bull. Johns Hopkins Hosp.* **75,** 359.

Jones, H. W., and Weil, P. G. (1938). *J. Amer. Med. Ass.* **111,** 519.

Josimovich, J. B., and MacLaren, J. A. (1962). *Endocrinology* **71,** 209.

Josimovich, J. B., Kosor, B., and Mintz, H. A. (1969). *Foetal Autonomy, Ciba Found. Symp.* p. 117.

Josimovich, J. B., Kosor, B., Boccella, L., Mintz, D. H., and Hutchinson, D. L. (1970). *Obstet. Gynecol.* **36,** 244.

Jost, A., Jacquot, R., and Cohen, A. (1962). *In* "The Human Adrenal Cortex" (A. R. Currie, T. Symington, and J. K. Grant, eds.), p. 569. Livingstone, Edinburgh.

Kahmann, H. K. (1970a). *Ned. Tijdschr. Geneesk.* **114,** 736.

Kahmann, H. K. (1970b). *Ned. Tijdschr. Verlosk. Gynaecol.* **70,** 305.

Kahmann, H. K., Kreutzer, H., Meulendijk, P., and Van Leusden, H. A. (1968). *J. Reprod. Fert.* **16,** 324.

Kahmann, H. K., Kreutzer, H., Meulendijk, P., and Van Leusden, H. A. (1969a). *Ned. Tijdschr. Verlosk. Gynaecol.* **69,** 148.

Kahmann, H. K., Kreutzer, H., Meulendijk, P., and Van Leusden, H. A. (1969b). *Ned. Tijdschr. Geneesk.* **113,** 1086.

Kaivola, S., Pesonen, S., Widholm, O., and Zilliacus, H. (1967). *Ann. Chir. Gynaecol. Fenn.* **56,** 111.

Kankaanrinta, T. (1963). *Scand. J. Clin. Lab. Invest.* **15,** Suppl., 74.

Kaplan, S. L., and Grumbach, M. M. (1965a). *Science* **147,** 751.

Kaplan, S. L., and Grumbach, M. M. (1965b). *J. Clin. Endocrinol. Metab.* **25,** 1370.

Kaplan, S. L., Gurpide, E., Sciarra, J. J., and Grumbach, M. M. (1968). *J. Clin. Endocrinol. Metab.* **28,** 1450.

Katz, S. R., Dancis, J., and Levitz, M. (1965). *Endocrinology* **76,** 722.

Kellar, R., Matthew, G. D., MacKay, R., Brown, J. B., and Roy, E. J. (1959). *J. Obstet. Gynaecol. Brit. Emp.* **66,** 804.

Keller, M. (1953). *Gynaecologia* **136,** 358.

Keller, P. J. (1966). *Gynaecologia* **163,** 159.

Kerr, M. G., Roy, E. J., Harkness, R. A., Short, R. V., and Baird, D. T. (1966). *Amer. J. Obstet. Gynecol.* **94,** 214.

Khoo, S. K., and MacKay, E. V. (1970). *Med. J. Aust.* **1,** 896.

Kim, M. H., Borth, R., McCleary, P. H., Woolever, C. A., and Young, P. C. M. (1971). *Amer. J. Obstet. Gynecol.* **110,** 658.

Kitchell, R. I., and Wells, L. J. (1952). *Anat. Rec.* **112,** 561.

Kloosterman, G. J., and Huis in 't Veld, L. G. (1961). *Ned. Tijdschr. Verlosk. Gynaecol.* **61,** 307.

Klopper, A. (1964). *In* "Research on Steroids" (C. Cassano, ed.), Vol. I, p. 119. Il Pensiero Scientifico, Roma.

Klopper, A. (1965). *In* "Research on Steroids" (C. Cassano, ed.), Vol. II, p. 63. Il Pensiero Scientifico, Roma.

Klopper, A. (1966). *Abh. Deut. Akad. Wiss. Berlin* p. 247.

Klopper, A. (1968). *Obstet. Gynecol. Surv.* **23,** 819.

Klopper, A. (1969). *In* "Foetus and Placenta" (A. Klopper and E. Diczfalusy, eds.), pp. 471–555. Blackwell, Oxford.

Klopper, A. (1970). *Amer. J. Obstet. Gynecol.* **107,** 807.

Klopper, A., and Billewicz, W. (1963). *J. Obstet. Gynaecol. Brit. Commonw.* **70,** 1024.

Klopper, A., and Diczfalusy, E., eds. (1969). "Foetus and Placenta." Blackwell, Oxford.

Klopper, A., and MacNaughton, M. C. (1959). *J. Endocrinol.* **18,** 319.

Klopper, A., and MacNaughton, M. C. (1965). *J. Obstet. Gynaecol. Brit. Commonw.* **72,** 1072.

Klopper, A., and Michie, E. M. (1956). *J. Endocrinol.* **13,** 360.

Klopper, A., and Stephenson, R. (1966). *J. Obstet. Gynaecol. Brit. Commonw.* **73,** 282.

Klopper, A., Turnbull, A. C., and Anderson, A. B. (1966). *J. Obstet. Gynaecol. Brit. Commonw.* **73,** 390.

Knowlton, A. I., Mudge, G. H., and Jailer, J. W. (1949). *J. Clin. Endocrinol. Metab.* **9,** 514.

Kock, H., Van Leusden, H. A., Seelen, J., and Van Kessel, H. (1965). *Ned. Tijdschr. Geneesk.* **109**, 633.

Kulin, H. E., Metzl, K., and Peterson, R. (1966). *J. Pediat.* **69**, 648.

Lachowicz, L. (1969). *Pol. Med. J.* **8**, 238.

Lajos, L., and Szontagh, F. E. (1950). *Zentralbl. Gynaekol.* **72**, 1035.

Langer, G., and Hockstaedt, B. (1959). *Int. J. Fert.* **4**, 242.

Langmade, C. G., Notrica, S., Demetriou, J., and Ware, A. (1961). *Amer. J. Obstet. Gynecol.* **81**, 1149.

Lanman, J. F. (1953). *Medicine (Baltimore)* **32**, 389.

Lanman, J. F. (1962). *In* "The Human Adrenal Cortex" (A. R. Currie, T. Symington, and J. K. Grant, eds.), p. 553. Livingstone, Edinburgh.

Laumas, K. R., Malkani, P. K., Koshti, G. S., and Hingorani, V. (1968). *Amer. J. Obstet. Gynecol.* **101**, 1062.

Lauritzen, C. (1969). *Arch. Gynaekol.* **207**, 401.

Lauritzen, C., and Lehmann, W. D. (1967). *J. Endocrinol.* **39**, 173.

Lauritzen, C., and Lehmann, W. D. (1971). *Acta Endocrinol. (Copenhagen),* Suppl. **155**, 186.

Lebech, P. E. (1971). *Acta Endocrinol. (Copenhagen),* Suppl. **155**, 134.

Lenters, G. J. (1958). Ph.D. Thesis, Groningen. Wolters, Groningen.

Levitz, M. (1966). *J. Clin. Endocrinol. Metab.* **26**, 773.

Liggins, G. C. (1968). *J. Endocrinol.* **42**, 323.

Liggins, G. C. (1969). *Foetal Autonomy, Ciba Found. Symp.* p. 218.

Liggins, G. C., Holm, L. W., and Kennedy, P. C. (1966). *J. Reprod. Fert.* **12**, 419.

Liggins, G. C., Kennedy, P. C., and Holm, L. W. (1967). *Amer. J. Obstet. Gynecol.* **98**, 1080.

Lindell, A. (1956). *Acta Obstet. Gynecol. Scand.* **35**, 136.

Little, W. A. (1962). *Amer. J. Obstet. Gynecol.* **84**, 220.

Lloyd, C. W., Hughes, E. C., Lobotsky, J., and Rienzo, J. (1951). *J. Clin. Endocrinol. Metab.* **11**, 786.

Loraine, J. A. (1950). *Quart. J. Exp. Physiol.* **36**, 11.

Loraine, J. A. (1956). *Vitam. Horm. (New York)* **14**, 305.

Loraine, J. A. (1958). "The Clinical Application of Hormone Assay." Livingstone, Edinburgh.

Loraine, J. A., and Mathew, G. D. (1950). *J. Obstet. Gynaecol. Brit. Emp.* **57**, 542.

Loraine, J. A., and Mathew, G. D. (1953). *J. Obstet. Gynaecol. Brit. Emp.* **60**, 640.

Lundvall, F., and Stakemann, G. (1966). *Acta Obstet. Gynecol. Scand.* **45**, 301.

Lundvall, F., and Stakemann, G. (1969). *Acta Obstet. Gynecol. Scand.* **48**, 497.

Lurie, A. O., Reid, D. E., and Villee, C. A. (1966). *Amer. J. Obstet. Gynecol.* **96**, 670.

Luukkainen, T., and Adlercreutz, H. (1967). *Proc. Int. Congr. Horm. Steroids, 2nd, 1966* Int. Congr. Ser. No. 132, p. 126.

McCarthy, C., and Pennington, G. W. (1964a). *Amer. J. Obstet. Gynecol.* **89**, 1069.

McCarthy, C., and Pennington, G. W. (1964b). *Amer. J. Obstet. Gynecol.* **89**, 1074.

McCormick, J. B. (1954). *Obstet. Gynecol.* **3**, 58.

MacDonald, P. C., and Siiteri, P. K. (1964). *Endocrinology* **24**, 685.

MacDonald, P. C., and Siiteri, P. K. (1965). *J. Clin. Invest.* **44**, 465.

Mackay, E. V., Macafee, C. A. J., and Anderson, C. (1967). *Aust. N. Z. J. Obstet. Gynaecol.* **7**, 94.

Mackay, E. V., Macafee, C. A., and Anderson, C. (1968). *Aust. N. Z. J. Obstet. Gynaecol.* **8**, 17.

McKean, C. M. (1960). *Amer. J. Obstet. Gynecol.* **80**, 596.

MacLeod, S. C., Brown, J. B., Beischer, N. A., and Smith, M. A. (1967). *Aust. N. Z. J. Obstet. Gynaecol.* **7**, 25.

MacNaughton, M. C. (1965). *J. Obstet. Gynaecol. Brit. Commonw.* **72**, 249.

MacNaughton, M. C. (1967). *Amer. J. Obstet. Gynecol.* **97**, 998.

MacNaughton, M. C., and Greig, M. (1965). *J. Obstet. Gynecol. Brit. Commonw.* **72**, 1029.

MacNaughton, M. C., and Michie, E. M. (1960). *In* "Advance Abstracts of Short Communications" (F. Fuchs, ed.), p. 669. Periodica, Copenhagen.

MacNaughton, M. C., Coutts, J. R. T., and Browning, M. C. K. (1970). *Proc. Roy. Soc. Med.* **63**, 1087.

MacRae, D. J. (1965). *J. Obstet. Gynaecol. Brit. Commonw.* **72**, 1038.

Maeyama, M., Nakagawa, T., Tuchida, Y., and Matuoka, H. (1969). *Steroids* **13**, 59.

Magendantz, H. G., Klausner, D., Ryan, K. J., and Yen, S. S. (1968). *Obstet. Gynecol.* **32**, 610.

Maguin, P., Villiers, H., Felman, D., and Theoleyre, J. (1967). *Gynecol. Obstet.* **66**, 117.

Malpas, P. J. (1938). *J. Obstet. Gynecol. Brit. Emp.* **45**, 932.

Mancuso, S. (1962). *Minerva Ginecol.* **14**, 717.

Mandelbaum, B., and Evans, I. N. (1969). *Amer. J. Obstet. Gynecol.* **104**, 365.

Mandelbaum, B., Ross, M., and Evans, T. N. (1970). *Obstet. Gynecol.* **35**, 570.

Martin, J. D., and Hahnel, R. J. (1964). *J. Obstet. Gynecol. Brit. Commonw.* **71**, 260.

Mathieu, A. (1939). *Amer. J. Obstet. Gynecol.* **37**, 654.

Matthies, D. L., and Diczfalusy, E. (1968). *Excerpta Med. Int. Congr. Ser.* **170**, 34.

Merkatz, I. R., New, M. I., Peterson, R. E., and Seaman, M. P. (1969). *J. Pediat.* **75**, 977.

Meyer, R. (1912). *Virchows Arch. Pathol. Anat. Physiol.* **210**, 158.

Michie, E. (1966). *Acta Endocrinol. (Copenhagen)* **51**, 535.

Michie, E. (1967). *J. Obstet. Gynaecol. Brit. Commonw.* **74**, 896.

Michie, E., Hobson, B. M., and Gasson, P. W. (1966). *J. Obstet. Gynaecol. Brit. Commonw.* **73**, 783.

Midgley, A. R., and Jaffe, R. B. (1968). *J. Clin. Endocrinol. Metab.* **28**, 1712.

Migeon, C. J., Prystowsky, H., Grumbach, M. M., and Byron, M. C. (1956). *J. Clin. Invest.* **35**, 488.

Mikhail, G., Wiqvist, N., and Diczfalusy, E. (1963a). *Acta Endocrinol. (Copenhagen)* **42**, 519.

Mikhail, G., Wiqvist, N., and Diczfalusy, E. (1963b). *Acta Endocrinol. (Copenhagen)* **43**, 213.

Mitchell, F. L. (1967). *Vitam. Horm. (New York)* **25**, 191.

Moeri, E. (1951). *Acta Endocrinol. (Copenhagen)* **8**, 259.

Møller, K. J. A., and Fuchs, F. (1965). *J. Obstet. Gynaecol. Brit. Commonw.* **72**, 1042.

Morrison, G., Meigs, R. A., and Ryan, K. J. (1965). *Steroids, Suppl.* **2**, 177.

Morrison, J., and Kilpatrick, N. (1969). *J. Obstet. Gynaecol. Brit. Commonw.* **76**, 719.

Müller, K., and Nielson, J. C. (1967). *Dan. Med. Bull.* **14**, 165.

Nakayama, I., Arai, K., Yanaihara, T., Tabei, T., Satoh, K., and Nagatomi, K. (1967). *Acta Endocrinol. (Copenhagen)* **55**, 369.

Neill, D. W., and Macafee, C. A. (1968). *J. Obstet. Gynaecol. Brit. Commonw.* **75**, 172.

Nelson, G. H. (1969). *S. Med. J.* **62**, 1085.

New, M. I. (1970). *Lancet* **1**, 83.

Nichols, J. (1969). *Lancet* **1**, 1151.

Nichols, J. (1970). *Lancet* **1**, 83.

Nichols, J., and Gibson, G. G. (1969). *Lancet* **2**, 1068.

Nilson, E. V. (1970). *Can. J. Med. Technol.* **32**, 45.

Nilsson, I., and Bengtsson, L. P. (1968). *Acta Obstet. Gynecol. Scand.* **47**, 213.

Nilsson, L. (1964). *Acta Obstet. Gynecol. Scand., Suppl.* **6**, 128.

Noto, T., Maile, J. B., and Riekers, H. (1964). *Amer. J. Obstet. Gynecol.* **90**, 859.

Oakey, R. E. (1970). *Vitam. Horm.* (*New York*) **28**, 1.

Oakey, R. E., Bradshaw, L. R., Eccles, S. S., Stitch, S. R., and Heys, R. F. (1967). *Clin. Chim. Acta* **15**, 35.

Papiernik-Berkhauer, E., and Hamelin, J. P. (1968). *Gynecol. Obstet.* **67**, 361.

Pattillo, R. A., Smith, T. C., Delfs, E., and Mattingly, R. F. (1966). *Amer. J. Obstet. Gynecol.* **96**, 337.

Payne, F. L. (1941). *Surg., Gynecol. Obstet.* **73**, 86.

Pearlman, W. H. (1957). *Biochem. J.* **67**, 1.

Pion, R. J. (1967). *Clin. Obstet. Gynecol.* **10**, 40.

Plotz, E. J., and Davis, M. E. (1957). *Proc. Soc. Exp. Biol. Med.* **95**, 92.

Plotz, E. J., Wiener, M., and Davis, M. E. (1963). *Amer. J. Obstet. Gynecol.* **87**, 1.

Porter, D. G. (1969). *Ciba Found. Study Group* [*Pap.*] **34**, 79–86.

Pose, S. V., and Fielitz, C. (1959). *In* "Oxytocin" (R. Caldeyro-Barcia and H. Heller, eds.), pp. 229–239. Pergamon, Oxford.

Rabau, E., and Szenjberg, L. (1955). *Gynaecologia* **139**, 158.

Rakoff, A. E. (1940). *Pa. Med. J.* **43**, 669.

Randall, C. L., Baetz, R. W., Hall, D. W., and Birtch, P. K. (1955). *Amer. J. Obstet. Gynecol.* **69**, 643.

Ratanasopa, V., Schindler, A. E., Lee, T. Y., and Herrmann, W. L. (1967). *Amer. J. Obstet. Gynecol.* **99**, 295.

Rawlings, W. J. (1965). *Fert. Steril.* **16**, 323.

Rebbe, H., and Alling Møller, K. J. (1966). *Acta Obstet. Gynecol. Scand.* **45**, 261.

Reid, S., Beischer, N. A., Brown, J. B., and Smith, N. A. (1968). *Aust. N. Z. J. Obstet. Gynaecol.* **8**, 189.

Reisfeld, R. A., Bergenstal, D. M., and Hertz, R. (1959). *Arch. Biochem. Biophys.* **81**, 456.

Rice, B. F., Barclay, D. L., and Sternberg, W. H. (1969). *Amer. J. Obstet. Gynecol.* **104**, 871.

Robson, T. B., and Gornall, A. G. (1955). *Can. Med. Ass. J.* **72**, 830.

Rourke, J. E., Marshall, L. D., and Shelley, T. F. (1968). *Amer. J. Obstet. Gynecol.* **100**, 331.

Roy, E. J., and Kerr, M. G. (1964). *J. Obstet. Gynaecol. Brit. Commonw.* **71**, 106.

Rubin, B., Dorfman, R. I., and Miller, M. (1946). *J. Clin. Endocrinol. Metab.* **6**, 347.

Runnebaum, B., and Zander, J. (1962). *Klin. Wochenschr.* **40**, 453.

Rushworth, A. G., Orr, A. H., and Bagshawe, K. D. (1968). *Brit. J. Cancer* **22**, 253.

Russell, C. S., Paine, C. G., Coyle, M. G., and Dewhurst, C. J. (1957). *J. Obstet. Gynaecol. Brit. Emp.* **64**, 649.

Russell, C. S., Dewhurst, C. J., and Blakey, D. H. (1960). *J. Obstet. Gynaecol. Brit. Emp.* **67,** 1.

Ryan, K. J. (1959). *J. Biol. Chem.* **234,** 2006.

Ryan, K. J. (1962). *Amer. J. Obstet. Gynecol.* **84,** 1695.

Saling, E. J. (1965). *Int. Fed. Gynaecol. Obstet.* **3,** 101.

Samaan, N., Yen, S. C. C., Gonzalez, D., and Pearson, O. H. (1966). *J. Clin. Endocrinol. Metab.* **26,** 1303.

Samaan, N., Yen, S. C. C., Gonzalez, D., and Pearson, O. H. (1968). *J. Clin. Endocrinol. Metab.* **28,** 485.

Samaan, N., Bradbury, J. T., and Goplerud, C. P. (1969). *Amer. J. Obstet. Gynecol.* **104,** 781.

Samaan, N., Gallagher, H. S., McRoberts, W. A., and Faris, A. M. (1971). *Amer. J. Obstet. Gynecol.* **109,** 63.

Samuels, L. T., Evans, G. T., and McKelvey, J. L. (1943). *Endocrinology* **32,** 422.

Sandberg, A. A., and Slaunwhite, W. R. (1958). *J. Clin. Endocrinol. Metab.* **18,** 253.

Saxena, B. N. (1971). *Vitam. Horm. (New York)* **29,** 95.

Saxena, B. N., Refetoff, S., Emerson, K., and Selenkow, H. A. (1968). *Amer. J. Obstet. Gynecol.* **101,** 874.

Saxena, B. N., Emerson, K., and Selenkow, H. A. (1969). *N. Engl. J. Med.* **281,** 225.

Schindler, A. E., and Herrmann, W. L. (1966). *Amer. J. Obstet. Gynecol.* **95,** 301.

Schindler, A. E., and Ratanasopa, V. (1968). *Acta Endocrinol. (Copenhagen)* **59,** 239.

Schindler, A. E., Ratanasopa, V., Lee, T. Y., and Herrmann, W. L. (1967). *Obstet. Gynecol.* **29,** 625.

Schofield, B. M. (1964). *J. Endocrinol.* **30,** 347.

Schwarz, R. H., Fields, G. A., and Kyle, G. C. (1969). *Obstet. Gynecol.* **34,** 787.

Schwers, J., Eriksson, G., and Diczfalusy, E. (1965a). *Acta Endocrinol. (Copenhagen)* **49,** 65.

Schwers, J., Govaerts-Videtsky, M., Wiqvist, N., and Diczfalusy, E. (1965b). *Acta Endocrinol. (Copenhagen)* **50,** 597.

Sciarra, N. (1970). *J. Obstet. Gynaecol. Brit. Commonw.* **77,** 420.

Sciarra, J. J., Sherwood, L. M., Varma, A. A., and Lundberg, W. B. (1968). *Amer. J. Obstet. Gynecol.* **101,** 413.

Scommegna, A. (1969). *Obstet. Gynecol. Surv.* **24,** 387.

Scommegna, A., and Chattoraj, S. C. (1967). *Amer. J. Obstet. Gynecol.* **99,** 1087.

Scommegna, A., and Chattoraj, S. C. (1968). *Obstet. Gynecol.* **32,** 277.

Scommegna, A., Nedoss, B. R., and Chattoraj, S. C. (1968). *Obstet. Gynecol.* **31,** 526.

Seegar, G., and Delfs, E. (1940). *J. Amer. Med. Ass.* **115,** 1267.

Selenkow, H. A. (1969). *N. Engl. J. Med.* **281,** 1308.

Sharp, A. H., and Wood, C. (1966). *Aust. N. Z. J. Obstet. Gynecol.* **6,** 321.

Shearman, R. P. (1959). *J. Obstet. Gynaecol. Brit. Emp.* **66,** 1.

Shearman, R. P., and Garrett, W. J. (1963). *Brit. Med. J.* **1,** 292.

Short, R. (1969). *Ciba Found. Study Group [Pap.]* **34,** 115–116.

Siegler, A. M., Zeichner, S., Rubenstein, I., Wallace, E. Z., and Carter, A. C. (1959).

Siiteri, P. K., and MacDonald, P. C. (1963). *Steroids* **2,** 713.

Siiteri, P. K., and MacDonald, P. C. (1966). *J. Clin. Endocrinol. Metab.* **26,** 751.

Simmer, H. H., Easterling, W. E., Pion, R. J., and Dignam, W. J. (1964). *Steroids* **4,** 125.

Simmer, H. H., Dignam, W. J., Easterling, W. J., Frankland, M. V., and Naftolin, F. (1966). *Steroids* **8**, 179.

Simmons, E., and Israelstam, D. M. (1968). *J. Obstet. Gynaecol. Brit. Commonw.* **75**, 477.

Singer, W. (1970). *Lancet* **1**, 237.

Singer, W., Desjardins, P., and Friesen, H. G. (1970). *Obstet. Gynecol.* **36**, 222.

Smith, E. R., and Kellie, A. E. (1967). *Biochem. J.* **104**, 83.

Smith, G. V., and Smith, O. W. (1934). *Amer. J. Physiol.* **107**, 128.

Smith, G. V., and Smith, O. W. (1939). *Amer. J. Obstet. Gynecol.* **36**, 618.

Smith, G. V., and Smith, O. W. (1948). *Physiol. Rev.* **28**, 1.

Smith, K., Greene, J. W., and Touchstone, J. C. (1966). *Amer. J. Obstet. Gynecol.* **33**, 365.

Soiva, K., Grönroos, P., and Rauramo, I. (1968). *Ann. Chir. Gynaecol. Fenn.* **57**, 67.

Solomon, S., and Younglai, E. V. (1969). *In* "Foetus and Placenta" (A. Klopper and E. Diczfalusy, eds.), pp. 249–298. Blackwell, Oxford.

Solomon, S., Watanabe, M., Dominguez, O. V., Gray, M. J., Meeker, C. I., and Sims, E. A. H. (1964). *In* "Placental Steroidogenesis" (F. Polvani and A. Bompiani, eds.), pp. 32–42. Karger, Basel.

Sommerville, I. F. (1969). *Ciba Found. Study Group [Pap.]* **34**, 42–48.

Sommerville, I. F., and Marrian, G. F. (1950). *Biochem. J.* **46**, 290.

Southren, A. L., Weingold, A. B., Kobayashi, Y., Sherman, D. H., Grimaldi, R., and Gold, E. M. (1968). *Amer. J. Obstet. Gynecol.* **101**, 899.

Spadoni, L. R., Horst, H., Bray, R. E., and Herrmann, W. L. (1966). *Obstet. Gynecol.* **28**, 830.

Speert, H. (1954). *Amer. J. Obstet. Gynecol.* **68**, 665.

Spellacy, W. N. (1969). *N. Engl. J. Med.* **281**, 1308.

Spellacy, W. N., and Teoh, E. S. (1969). *Surg. Forum* **20**, 409.

Spellacy, W. N., Carlson, K. L., and Birk, S. A. (1966). *Amer. J. Obstet. Gynecol.* **96**, 1164.

Spellacy, W. N., Cohen, W. D., and Carlson, K. L. (1967). *Amer. J. Obstet. Gynecol.* **97**, 560.

Spellacy, W. N., Teoh, E. S., and Buhi, W. C. (1970). *Clin. Res.* **18**, 36.

Spellacy, W. N., Teoh, E. S., Buhi, W. C., Birk, S. A., and McCreary, S. A. (1971). *Amer. J. Obstet. Gynecol.* **109**, 588.

Staffeldt, K. (1966). *Geburtsh. Frauenheilk.* **26**, 975.

Stitch, S. R., Sevell, M. J., and Oakey, R. E. (1966). *Lancet* **1**, 1344.

Strand, A. (1956). *Acta Obstet. Gynecol. Scand.* **35**, 76.

Strand, A. (1966). *Acta Obstet. Gynecol. Scand., Suppl.* **1**, 125.

Strickler, H. S., Holt, S. S., Acevedo, H. F., Saier, E., and Grauer, R. C. (1967). *Steroids* **9**, 193.

Suwa, S., and Friesen, H. (1969). *Endocrinology* **85**, 1037.

Szarka, S. (1930). *Zentralbl. Gynaekol.* **54**, 2211.

Szenjberg, L., and Rabau, E. (1950). *Gynaecologia* **130**, 221.

Tähkä, H. (1951). *Acta Pediat. (Stockholm), Suppl.* **81**, 1.

Talbert, L. M., and Easterling, W. E. (1967). *Amer. J. Obstet. Gynecol.* **99**, 923.

Talbert, L. M., Easterling, W. E., and Roberson, W. E. (1969). *S. Med. J.* **62**, 1090.

Tashima, C. K. (1965). *J. Clin. Endocrinol. Metab.* **25**, 1493.

Taubert, H. D., and Haskins, A. L. (1963). *Obstet. Gynecol.* **22**, 405.

Taylor, E. S., Bruns, P. D., Hepner, H. J., and Drose, V. E. (1958). *Amer. J. Obstet. Gynecol.* **76**, 983.

Taylor, E. S., Hassner, H., Bruns, P. D., and Drose, V. E. (1963). *Amer. J. Obstet. Gynecol.* **85**, 10.

Taylor, E. S., Bruns, P. D., and Drose, V. E. (1965). *Clin. Obstet. Gynecol.* **8**, 550.

Taylor, H. C., and Scandron, E. E. (1939). *Amer. J. Obstet. Gynecol.* **37**, 963.

Telegdy, G., Weeks, J. W., Wiqvist, N., and Diczfalusy, E. (1970). *Acta Endocrinol. (Copenhagen)* **63**, 105.

Ten Berge, B. S. (1961). *Cerebral Palsy Bull.* **3**, 323.

Ten Berge, B. S., Weeke, A., and Groen, A. (1957). *Arch. Gynaekol.* **189**, 140.

Tenhaeff, D., and Karajiannis, G. (1968). *Muenchen. Med. Wochenschr.* **110**, 2142.

Teoh, E. S. (1967). *J. Obstet. Gynaecol. Brit. Commonw.* **74**, 80.

Teoh, E. S., and Sivasamboo, R. (1968). *J. Obstet. Gynaecol. Brit. Commonw.* **75**, 724.

Thierstein, S. T. (1965). *Nebr. State Med. J.* **50**, 435.

Timonen, S., and Hirvonen, E. (1964). *Ann. Chir. Gynaecol. Fenn.* **53**, 96.

Timonen, S., and Tervilä, L. (1968). *Ann. Chir. Gynaecol. Fenn.* **57**, 447.

Timonen, S., Hirvonen, E., and Sokkanen, R. (1965). *Acta Endocrinol. (Copenhagen)* **49**, 393.

Tivenius, L. (1959). *Acta Med. Scand.* **164**, 147.

Toaff, R., Ayalon, D., Lunenfeld, B., and Eshkol, A. (1965). *J. Obstet. Gynaecol. Brit. Commonw.* **72**, 236.

Troen, P., Nilsson, B., Wiqvist, N., and Diczfalusy, E. (1961). *Acta Endocrinol. (Copenhagen)* **38**, 361.

Trolle, D. (1955a). *Acta Endocrinol. (Copenhagen)* **19**, 373.

Trolle, D. (1955b). *Acta Endocrinol. (Copenhagen)* **19**, 217.

Tulsky, A. S., and Koff, A. K. (1957). *Fert. Steril.* **8**, 118.

Turkington, R. W., and Topper, Y. (1966). *Endocrinology* **79**, 175.

Turnbull, A. C., and Anderson, A. B. M. (1969). *Ciba Found. Study Group [Pap.]* **34**, 106–113.

Turnbull, A. C., Anderson, A. B., and Wilson, G. R. (1967). *Lancet* **2**, 627.

Van der Molen, H. J., and Hart, P. G. (1961). *Ned. Tijdschr. Verlosk. Gynaecol.* **61**, 391.

Van Leusden, H. A. (1969). "Foetoplacentaire Endocrinologie." Dekker en v.d. Vegt, Nijmegen.

Van Leusden, H. A. (1970a). *Ned. Tijdschr. Verlosk. Gynaecol.* **70**, 349.

Van Leusden, H. A. (1970b). *Ned. Tijdschr. Geneesk.* **114**, 741.

Van Leusden, H. A. (1970c). *Excerpta Med. Found. Int. Congr. Ser.* **210**, 78.

Van Leusden, H. A. (1971). *Excerpta Med. Found. Int. Congr. Ser.* **219**, 823–827.

Van Leusden, H. A. (1972a). "De bewaking van het kind in utero." Stafleu, Leiden.

Van Leusden, H. A. (1972b). *Eur. J. Obstet. Gynecol.* **2** (in press).

Van Leusden, H. A. (1972c). Unpublished data.

Van Leusden, H. A., and Siemerink, M. (1969). *Acta Endocrinol. (Copenhagen)* **61**, 68.

Van Leusden, H. A., and Villee, C. A. (1966). *J. Clin. Endocrinol. Metab.* **26**, 842.

Van Leusden, H. A., and Villee, C. A. (1967). *Proc. Int. Congr. Horm. Steroids, 2nd, 1966* Int. Congr. Ser. No. 132, p. 601.

Van Leusden, H. A., Houtzager, H. L., and Mastboom, J. C. (1967). *Acta Endocrinol. (Copenhagen), Suppl.* **119**, 78.

Van Wering, R. F. (1969). *Ned. Tijdschr. Geneesk.* **113**, 1370.

Vedra, B., and Horska, S. (1969). *Arch. Gynaekol.* **208,** 1.

Venning, E. H., and Browne, J. S. L. (1940). *Endocrinology* **27,** 707.

Venning, E. H., Sybulski, S., Pollak, V. E., and Ryan, R. J. (1959). *J. Clin. Endocrinol. Metab.* **19,** 1486.

Vermelin, H., Ribon, M., and Ribon, C. (1957). *Bull. Fed. Soc. Gynaecol. Obstet. Lang. Fr.* **9,** 210.

Vesell, M., and Goldman, S. (1944). *Amer. J. Obstet. Gynecol.* **42,** 272.

Waldstein, E. (1929). *Zentralbl. Gynaekol.* **53,** 1305.

Wallace, S. J., and Michie, E. (1966). *Lancet* **2,** 560.

Warburton, D., and Fraser, F. C. (1959). *Clin. Obstet. Gynecol.* **2,** 22.

Warren, J. C., and Cheatum, S. G. (1967). *J. Clin. Endocrinol. Metab.* **27,** 433.

Watts, R. M., and Adair, F. L. (1943). *Amer. J. Obstet. Gynecol.* **46,** 183.

Wei, P. Y., Ouyang, P. C., Lee, T. Y., and Chen, J. S. (1968). *Amer. J. Obstet. Gynecol.* **102,** 8.

Welshman, S. G., Armstrong, M. J., and Bell, J. F. (1969). *Clin. Chim. Acta* **26,** 339.

White, P. (1949). *Amer. J. Med.* **7,** 609.

White, P. (1952). *In* "Treatment of Diabetes Mellitus" (E. P. Joshlin, ed.), p. 676. Kimpton, London.

WHO Scientific Group. (1966). *Bull. WHO* **34,** 765.

WHO Scientific Group. (1971). *World Health Organ., Tech. Rep. Ser.* **471.**

Wide, L. (1962). *Acta Endocrinol. (Copenhagen), Suppl.* **70,** 1.

Wide, L. (1967). *Advan. Obstet. Gynecol.* **1,** 56.

Wide, L., and Gemzell, C. A. (1960). *Acta Endocrinol. (Copenhagen)* **35,** 261.

Wide, L., and Hobson, B. (1967). *Acta Endocrinol. (Copenhagen)* **54,** 105.

Wiest, W. G., Fujimoto, G. I., and Sandberg, A. A. (1955). *Fed. Proc., Fed. Amer. Soc. Exp. Biol.* **14,** 304.

Wilken, H., Stark, K. H., and Junge, W. D. (1966). *Z. Geburtsh. Gynaekol.* **166,** 97.

Wilson, R. B., Albert, A., and Randall, M. (1949). *Amer. J. Obstet. Gynecol.* **58,** 960.

Wodrig, W., and Göretzlehner, W. (1964). *Z. Geburtsh. Gynaekol.* **162,** 89.

Wray, P. M., and Russel, C. S. (1964). *J. Obstet. Gynaecol. Brit. Commonw.* **71,** 97.

Würtele, A. (1962). *Z. Geburtsh. Gynaecol.* **159,** 287.

Würtele, A. (1963). *Arch. Gynaekol.* **198,** 131.

Wyss, H. I. (1968). *Gynaecologia* **167,** 357.

Wyss, H. I., and Meyer, C. M. (1966). *Gynaecologia* **161,** 75.

Yagami, Y., and Ito, Y. (1965). *J. Jap. Obstet. Gynecol. Soc.* **12,** 82.

Yen, S. S. C., Samaan, N., and Pearson, D. H. (1967). *J. Clin. Endocrinol. Metab.* **27,** 1341.

Yen, S. S. C., Pearson, O., and Rankin, J. S. (1968). *Obstet. Gynecol.* **32,** 86.

Yogo, I. (1969). *Endocrinol. Jap.* **16,** 215.

Yoshimi, T., Strott, C. A., Marshall, J. R., and Lipsett, M. B. (1969). *J. Clin. Endocrinol. Metab.* **29,** 225.

Yousem, H., Seitchik, J., and Solomon, D. (1966). *Obstet. Gynecol.* **28,** 491.

Zander, J. (1954). *Nature (London)* **174,** 406.

Zander, J. (1959). *In:* "Recent Progress in the Endocrinology of Reproduction" (C. W. Lloyd, ed.), p. 255. Academic Press, New York.

Zarrow, M. X., Anderson, N. C., and Callantine, M. R. (1963). *Nature (London)* **198,** 690.

Zondek, B. (1929). *Zentralbl. Gynaekol.* 53, 834.

Zondek, B. (1935). "Hormone des Ovariums und des Hypophysenvorderlappens," 2nd ed. Springer-Verlag, Berlin and New York.

Zondek, B. (1937). *J. Amer. Med. Ass.* 108, 607.

Zondek, B. (1942). *J. Obstet. Gynaecol. Brit. Emp.* 49, 397.

Zondek, B. (1954). *Recent Progr. Horm. Res.* 10, 395.

Zondek, B., and Goldberg, S. (1957). *J. Obstet. Gynaecol. Brit. Emp.* 64, 1.

Zondek, B., and Pfeifer, V. (1959). *Acta Obstet. Gynecol. Scand.* 38, 742.

Zucconi, G., Lisboa, B. P., Simonitisch, E., Roth, L., Hagen, A. A., and Diczfalusy, E. (1967). *Acta Endocrinol. (Copenhagen)* 56, 413.

Zuckermann, J. E., Fallon, V., Tashjian, A. H., Levine, L., and Friesen, H. G. (1970). *J. Clin. Endocrinol. Metab.* 30, 769.

Author Index

Numbers in italics refer to the pages on which the complete references are listed.

A

Aakvaag, A., 236, *278*
Abbott, M. T., 17, *37, 42, 43*
Abdul Enein, M. A., 286, *345*
Abe, K., 111, *164*
Abramovich, D. R., 259, *271,* 309, *345*
Abrams, C. L., 297, *350*
Abrams, R. M., 115, 116, *160*
Acevedo, H. F., 299, 324, 331, 334, 337, 340, *345, 358*
Adams, C. E., 231, *271*
Adams, W. M., 257, *271*
Adlercreutz, H., 300, 302, *345, 354*
Ahren, K., 150, *151*
Ainsworth, L., 237, 240, 245, *271*
Aitken, E. H., 249, *271*
Ajika, K., 91, *157*
Akasu, F., 308, *345*
Albert, A., 285, *350, 360*
Alberts, M., 259, *272*
Albracht, S. P. J., 63, *81*
Alder, R. M., 331, *345*
Aleem, F. A., 309, 312, 314, 316, *345*
Alexander, D. P., 257, *271*
Alexander, M. H., 265, *271*
Alfheim, A., 314, *351*
Alfin-Slater, R. B., 54, *78*
Allam, H., 305, *345*
Allen, J. R., 255, *275*
Allen, W. M., 229, 231, 235, 237, 241, 262, 263, *271, 274, 276, 277,* 329, 336, *345*
Allende, J. E., 2, *38*
Alling Møller, K. J., 305, *356*
Alonso, C., 305, *349*
Amati, G., 305, *345*
Amenomori, Y., 170, 171, 173, 175, 176, 178, *216, 217, 221*
Amoroso, E. C., 228, 230, 245, 251, *271*
Amoss, M. S., 105, 106, 111, 124, 137, *151, 159*
Anden, N. E., 185, *216*
Anderson, A. B. M., 252, 254, 258, 259,

272, 277, 278, 315, 320, 329, 340, *345, 353, 359*
Anderson, C., 304, *354*
Anderson, L. L., 237, 241, *274*
Anderson, N. C., 235, *279,* 330, *360*
Andreoli, C., 327, *348*
Angers, M., 306, 328, *350*
Angevine, D. M., 309, *345*
Anker, R. M., 31, *43*
Ansay, M., 21, 36, *40*
Antunez-Rodriguez, J., 96, 99, 104, 114, 116, 124, *153, 158, 159*
Anuman-Rajadhon, Y., 300, *351*
Aoba, H., 316, 317, *345*
Aono, T., 145–146, *164*
Arai, K., 259, *276,* 309, *355*
Ardai, Y., 120, *151*
Archibald, F. M., 47, *81*
Arimura, A., 85, 97, 99, 100, 101, 102, 104, 105, 106, 107, 108, 110, 111, 112, 113, 116, 117, 118, 119, 121, 122, 123, 124, 125, 126, 127, 128, 130, 131, 132, 133, 134, 135, 136, 137, 138, 140, 141, 142, 143, 145, *151, 152, 153, 157, 158, 159, 160, 161, 163, 164,* 197, *221*
Armentrout, R. W., 106, 109, *154*
Armstrong, D. T., 92, *160*
Armstrong, M. J., 304, 318, *360*
Arnold, W., 111, *155*
Aro, H., 9, *41*
Aronson, R. B., 2, 8, 10, 15, *41*
Arras, B. J., 299, 324, 331, 337, 340, *345*
Aschheim, P., 96, 99, *153*
Aschheim, S., 84, 86, *164*
Asdell, S. A., 256, 265, *272*
Assenmacher, I., 89, 93, *152*
Astrada, J. J., 114, *152*
Atkinson, L. E., 113, 145, *156, 159*
Aubert, M. L., 295, *350*
Aubry, R. H., 290, 291, 292, 312, 313, 315, 316, 318, *345*
Auliac, P. B., 47, *78*
Averill, R. L. W., *216*

363

Clucas, I. J., 32, *38*
Cmuchalova, B., 34, *38*
Coble, Y. D., 212, *217*
Coburn, W. A., 332, *345*
Coch, J. A., 267, *272*
Cohen, A., 310, *352*
Cohen, A. I., 96, 97, 99, 100, 101, 102, 120, 124, 125, *153, 162, 164*
Cohen, L., 315, 318, 319, *349*
Cohen, M., 298, *347*
Cohen, S., 299, *347*
Cohen, W. D., 294, *358*
Cohere, G., 196, *217*
Cohn, E. J., 86, *155*
Cohn, M., 35, *42*
Colas, A., 259, *272*
Colbeau, A., *79*
Coldwell, A. L., 233, *279*
Cole, H. S., 297, 315, *347*
Cole, J. W., 111, *155*
Collip, J. B., 231, 237, 250, 251, *278*
Colonge, A., 85, *153*
Comline, R. S., 257, 258, *272*
Comstock, J. P., 35, *39*
Condon, G. P., 314, *350*
Connon, A. F., 291, *347*
Conrad, J. T., 263, *273*
Conrad, S. H., 236, *273, 277*, 326, 327, *347*
Constable, 22, 23, 24, 25, 26, 27, 28, 29, 33, *37, 38*
Conte, F. A., 297, *350*
Contopoulas, A. N., 90, *153*
Convey, E. M., 214, *217*
Cooper, D. Y., 63, *80*
Cooper, W., 328, *350*
Coppola, J. A., 183, *217*
Corbin, A., 97, 114, 120, 121, *153*
Corker, C. S., 113, 145, *153*
Corner, G. W., 229, *271*, 329, 336, *345*
Cortes, W. T., 303, *348*
Corwin, L. M., 59, 60, *79*
Coscia, A., 238, *278*
Cottini, E. P., 297, *349*
Courey, N. G., 303, *347, 348*
Courrier, R., 85, 96, 99, *153*, 230, 232, 237, *273*
Coutts, J. R. T., 307, 334, 335, *348, 355*
Cox, D. F., 265, *273*
Cox, E. V., 31, *38*
Cox, R. I., 249, *273*

Coyle, M. G., 311, 314, 316, 318, 326, 328, 332, 337, 339, *347, 348, 350, 356*
Crandall, W. R., 263, *273*
Crane, F. L., 52, *79*
Creamer, D. W., *348*
Crighton, D. B., 121, 148, *153, 163*
Critchlow, V., 93, *153*
Cross, B. A., 172, *217*, 267, *272*
Croxatto, H. B., 118, 124, 136, 137, *156*
Crystle, C. D., 294, *349*
Csapo, A. I., 229, 231, 233, 234, 235, 237, 241, 243, 251, 254, 262, 263, 264, *273, 274, 276*, 329, 330, 340, *348*
Cummings, R. V., 299, 304, *348*
Cunningham, L. W., 35, *38, 41*
Cunningham, W. P., 52, *79*
Curie, B. L., 111, *153*
Curnow, R. N., 264, *272*
Currie, A. R., 295, *348*
Currie, B. L., 111, *152*

D

Daane, T. A., 126, 146, *153, 160*
Daems, W. T., 51, *79*
Daenen, M., 237, 240, 245, *271*, 310, *348*
Dässler, C. G., 310, 339, *348*
Dahlstrom, A., 182, *217*
Dancis, J., 314, *350, 353*
Daniel, E. E., 234, *273*
Daniëlsson, M., 284, 292, *348*
Danielli, J. F., 46, *79*
Daniels, E. L., 114, 120, 121, *153*
Danon, A., 184, *217*
Daughaday, W. H., 94, *160*, 186, 198, *216*, 297, *345*
David, M., 97, 120, *153*
Davidson, C. J., 31, *39*
Davidson, J. M., 89, 90, 113, 114, 115, 116, 117, 145, *153, 164*
Davies, I. J., 240, 244, 247, 249, *273*
Davis, J. C., 311, *352*
Davis, M. E., 325, 326, 328, *348, 356*
Davis, N. R., 25, *38*
Davson, H., 46, *79*
Deanesly, R., 228, 231, 237, 238, *273, 274*
Debackere, M., 267, *273*
Debeljuk, L., 85, 102, 105, 106, 108, 111, 112, 116, 117, 118, 122, 123, 124, 128, 129, 131, 132, 133, 136, 137, 138, 144, 145, 147, *151, 153, 163, 164*
DeDella, C., 244, *276*

Midtvedt, T., 15, 16, *41*
Migeon, C. J., 257, 259, 260, 310, *272, 275, 276, 277, 355*
Mikhail, G., 237, 241, *276*, 314, 327, *355*
Milgrom, E., 244, *276*
Miller, E. J., 24, *40, 41*
Miller, M., 290, 314, *356*
Miller, M. C., III, 125, 126, 139, 140, 141, *157, 164*
Miller, R. L., 11, *41*
Milmore, J. E., 121, *153*
Minaguchi, H., 118, 122, *159*, 167, 179, 187, 191, 193, 216, *217, 219*
Minn, H. N., 238, *274*
Mintz, D. H., 258, *272*
Mintz, H. A., 294, 296, 297, 298, *352*
Mishkinsky, J., 180, 189, *219*
Mitchell, F. L., 326, *348, 355*
Mitoma, C., 21, 27, *41*
Mittler, J. C., 85, 96, 101, 106, 120, 123, 124, 125, 126, 127, 133, *159, 162*
Miyake, Y., 64, *80*
Mizuno, H., 182, *219*
Mlytz, H., 290, *351*
Moeri, E., 311, *355*
Moguilevsky, J. A., 119, *158, 159, 162*
Molenaar, I., 65, 66, 67, 68, 69, 71, 73, 75, 76, *80, 81*
Molitch, M., 215, *218*
Møller, K. J. A., 332, *355*
Monahan, M., 111, *159*
Monroe, S. E., 124, 128, 145, *159, 160*
Montuori, E., 252, *277*
Moore, C. R., 85, 114, *159*
Moraca, J. I., 331, *345*
Morgan, P. H., 35, *41*
Morgan, R., 111, *155*
Morré, D., 47, 48, *80*
Morris, J., 286, 305, 317, 334, *345, 347, 351*
Morrison, G., 236, *276*, 327, *355*
Morrison, J., 304, *355*
Morton, L. F., 22, 23, 24, 25, 27, 28, 29, 33, *38*
Moschetto, Y., 99, *152*
Moscowitz, C., 262, *273*
Mosier, H. D., 259, *276*
Moszkowska, A., 122, *159*
Motta, M., 113, 115, 119, 120, *159*
Moulé, Y., 80
Mudge, G. H., 327, *353*

Müller, K., 313, *355*
Müller, P. K., 3, 36, *41*
Muller, E. E., 97, 99, 100, 101, 125, 134, *151, 161, 162*
Mulveny, T., 2, 10, *42*
Muñoz, A. J., 29, *40*
Munson, P. L., *219*
Murrell, E. A., 56, 57, *79*
Mussini, E., 18, *41*
Muthy, J. R., 56, 57, *79*
Myamoto, M., 119, *163*

N

Nachbaur, J., *79*
Nadler, R. D., 118, *154*
Närvänen, S., 328, *347*
Naeye, R. L., 259, *276*
Naftolin, F., 113, 141, 145, *152, 153, 156, 159*, 259, *273*, 301, *358*
Nagasawa, H., 166, 176, 198, 202, 216, *219, 220, 221*
Nagata, N., 111, *164*
Nagatomi, K., 259, *276*, 309, *355*
Nagle, R. G., 288, *346*
Nair, P. P., 59, 75, 76, *80*
Nair, R. M. G., 85, 89, 102, 104, 105, 106, 108, 110, 111, 124, 129, 131, 132, *159, 162, 163*
Naito, H., 60, *80*
Nakagawa, T., 310, *355*
Nakayama, I., 309, *355*
Nakayama, T., 259, *276*
Nalbandov, A. V., 99, 123, 124, *155, 160, 164*
Nallar, M. D., 178, *218*
Nallar, R., 100, 114, 116, 123, *153, 155, 159*
Namtredt, M. J., 61, *81*
Nason, A., 59, 75, 76, *80*
Nedoss, B. R., 301, 302, 304, *357*
Needham, D. M., 244, *276*
Negro-Vilar, A., 120, 121, *159, 160*, 188, 189, 215, *221*
Neill, D. W., 309, 312, 314, 316, *345, 356*
Neill, J. D., 145, *160*, 169, *220*, 231, 237, 242, *276*
Nellor, J. E., 235, *277*
Nelson, D. M., 123, *155*
Nelson, G. H., 318, *356*
Nelson, W. O., 231, *277*

Subject Index

388